COVID-19 and WORLD ORDER

ABOUT THE EDITORS

Hal Brands is the Henry A. Kissinger Distinguished Professor of Global Affairs at the Johns Hopkins University School of Advanced International Studies (SAIS) and a scholar at the American Enterprise Institute. A columnist for Bloomberg Opinion, he is also the author or editor of several books, including *American Grand Strategy in the Age of Trump, Making the Unipolar Moment: U.S. Foreign Policy and the Rise of the Post–Cold War Order*, and *What Good Is Grand Strategy? Power and Purpose in American Statecraft from Harry S. Truman to George W. Bush*. His newest book, *The Lessons of Tragedy: Statecraft and World Order*, was coauthored by Charles Edel.

Francis J. Gavin is the Giovanni Agnelli Distinguished Professor and the inaugural director of the Henry A. Kissinger Center for Global Affairs at the Johns Hopkins University School of Advanced International Studies (SAIS). Gavin is also the chairman of the Board of Editors of *Texas National Security Review*. He is the author of *Gold, Dollars, and Power: The Politics of International Monetary Relations, 1958–1971* and *Nuclear Statecraft: History and Strategy in America's Atomic Age*. His latest book, *Nuclear Weapons and American Grand Strategy*, was published in 2020.

COVID-19

AND

WORLD ORDER

THE FUTURE OF CONFLICT, COMPETITION, AND COOPERATION

EDITED BY

Hal Brands | Francis J. Gavin

Johns Hopkins University Press

Baltimore

In collaboration with and appreciation of the book's coeditors, Professors Hal Brands and Francis J. Gavin of the Henry A. Kissinger Center for Global Affairs at Johns Hopkins SAIS, Johns Hopkins University Press is pleased to donate funds to the Maryland Food Bank, in support of the university's food distribution efforts in East Baltimore during this period of food insecurity because of COVID-19 pandemic hardships.

Johns Hopkins University Press
2715 North Charles Street
Baltimore, Maryland 21218-4363
www.press.jhu.edu

Library of Congress Control Number: 2020942747
A catalog record for this book is available from the British Library.

ISBN-13: 978-1-4214-4075-0 (open access)
ISBN-13: 978-1-4214-4073-6 (pbk. : alk. paper)
ISBN-13: 978-1-4214-4074-3 (electronic)

Special discounts are available for bulk purchases of this book. For more information, please contact Special Sales at specialsales@press.jhu.edu.

Johns Hopkins University Press uses environmentally friendly book materials, including recycled text paper that is composed of at least 30 percent post-consumer waste, whenever possible.

Contents

Foreword

In the heart of Frankfurt, Germany, stands the IG Farben building. Completed in 1930, this massive and seemingly indestructible triumph of modernist design was named for its first owners, the IG Farben Company, at the time Germany's largest chemical conglomerate. Within the decade, IG Farben became deeply entangled with the Nazis and was eventually complicit in many of the worst atrocities of Hitler's Germany, including the manufacture of the notorious Zyklon B gas used in concentration camps.

Following the Allied invasion of Frankfurt in March 1945, the building was evacuated and the corporation's executives arrested. When General Dwight D. Eisenhower touched ground and saw that the IG Farben headquarters was one of the few structures in the city to have survived the assault, he decided to make it the center for Allied operations. From his office on the first floor, he not only oversaw the end of the war but also began the meticulous task of rebuilding democracy in Germany out of the ashes of violent dictatorship—an endeavor that, in turn, seeded the ground for a new liberal world order to emerge.

Today, the Farben building exemplifies the very best of that world. A part of the Goethe University in Frankfurt, it serves as the entry point to the university's sprawling, modern campus. No longer merely a monument to human evil, it is a portal to free inquiry, vigorous debate, and the exchange of ideas that allow global society to thrive, and—in times like ours—to survive.

The story of the Farben building serves as a metaphor for the trajectory of our world over the past century, embodying the victory over brutal fascism and genocide; the construction of an international system committed to creating a more just, peaceful, and prosperous world; and the difficult, ongoing work of sustaining that project through institutions that forge partnerships and lay the foundation to address global society's most daunting problems.

Yet, as observers and scholars have carefully documented, that order is fracturing. Soaring economic inequality and rapid demographic change have fueled populist resentment, ethno-nationalism, and a sweeping distrust in national and international institutions alike. In parallel, massive shifts in technology and communication have heightened the avenues for surveillance and enabled the proliferation of disinformation. And with the increasing prominence of China on the world stage, along with new waves of authoritarianism cresting across the globe, it is clear that we inhabit a multipolar world whose aims and values no longer necessarily align with those of liberal democracy. At this moment, 54% of the world's population now lives under some form of authoritarian rule.

The COVID-19 pandemic has only accelerated these trend lines. The United States' failures to control effectively and mitigate the virus are reflective of its diminished role as a geopolitical leader, while China's admittedly flawed but far more deliberate response has only affirmed its centrality in the 21st-century world order. Meanwhile, the European Union can no longer claim to be a body composed of democratic states. In the early days of the pandemic, Prime Minister Viktor Orbán of Hungary used the virus as a pretext for seizing emergency powers that all but extinguished what little remained of Hungary's once promising democracy, consolidating Hungary's position as the first authoritarian state to be an EU member nation—something virtually inconceivable a generation ago.

COVID-19 marks a moment of reckoning for our era. While this disease, thankfully, is not likely to claim as many lives as the period from 1939 to 1945 did, its impacts on the global economy, on democracy, on public health, on food security, and on governance will reverberate for years to come. It is a multidimensional emergency that requires the efforts of all disciplines: a public health crisis that demands new tools to prevent the spread of this devastating disease and to conduct effective testing and tracing; a medical crisis that necessitates new modalities of treatment to heal those who are afflicted; and, in the recent words of an open letter whose signatories include former US Secretary of State Madeleine Albright, a "political crisis that threatens the future of liberal democracy."*

As the past has shown us, a moment of upheaval like this one—when so much upon which we have come to rely seems ruptured—is not the time to resign ourselves to despair nor to abandon the norms, institutions, and alliances that have upheld the modern world order for nearly eighty years. There is the possibility for renewal. But, like the Farben building in Frankfurt, these foundational structures must be reimagined and infused with new ideas for a new era.

* National Endowment for Democracy, "A Call to Defend Democracy," June 25, 2020, https://www.ned.org/covid-19-crisis-threatens-democracy-leading-world-figures-warn-joint -statement-press-release/.

Higher education will be integral to that endeavor. Time and again across the past century, the world's great universities have been vital partners in making, sustaining, and revitalizing the world order. One need not look far for an example. In 1943, just two years before General Eisenhower arrived in Frankfurt, two government officials named Paul Nitze and Christian Herter in Washington, DC—one a Republican, the other a Democrat—recognized the need for a graduate school that would combine the rigor and analytic power of the academy with the burgeoning field of international affairs. They called it the School of Advanced International Studies (SAIS), and it graduated its first class in June 1945, a mere month after the fall of Nazi Germany. In short order, the new school's faculty, students, and alumni—alongside experts from across government, military, and industry—proved instrumental in designing the treaties, the frameworks, and the organizations (the United Nations and North Atlantic Treaty Organization among them) that defined and sustained the international order that emerged in the wake of World War II. Now, with the publication of this volume, SAIS is once more helping to take up the core questions confronting our global community at a critical juncture in our history.

This book is the product of a two-day virtual forum hosted by Johns Hopkins SAIS in June 2020 that gathered a multidisciplinary group of exceptional scholars, thinkers, and leaders to consider collectively the future of our world order after COVID-19. The proceedings were viewed by thousands of people around the globe, from interested citizens to renowned scholars to national security experts to elected officials. Anyone who has ever organized an academic conference knows that attracting such an audience is no easy feat. To do so virtually and in the middle of a pandemic is even more astonishing.

Its success speaks to the truly Herculean efforts of editors and SAIS faculty Hal Brands and Frank Gavin, alongside their able teams and the extraordinary roster of contributors to this volume. But it also indicates the genuine hunger of a wide international audience for a sophisticated, meaningful, and collaborative conversation about the future of the geopolitical landscape, one that faces head-on the vital questions of this era: How are we going to confront the massive challenges posed by new centers of global power? How are we going to adapt and reimagine our institutions to ensure that they will continue to promote human flourishing and be responsive to the needs of the most vulnerable and marginalized among us? And how can we ensure that we do not stray from the essential democratic values that have defined the modern order since its origins?

The contributors to this book offer an array of bracing answers that will certainly be of great interest and use to policy makers who are implementing new measures to confront this crisis, to the students who are returning to classrooms or attending seminars virtually, and to faculty who are teaching the next generation about and in the midst of COVID-19. This global pandemic is, in so many ways, unprecedented in our lifetimes, and it will require unprecedented solutions that will profoundly reshape our world. Yet the tools for arriving at these solutions are the same as they have ever been: free inquiry, critical thought, and the passionate contestation of ideas tempered always by reason. It is my sincere hope that this robust and timely collection will inspire more of all three as we advance—steadily and slowly—into a post-COVID world.

RONALD J. DANIELS, PRESIDENT OF JOHNS HOPKINS UNIVERSITY
Adapted from opening remarks given at the World Order after COVID-19 Forum, a Johns Hopkins University Virtual Event, held by the School of Advanced International Studies and the Henry A. Kissinger Center for Global Affairs, June 30, 2020

Acknowledgments

This book is a reflection of the institution that produced it. The project was initially conceived by the president of Johns Hopkins University, Ronald J. Daniels, a visionary academic leader who has long excelled at bringing academic knowledge to bear on policy challenges. It grew out of a global, online conference that brought together participants from many of the disciplines and schools that make up the university.

We are extraordinarily grateful for the efforts of our friends from around campus in orchestrating an outstanding event on such a short timeline, including Christopher Austin, Cybele Bjorklund, Rachel Dawson, Sean McComas, Jodi Miller, Stephen Ruckman, and Grant Shreve from the President's office; Kristin Blanchfield, Allison Crean, Susan deMuth, Gwen Harley, Stephanie Muller, and Laura Savettiere from Development and Alumni Relations; and Andrew Green, Karen Lancaster, Marianne von Nordeck, and Jill Rosen from University Communications. A special thanks goes to Hiro Amano of Open Range Video and Gus Sentementes, the Director of Social Media and Analytics. Working nights and weekends, Hiro and Gus pulled off what we thought impossible in the age of Zoom exhaustion: a high-end, engaging, technically flawless production. And they did it with warmth and good cheer. Not least, we are grateful to Larry Summers, Angus Burgin, James Miller, Alina Polyakova, Gary Roughead, Jake Sullivan, and Alexandre White, who played key intellectual roles in the conference as presenters or chairs of panels. They may not have written chapters for this book, but their insights are nonetheless reflected in its pages.

We also owe thanks to our particular part of JHU: The School of Advanced International Studies headed by Dean Eliot Cohen. We are grateful to the whole SAIS family for their remarkable support, and especially the amazing work of the communications and events teams, including Debbie Aguilar, Miji Bell, Moe Elahi, Sonya Holmes, Jacquelyn Kasuya, Pedro Matias, Brittani Menina, Christopher Peña, Kensei Tsubata, and Lindsey Waldrop.

This book has been produced in record time: a little over four months from conception to production. This could not have been accomplished without the extraordinary efforts of Johns Hopkins University Press, in particular Barbara Kline Pope, Heidi M. Vincent, Kathryn Marguy, and especially Kelley Squazzo.

The Henry A. Kissinger Center for Global Affairs is actually a very small operation. Our remarkable colleagues, however, punch well above their weight. Lyndsay Howard, who runs our America and the Future of World Order Project, dropped everything to take command of the daunting logistics. Lyndsay, aided by the excellent Travis Zahnow, was our Count Carnot, the "organizer of victory." Diane Bernabei, Megan Ophel, and Zachary Wheeler were, as they always are, indispensable.

There is one person for whom we are especially grateful: Kissinger Center Associate Director Christopher Crosbie. As anyone who has dealt with him knows, no one works more tirelessly, with greater intelligence, integrity, and, given the incredible stress of working with us, great warmth and humor, than Chris. None of this would have happened without him.

HAL BRANDS

FRANCIS J. GAVIN

COVID-19 and WORLD ORDER

COVID-19 and World Order

Hal Brands and Francis J. Gavin

The coronavirus crisis was a shock, but should not have been a surprise. Public health experts had been warning about the dangers of viral pandemics for years. SARS, H1N1, Ebola, and MERS had highlighted the risks of diseases that raced across borders and the need for effective national and global responses. Not long before the first reported cases of COVID-19 in Wuhan, China, both the Johns Hopkins Center for Health Security and the Kissinger Center for Global Affairs Senior Fellow Dr. Kathleen Hicks had organized separate exercises that highlighted how profoundly a fast-moving virus could endanger the international system and US national security.[1]

Yet these warnings went largely unheeded and the world was not prepared to react effectively when the crisis began. COVID-19 overwhelmed national and international efforts to contain the pandemic while exposing deep flaws in the global public health infrastructure. The institutions most responsible for public health—the World Health Organization (WHO) for the world, the Centers for Disease Control and Prevention (CDC) for the United States—have not performed well. As we write, the world has seen more than 18 million confirmed cases of COVID-19 and rising. The United States has been especially hard hit, with over

Hal Brands is the Henry A. Kissinger Distinguished Professor at the Johns Hopkins School of Advanced International Studies (SAIS). Francis J. Gavin is the Giovanni Agnelli Distinguished Professor and the inaugural director of the Henry A. Kissinger Center for Global Affairs at SAIS.

5 million confirmed cases and the spread still not under control.[2] The science and epidemiological knowledge surrounding the virus is evolving, new therapies are being developed, and intensive efforts to create an effective vaccine all provide some hope. Until then, COVID-19 will dominate the international landscape.

Even after the virus is contained, the consequences will be with us for some time. This is because the pandemic arrived at an especially troubling moment for the world. In the past few years, many have commented on the fraying of international arrangements to provide for a stable, peaceful, and prosperous world order.[3] What had been feared for some time was now seen as a stark reality: many of the norms, institutions, and practices that upheld the liberal international order and marked American leadership since the end of the Cold War and, in some cases, the end of the Second World War, were under enormous stress. The causes are many and interconnected: the reemergence of great-power political rivalry, marked by the worsening and increasingly toxic relationship between the two largest powers, the United States and China; the increase in populism and nationalism, as well as a seeming loss of faith in democracy as authoritarianism increases its grip on many parts of the world; the dizzying and disorienting effects of new technology; and numerous other causes. These challenges have manifested as a polarized United States grows increasingly uncertain about its role in the world, as many around the world lose faith in the benefits of globalization and interdependence, and as a raft of new transnational concerns, ranging from climate change to disinformation, reveal the shortcomings of existing international institutions.

The crisis does provide an opportunity, however. This volume is a multidisciplinary effort to assess the current state of world order, analyze the effects of the COVID crisis, and offer insights and ideas for the future. The crisis has made clear that much work needs to be done to improve our national and global public health capabilities and institutions and to elevate the threat of disease and pandemic to a higher priority in our national and international security frameworks. This book, however, is premised on something more: the idea that the crisis highlights a number of other pressing national and global challenges, in areas ranging from climate change to relations with China. We believe this crisis is potentially a crucial pivot point, providing an opportunity to rethink—and perhaps revitalize—our current international system. This book begins a much-needed conversation about how to shape international relations in a post-COVID world.

World Orders, Old and New

Historically, efforts to construct effective international arrangements emerge after periods of war, crisis, and turmoil.[4] The Peace of Westphalia ended the vicious wars of religion that had plagued Europe and constructed a comparatively stable system based on the balance of power among nation-states. The 1814–1815 Congress of Vienna was marked by the masterful diplomacy of Count Metternich of Austria and Lord Castlereagh of Great Britain, who worked with other European leaders to tame the wars and ideological fervor unleashed by the French Revolution.[5] These efforts arguably kept the peace in Europe until the Crimean War and prevented any one European power from dominating the continent until the start of the 20th century.

What was left of the Concert system collapsed with World War I, leading to a series of efforts over the succeeding decades to rebuild world order. The Versailles conference after the First World War was inspired by American President Woodrow Wilson's desire to build a peace based on national self-determination, open diplomacy, the ends of arms races, and collective security through a League of Nations—the cures, he believed, to the pathologies of imperialism, militarism, and cutthroat diplomacy that had brought on the conflict. This vision failed as the United States retreated from the system Wilson proposed while lingering and unresolved grievances from the war poisoned the international climate. A global depression, the rise of violent, revolutionary regimes, and the onset of the Second World War destroyed the system created at Versailles and revealed the desperate need for effective mechanisms to generate world order.[6]

Learning from this failure, American planners worked with their allies to start constructing the postwar order before the war even ended. Conferences between the three major players—the United States, the Soviet Union, and Great Britain—at Tehran, Yalta, and Potsdam mixed plans to win the war with efforts to coordinate the postwar peace. International meetings at Bretton Woods and Dumbarton Oaks designed global institutions such as the International Monetary Fund, the World Bank, and the United Nations.[7] American officials hoped for a seamless, integrated world order that would bring the leading nations together in avoiding war and maintaining a secure, prosperous peace.[8]

Yet the Cold War spoiled this vision of "One World," and what emerged in the years and decades that followed was not one order but several. In the economic realm, the so-called Bretton Woods order, which was focused on the capitalist world, created a system that encouraged revitalized global trade but prioritized domestic reconstruction, regional integration, and stability. This system frayed in the 1960s and 1970s, and after a time marked by some disorder, was replaced by the more open, globalized system we have now, based on flexible and market-determined currencies, large-scale global investment and trade, and the dominance of dollar-denominated banking and finance.[9] International security evolved in unexpected directions as well. The United Nations system, premised on state sovereignty and universal principles, was overshadowed by a bipolar system that saw intense ideological and geopolitical rivalry between two rival superpower blocs led by the Soviet Union and the United States.[10] The United States ended up leading a secure, prosperous international order—but one that was limited to the "free world" rather than the entire world.

The superpowers nonetheless cooperated to create a third order: a very successful nuclear order, based upon their shared interest in limiting the dangers posed by the "absolute weapon." This order was built around a series of bilateral and global arms control treaties—including the 1963 Partial Test Ban Treaty, the 1968 Nuclear Nonproliferation Treaty, and the 1972 Antiballistic Missile and Strategic Arms Limitation Treaties—as well as less formalized norms and practices, from tolerance of satellite overflights by the enemy (necessary to reduce the danger of surprise attack) and an implicit understanding, which evolved over time, that nuclear weapons were not merely powerful bombs but were in a category all their own.[11] Though it came under constant pressure, this element of order—rivals working to manage and limit the dangers of new technologies—was more successful than anyone expected and perhaps provides a model for contemporary challenges.

The unexpected end of the Cold War and the rapid demise of the Soviet Union highlighted both the success of these postwar arrangements and the need to rethink world order for a new era. It was also a time of great intellectual creativity, as scholars such as John Mearsheimer, Francis Fukuyama, John Ikenberry, Charles Krauthammer, and Samuel Huntington offered innovative conceptual frames to understand a rapidly changing world.[12] Events moved quickly. Germany was peacefully reunified and the European Union project flourished; democracies emerged around the world, and some long-simmering conflicts and civil wars were resolved peacefully.[13] The United States, working through the United Nations, built an impressive coalition to enforce collective security and expel Iraq from Kuwait. To the surprise of many, some elements of the postwar era, such as the North Atlantic Treaty Organization, were not only maintained but expanded. Other institutions, such as the International Monetary Fund, were reimagined. Over time, still other institutions, such as the World Trade Organization (WTO) and Group of

Twenty (G20) were inaugurated. The post–Cold War era was marked by a combination of multilateralism and American ideals and power, as the United States found itself in a commanding position in world affairs. To the extent that there was a single world order, it was largely an expansion and modification of the liberal system that had taken root in the non-communist world after World War II.[14] As this system took on increasingly global dimensions, it was a time of hope and promise.

That period of optimism now seems like a distant memory. The 9/11 attacks on the United States, followed by difficult, controversial wars in Iraq and Afghanistan, exposed new sources of insecurity. The war in Iraq, in particular, drained US energies and shook international support for American power. The 2007–9 financial crisis pummeled the global economy and undermined faith in the market. Populism rose and the movement toward democracy weakened.[15] As China's economy boomed, that country did not, as many had hoped, embrace liberal principles, but instead challenged both regional and global norms and institutions while descending deeper into authoritarianism. Information technology, once seen as a liberating force, showed its darker side through cyberattacks and disinformation campaigns; climate change loomed as a potentially existential challenge. Both the vote of the United Kingdom to leave the European Union (Brexit) and the unexpected election of Donald J. Trump as US president on a campaign of "America First" made 2016 the year when it was clear the existing world order was imperiled. The principles and values that many believed were the cornerstone of this order—openness and innovation, democratic practice and tolerance, interdependence and globalization—were viewed with suspicion by large swaths of America and the world.

As the chapters in this volume demonstrate, COVID-19 highlighted and exacerbated many of the strains that were already testing the post–Cold War system. The pandemic was so disruptive because it exploded in a world that was already increasingly disordered. The question of how to reconstruct world order after COVID involves dealing with not just the disease but also the underlying problems it revealed. How should we diagnose and understand these challenges to world order, and what principles and policies should shape our efforts moving forward?[16] Answering these questions is the purpose of this book.

World Order after COVID

This volume is an undertaking of the Henry A. Kissinger Center for Global Affairs at Johns Hopkins University School of Advanced International Studies (SAIS). Inspired by its namesake, the renowned diplomat and scholar Henry Kissinger, the Center is dedicated to better understanding and applying the lessons of history in order to make sense of an increasingly complex world. Since its inception in 2016, the Center and its scholars have engaged deeply with questions of world order. The COVID-19 crisis has offered an opportunity to convene global experts from Johns Hopkins University and other leading institutions to understand a landmark crisis and plot a course for the future.

This volume draws upon that expertise to address issues ranging from global public health and climate change to international institutions and great-power rivalry. The particular challenge of our moment is that it is impossible to grapple with questions of world order without considering "hard" and "soft" security issues, novel transnational challenges and timeless geopolitical contests, and politics within states as well as politics between them. As always, addressing any of these subjects requires a historical perspective as well as an eye to the future.

Part I of this book thus focuses on *Applied History and Future Scenarios*. It includes essays that use the past to highlight overlooked or misunderstood dynamics of the current crisis and that push us to think imaginatively about the future. These intellectual tasks are particularly important in times of radical uncertainty: in these moments, grounding ourselves in history, or systematically assessing the different paths the future might take, yields the greatest payoff.

Jeremy A. Greene and Dora Vargha employ a historical mindset to address the most basic question we confront today: When will we move from a "world of COVID" to a "world after COVID"? The answer they offer is that we are unlikely to see any single moment that marks the end of the pandemic. Rather, there will be a gradual recession of danger that never fully goes away and that probably will not match the easing of restrictions put in place to deal with that danger. Margaret MacMillan asks why we are so often surprised by catastrophes that might have been predicted, why some leaders and societies cope better than others, and how we can deal with the lasting consequences of great shocks—issues we can better understand by revisiting the trajectory of major upheavals in the past. Using history as a guide, Philip Bobbitt considers why many faddish predictions about the post-COVID world may be wrong and offers his own future scenario—that of a deepening crisis of constitutional order in major nation-states—as a way of pushing us to prepare for an uncertain future.

Part II deals with *Global Public Health and Mitigation Strategies*. These issues are now of incontestable importance to world order because of the horrific human toll pandemics can take and the way that epidemiological catastrophes can trigger economic and geopolitical ones. There is no guarantee, after all, that the end of

COVID will bring a respite from aggressive global disease. It might mark the beginning of a new era of even more catastrophic outbreaks.

In response to this danger, Tom Inglesby offers a detailed program for making pandemics lose their power, and in doing so reminds us that the dichotomy between unilateral and multilateral responses is a false one. Lainie Rutkow argues that policy makers must not, in the aftermath of the crisis, lose the sense of urgency that a pandemic creates. Rather, they must raise the profile of public health measures that are often invisible until a crisis breaks, while cultivating new collaborations and networks within and between nations. Finally, Jeffrey P. Kahn, Anna C. Mastroianni, and Sridhar Venkatapuram consider the ethics of global health in a post-COVID world. In their view, the crisis reveals the limitations of bioethics as a field and underscores the need for a more holistic conception of what makes a global health system morally just. Without such a shift, we will be ill-equipped to address global health challenges that can wreak havoc on the entire world.

Part III moves to *Transnational Issues: Technology, Climate, and Food.* In each of these areas, purely national solutions to accelerating challenges are unworkable. And in each of these areas, COVID-19 has highlighted the urgency of action.

For Johannes Urpelainen, a pandemic is a terrible thing to waste. He contends that the crisis, by temporarily suppressing global emissions, has created an opportunity to invest heavily in green technologies and perhaps head off the worst impacts of climate change. Jessica Fanzo reminds us that COVID will dramatically worsen food insecurity around the world—a development likely to heighten political instability, geopolitical conflict, and other forms of strife. "Without food security," she tells us, "there is no world order." Finally, Christine Fox and Thayer Scott point out that COVID has intensified the technological rivalry between the United States and China and that Washington must deepen its collaboration with other democracies if it is to manage the consequences of a technological revolution that creates as many risks as opportunities.

Part IV covers *The Future of the Global Economy.* In hindsight, we are likely to remember COVID-19 as an economic crisis as much as an epidemiological one. For it not only brought the global economy to a standstill—triggering the most rapid, if perhaps temporary, de-globalization the world has ever seen—but also revealed the weaknesses of existing international institutions for managing the global economy and the dangerous dependencies globalization had created.

Benn Steil argues that the pre-COVID economic order is probably not coming back. But instead of reverting to isolationism or persisting in the search for a single, integrated global economic order, the United States should consider the "two worlds" approach it took during the Cold War. This means limiting reliance on the authoritarian world while deepening American integration with other democracies. John Lipsky examines why institutions, such as the G20, worked relatively well in dealing with the fallout from the global financial crisis but have performed so poorly in handling the economic dimensions of the pandemic and what this tells us about the future of global economic governance.

Lipsky's essay serves as a bridge to part V, which covers *Global Politics and Governance*. For those who believe in the virtues of the liberal international order, the most shocking aspect of the COVID crisis is surely the degree to which many of the order's key institutions—from the WHO to the G7—underperformed or proved incapable of constructive action. Failures of governance at the domestic level were accompanied by failures of governance at the global level. Any post-COVID effort at world order will have to begin with an understanding of what went wrong.

Anne Applebaum points to a variety of factors—the abdication of American leadership, the determined Chinese effort to capture international institutions, and the fact that bodies created in the 20th century may lack the speed and agility the current moment requires. Fixing the system may require fundamentally rethinking what role we expect deeply entrenched, bureaucratic entities to play in global politics. Henry Farrell and Hahrie Han believe that the liberal institutional order was collapsing even before the crisis began because of a growing deficit of democratic accountability. They, too, argue for a fundamental reimagining that reconnects the international system with the publics it is meant to serve. Janice Gross Stein asserts that the world is becoming more contested and competitive after COVID and that consensus-based institutions are unlikely to perform well in such a world. If international governance is to work, it will have to go "off-site," into informal networks and plurilateral coalitions working outside of existing bodies. Finally, James B. Steinberg argues that the best way of salvaging some order from potential chaos is by rebuilding a system that emphasizes arrangements for addressing shared challenges, sets rules and norms for emerging technologies, engages public and civil society, and safely manages a competitive US-China relationship.

Part VI is also about high politics, focusing on *Grand Strategy and American Statecraft*. World orders are, to a great extent, a reflection of the policies and values of the most powerful global actors. And if COVID has revealed significant weaknesses in the post–Cold War order, it has also raised profound questions about what grand strategy the United States should pursue in the future—or whether it even wishes to lead that order.

Interestingly, the authors in this section mostly offer glass-half-full interpretations, while contending that American grand strategy should adapt but not change fundamentally. Hal Brands, Peter Feaver, and William Inboden argue that the pandemic need not make the world far more menacing for the United States. It could, rather, create opportunities to pursue a smarter, more geopolitically savvy globalization, to reinvest in partnerships with liberal democracies, and to forge a stronger counterbalancing coalition against a neo-totalitarian China. That will, of course, require more enlightened American leadership than is currently in evidence; it will also require that the United States address dangers from pandemics and other "soft" security threats without hollowing out its capability to meet "hard" security challenges. Similarly, Thomas Wright calls for the United States to resist the understandable urge to fundamentally reorient its grand strategy toward transnational issues. The better option would be a "free world" strategy focused on improving the resilience and solidarity of the world's democracies against great-power revisionism and resurgent authoritarianism.

Kori Schake also offers a moderately optimistic take, arguing that the pandemic could ultimately result in a renaissance of American global engagement, the strengthening of the domestic foundations of US power, and stronger efforts by free societies to deal with China's rise. Finally, Kathleen H. Hicks sees the crisis as an opportunity to revisit core elements of American grand strategy and improve the mix of tools the United States uses to protect and pursue its interests in the world. Hicks is also relatively bullish on the long-term strength of democracies, seeing the protests for racial justice as a sign that political will and even consensus is emerging for much-needed change.

Looming over so many of these issues is the topic covered in part VII: *Sino-American Rivalry*. If before the crisis China and America already seemed headed for a deep and prolonged competition—a new Cold War, as some have termed it—that trajectory seems all the more pronounced since the pandemic struck.[17] Positions have hardened on both sides of the Pacific; the hostility has become palpable, even as the reality of interdependence has never been clearer.

Elizabeth Economy offers a stark assessment of the challenge that Xi Jinping's China poses to the existing world order. She argues that while the United States has increasingly embraced a strategy of competing with, and even containing, Beijing, that strategy is unlikely to succeed unless Washington also reinvests in a broader concept of a world order centered on democratic values and solidarity among the liberal democracies. Graham Allison calls instead for America to seek a "rivalry partnership" with Beijing, in which the two competitors seek to make a world "safe for diversity" and find common ground in areas where their interests overlap. Eric Schmidt contends that technology has become the central axis of great-power rivalry and outlines an agenda meant to allow the United States to win this new "great game" without forgoing all the advantages of interchange and interdependence. Finally, Niall Ferguson rounds out the volume by arguing that a new cold war is very much under way. He believes that the Trump administration has actually done fairly well in positioning the United States to win it, yet he reminds us that the choices of lesser powers ultimately did much to determine the outcome of the US-Soviet Cold War. Ferguson warns that many of America's allies are contemplating nonalignment in the present rivalry. If that happens, America will find it nearly impossible to prevail in a long competition with China—or sustain its concept of world order.

Themes and Insights

The authors cut across disciplinary lines and deal with subjects that inevitably overlap; they offer both complementary and contrasting viewpoints. The chapters cluster around a variety of themes and debates that bring together the volume as a whole. Here, we highlight a few issues of particular importance.

Will COVID-19 Remake World Order?

It is undeniable that COVID-19 is shaking up the world and laying bare the weaknesses of existing arrangements and institutions. But will COVID mark the end of one world order and the emergence of another? The answer, we believe, is not so simple.

It is not a coincidence that the biggest, most epochal shifts in world order often occur in the wake of major wars. Such cataclysms fatally rupture existing relationships and institutions; they reset the global distribution of power. By leveling the architecture of one world order, they create new possibilities for construction.

That COVID will have a similarly transformative effect seems unlikely. The pandemic has been monumentally traumatic, of course, and all bets are off if the world faces multiple, increasingly lethal outbreaks before a vaccine is developed. But short of that happening, COVID will probably not dramatically change the distribution of material power. To be sure, the United States has fared poorly from a public health perspective and has suffered a severe diminution—in the near term, at least—of its credibility and reputation for competence. Yet several aspects of the crisis—the role of the US Federal Reserve in stabilizing the world economy, the flight to the dollar, and others—actually testify to America's immense structural power. Moreover, it is far from clear that America's foremost challenger— China—will see its own long-term position enhanced, in part because of the way that the crisis has underscored that country's authoritarian pathologies and in part because one result of the pandemic may be a more concerted counterbalancing effort from the world's democracies.

When it comes to institutions, the pandemic has undoubtedly revealed deep-seated weaknesses within many prominent international bodies, from the WHO and WTO to the G7. The need for reform has become clear to all; so has the absence of well-developed institutional structures to deal with a variety of emerging challenges. This should not surprise us: much of our global governance architecture was created at a different time, in a different world, to deal with different challenges. Some of it is now out of date or ill-fitted for new global threats.

Those with long memories understand that there have been previous periods of institutional underperformance, failure, and adaptation within the context of particular orders. The roles and responsibilities of the International Monetary Fund and World Bank have shifted considerably since their creation; the General Agreement on Tariffs and Trade gave way to the World Trade Organization after the Cold War; ad hoc arrangements have often emerged to complement, rather than replace, existing bodies on issues such as nuclear proliferation. Viewed against this precedent, COVID may simply spur a period of much-needed institutional reform and evolution rather than a new start. Indeed, in several chapters in this volume, the authors indicate that, far from destroying the existing order, COVID could spur its reform and renewal. Perhaps that order will be somewhat narrower than it was after the Cold War: a number of contributors argue that the key is to lessen dependence on China while deepening cooperation among the democracies, a reversion to something like the "two worlds" approach of the postwar era. Although that change would be a significant departure from the post–Cold War era of global integration, it would actually take the United States back to its order-building roots, so to speak.

Could the crisis nonetheless force a significant change in our approach to world order by fundamentally altering how the United States and other countries perceive and prioritize key international threats? If COVID ends up killing, just within the United States, a number of people that is orders of magnitude higher than the number that died on 9/11, then surely "soft" security threats will rise in importance relative to "hard" security challenges such as terrorism and geopolitical rivalry. Perhaps the military balance of power is becoming passé—perhaps it simply is not that relevant in a world where small states have often done better than large states in suppressing the pandemic and where grave threats to human prosperity and flourishing do not respect geopolitical divides.[18]

Here too, though, the story is not so simple. COVID-19 may have elevated the threat posed by pandemics and other nontraditional threats. But the threat posed by more traditional dangers remains. COVID has created new temptations for authoritarian actors to undermine the politics and cohesion of democratic societies; it could well exacerbate state failure and instability in fragile regions throughout the world, including the always volatile greater Middle East. And the pandemic was accompanied by a marked increase in Chinese assertiveness, from Hong Kong to the South China Sea to South Asia and beyond, using tools from "wolf warrior" public diplomacy to outright military coercion.[19]

The real takeaway from COVID may be that hard and soft threats often work in tandem, potentially mixing and combining in powerful ways. Geopolitical rivalry may make transnational threats harder to combat; transnational threats can sharpen geopolitical rivalries and instability. America and other countries will not be able to ignore hard or soft threats in a post-COVID world because those challenges are so deeply interrelated.

BALANCING COMPETITION AND COOPERATION

This relates to a second theme: the uncertain balance of competition and cooperation. We may look back on COVID as the crisis that crystallized a protracted, high-stakes competition between the world's greatest powers—much as crises in Greece and Turkey in 1946–47 crystallized an emerging Cold War. The pandemic underscored that the world is fracturing rather than converging; great-power politics are taking on an increasingly zero-sum logic.[20] Yet we may also look back on COVID as the event that threw into relief the mutual vulnerability of even bitter rivals and the need for positive-sum cooperation between them. How—and whether—this balance between competition and cooperation gets struck will be a defining challenge of world order in the 21st century. It will pertain not just to pandemics, but to climate change, food security, migration, information and biotechnology, and other issues with the potential to fundamentally upset the human experience.

There are contrasting perspectives on how to address this dilemma. Some analysts argue that the world's democratic states should first focus on waging and winning the competition with China, because a favorable balance of power is the best guarantee of securing cooperation with rivals on favorable terms. It would be unwise, in this view, to mute Sino-American rivalry in hopes of gaining Chinese cooperation on pandemics or climate change. Rather, America and its allies should compete vigorously, confident that cooperation on shared interests can be compartmentalized, just as the superpowers managed to cooperate on arms control and smallpox eradication during the Cold War.[21]

Or perhaps this first view is too sanguine. US-Soviet cooperation on arms control and global disease emerged only after two decades of Cold War and early moves toward a superpower détente. Perhaps it will be necessary to limit Sino-American rivalry before positive-sum behaviors can take root. If this is the case, a determined effort to seize the geopolitical and ideological high ground could simply ensure that *all* issues come to be seen in zero-sum terms—as happened in the early stages of the COVID crisis.[22] And while the threat that China poses is very real, it remains somewhat more abstract than the human and economic carnage COVID has been wreaking on both countries and around the world. For some, the changed nature of the international system means that a failure by the great powers to subsume their differences to work on shared and potentially catastrophic global challenges will lead the world to ruin.

This book will not fully resolve which approach is best.[23] But the debate reminds us that the challenges of sustaining a peaceful, flourishing world in this century are particularly daunting, because the world is increasingly dividing along geopolitical and ideological lines even as it requires cooperation across them. And it shows that a form of American statecraft that is purely competitive in nature—one that does not feature a leading US role in catalyzing action on transnational challenges—will not meet the demands of global leadership.

The Future of Globalization and Innovation

COVID-19 is not simply a crisis of public health. It is an economic crisis—a self-induced coma, as it has been termed—unparalleled in modern history. Quarantines, shelter-in-place orders, and other restrictions caused growth to collapse and unemployment to surge. These measures also raised sharp questions about how long the resulting damage would last, which industries and countries would emerge with a competitive advantage, and what prospects there are for vibrant equitable economies—at the national and global levels—in the years to come.

Complicating matters is the fact that COVID occurred amid a growing dissatisfaction with the effects of globalization and interdependence. In the years after the Cold War, globalization had intensified and deepened. The process connected the world as never before, generated massive wealth, and pulled individuals around the world out of poverty. Yet domestically, offshoring also exacerbated de-industrialization and the loss of manufacturing jobs in the United States. Globally, massive increases in trade and financial flows generated turbulence and occasional crises, and left countries vulnerable to powerful global forces outside of their control. It was hoped that globalization would bring along with it liberal democracy, transparency, tolerance, and openness, but authoritarian governments—China's being the clearest example—cleverly found ways to capture economic benefits without making political or social sacrifices.

Anxiety about openness went hand-in-hand with anxiety about technological innovation. Much growth and even more interconnectedness have been driven by profound changes in technology, especially in the information sector. Only a decade ago, this technological revolution was viewed as almost entirely beneficial to humanity, but since then, we have seen some of its dark sides. Disinformation campaigns have deepened polarization within democracies while new technologies, such as facial recognition tools, empower authoritarian governments.[24] Artificial intelligence, robotics, machine learning, and biotechnology promise extraordinary benefits for humanity while also raising the threat of potentially vast dangers.[25]

We can take some comfort in the fact that we have been here before. Technological innovation has always been a source of danger as well as opportunity. The postwar economic order was never as smooth or seamless as we sometimes believe. The vaunted Bretton Woods system was prone to crises and collapsed altogether in the early 1970s, leading to years of ad hoc efforts to stabilize a turbulent system. When the Cold War ended, many countries around the world reduced trade barriers, liberalized their economies, and allowed foreign investment; the decades that followed witnessed impressive growth but also debilitating crises. The story of the post–World War II global economy is one of fantastic prosperity and severe, recurring challenges.

In this crisis, there is bad news and good news. The bad news is that globalization proved surprisingly fragile in the face of a raging pandemic—even countries within the European Union barred exports of critical goods and shut their borders. The good news is that certain aspects of the system have worked fairly well. Similar to the 2007–9 global financial crisis, the US Federal Reserve acted as the banker to the world during the pandemic, providing much-needed liquidity to avoid a depression (albeit with less global coordination). National governments, including the United States, initiated massive stimulus programs; the results were mixed but the outcome was surely better than it would have been absent these injections. There are also certain indications that governments may still respond to the crisis in mostly constructive ways. If the outcome of the pandemic is a reduction of specific dependencies on authoritarian regimes, an emphasis on economic resilience that nonetheless encourages deep integration between democracies, a greater pooling of resources among like-minded nations to develop and master the technologies of the future, and enhanced efforts to address inequalities both within and between countries—all possibilities to which authors in this volume point—then the crisis could be a source of renewal rather than a harbinger of a dark new age.

Politics, At Home and Abroad

One reason the COVID-19 crisis has been so jarring is that it seemed to worsen the deepening global crisis of governance. Fraying democratic norms, increased populism and nationalism, overmatched and ineffective government bureaucracies, and the growing reach of autocratic leaders have menaced the global order for several years.[26] The pandemic has, at least in the short term, accelerated many of these worrisome trends. American statecraft has long held that world order should be based on liberal ideas and democratic values. If so, reinvigorating and rethinking democratic politics at home may be a prerequisite to sustaining the influence of those values on the global stage.

While there are different views in the book on how the battle between democratic forms of governance and authoritarianism will play out, the future may not be as foreboding as some of the early indicators make it seem. As some contributors note, democracies such as New Zealand, Taiwan, Iceland, and Germany implemented especially effective measures to limit the coronavirus's spread. Countries with illiberal populists or authoritarian leaders in charge—Brazil, Iran, Russia, North Korea, Belarus—saw cases, hospitalizations, and deaths surge. Unfortunately, the world's leading democracy—the United States—fared poorly, due to the erratic presidency of Donald Trump as well as the disappointing performance of the federal bureaucracy. The contrast to the autocratic efficiency of China seems, at first glance, quite striking.

But the story is not all bad. The extent to which China's system has truly done better against COVID is hard to confirm with any precision, given the regime's systematic suppression of reliable information. Whatever progress Beijing has made has come at a high cost in violations of human rights and basic liberties, and failing to honestly communicate the severity of the virus's spread to other states and global authorities.[27] In the United States, the absence of national oversight has allowed certain state and local governments to demonstrate competence and vision. Elements of the nonprofit and private sector have exhibited qualities of nimbleness and adaptation. The extraordinary effort, ongoing as we write this, to develop both effective therapies and a mass-produced vaccine in record time is breathtaking.[28] America's deep, diverse, and innovative civil society provides a degree of resiliency, even in the face of federal underperformance, that autocracies find hard to mimic.

A number of contributors to this volume also point out that COVID-19 may force democracies to confront their limitations, as crises often do. COVID will equip democratic governments around the world with a greater understanding of the dangers of authoritarian disinformation campaigns. The pandemic has highlighted lingering issues of inequality and racial injustice in the United States and other democratic societies. Not least, it has revealed how deep political polarization and tribalism has too often gotten in the way of wise, coordinated policies.[29] It is clear that the United States and other democratic societies face a crisis of politics and governance. We must escape a terrible cycle: the worse our institutions and politics perform, the more people lose faith in governance and the more our politics becomes poisoned. If we are looking for something that will provide an impetus to the slow, messy, incremental process of reform needed to avert such an outcome, a global pandemic seems as good a candidate as any.

Crisis as Opportunity

We are living through a dark time. The world confronts overlapping national and global crises. Governments and international institutions often seem inadequate to the task. Aggressive authoritarianism and illiberalism often seem to be on the ascent. Aspects of the postwar and post–Cold War orders appear worn and outdated.

Here history can provide both consolation and inspiration. The world has seen other periods of great disorder and turbulence—even since World War II—that were arguably worse than our own. The current crisis has even revealed underlying strengths of the current world order. For example, the unprecedented sharing of scientific information and the drive for therapies and a vaccine remind us of the breathtaking economic, intellectual, and scientific advances that have occurred in recent decades.[30] Finally, history reminds us that times of crisis provide opportunities for creativity and reform. Innovation and technical breakthroughs often emerge from economic depressions (the bicycle was invented in Germany during an epidemic among horses in 1815!). Moments of crisis break inertia and create a fluidity that can be put to good purpose; they can foster the political will needed to confront entrenched pathologies. The extraordinary protests over racial injustice in June 2020, which rapidly spread around the world, reflect a collective national and global desire to bring real change. Proposals to reform global governance, enhance the solidarity of democratic nations, and invest in new efforts to confront looming threats reflect a similar impulse.

Can we make the most of the moment? The starting point is to think creatively about how we arrived at our current juncture and how we can make our way out of the accompanying uncertainty. Our hope is that this volume can guide decision makers in this endeavor.

NOTES

1. See appendix B: "2019 Global Security Forum Scenarios," in Samuel J. Brannen, Christian S. Haig, Katherine Schmidt, and Kathleen H. Hicks, "Twin Pillars: Upholding National Security and National Innovation in Merging Technological Governance," *CSIS*, Jan. 2020, https://csis-website-prod.s3.amazonaws.com/s3fs-public/publication/200123 _Brannen_TwinPillars_WEB_FINAL.pdf; and Samuel Brannen and Kathleen Hicks, "We Predicted a Coronavirus Pandemic: Here's What Policymakers Could Have Seen Coming," *Politico Magazine*, March 7, 2020, https://www.politico.com/news/magazine/2020/03/07 /coronavirus-epidemic-prediction-policy-advice-121172. The Johns Hopkins Center for Health Security, in partnership with the World Economic Forum and the Bill and Melinda Gates Foundation, held a global pandemic simulation, "Event 201," in October 2019, https://www.centerforhealthsecurity.org/event201/.

2. For up-to-date data on global COVID-19 cases, see the Johns Hopkins University COVID-19 Tracking Map, developed by Dr. Lauren Gardner and the Center for Systems Science and Engineering at JHU, https://coronavirus.jhu.edu/map.html.

3. Robert Kagan, *The Jungle Grows Back: America and Our Imperiled World* (New York: Borzoi Book, 2018); Hal Brands, *American Grand Strategy in the Age of Trump* (Washington, DC: Brookings Institution Press, 2018); Francis J. Gavin, "Pandemic and the Plight of American Public Policy," *War on the Rocks*, April 2, 2020, https://warontherocks.com/2020 /04/pandemic-and-the-plight-of-american-public-policy/; G. John Ikenberry, *A World Safe for Democracy: Liberal Internationalism and the Crises of the Global Order* (New Haven, CT: Yale University Press, 2020); and G. John Ikenberry, "The Next Liberal Order," *Foreign Affairs* (July/August 2020), https://www.foreignaffairs.com/articles/united-states/2020-06 -09/next-liberal-order.

4. Hal Brands and Charles Edel, The *Lessons of Tragedy: Statecraft and World Order* (New Haven, CT: Yale University Press, 2019); Henry Kissinger, *Diplomacy* (New York: Simon & Schuster, 1994); and G. John Ikenberry, *After Victory* (Princeton, NJ: Princeton University Press, 2001).

5. Henry Kissinger, *A World Restored* (Gloucester, UK: Peter Smith, 1973); and John Bew, *Castlereagh: A Life* (Oxford, UK: Oxford University Press, 2012).

6. Sally Marks, *The Illusion of Peace: International Relations in Europe 1918–1933* (New York: St. Martin's Press, 1976); and Adam Tooze, *The Deluge: The Great War, America and the Remaking of the Global Order, 1916–1931* (New York: Penguin Books, 2014).

7. Robert Dallek, *Franklin Roosevelt and American Foreign Policy, 1932–1945* (Oxford, UK: Oxford University Press, 1979; Henry Kissinger, *Diplomacy* (New York: Simon & Schuster, 1994); and Benn Steil, *The Battle of Bretton Woods: John Maynard Keynes, Harry Dexter White, and the Making of a World Order* (Princeton, NJ: Princeton University Press, 2013).

8. John Lewis Gaddis, *We Now Know: Rethinking Cold War History* (New York: Oxford University Press, 1997).

9. Harold James, *International Monetary Cooperation since Bretton Woods* (Washington, DC: International Monetary Fund, 1996); and Barry J. Eichengreen, Arnaug Mehl, and Livia Chitu, *How Global Currencies Work: Past, Present, and Future* (Princeton, NJ: Princeton University Press, 2018).

10. Marc Trachtenberg, *A Constructed Peace: The Making of the European Settlement, 1945–1963* (Princeton, NJ: Princeton University Press, 1999).

11. John Lewis Gaddis, *The Long Peace: Inquiries into the History of the Cold War* (New York: Oxford University Press, 1987); Francis J. Gavin, *Nuclear Statecraft: History and Strategy in America's Atomic Age* (Ithaca, NY: Cornell University Press, 2012); James Cameron, *The Double Game: The Demise of America's First Missile Defense System and the Rise of Strategic Arms Limitation* (Oxford, UK: Oxford University Press, 2017); and Hal Brands, "Non-Proliferation and the Dynamics of the Middle Cold War: The Superpowers, the MLF, and the NPT," *Cold War History* 7, no. 3 (2007): 389–423, https://doi.org/10.1080/1468 2740701474857.

12. Francis Fukuyama, "The End of History?" *The National Interest,* no. 16 (Summer 1989): 3–18, www.jstor.org/stable/24027184; Samuel P. Huntington, "The Clash of Civilizations?" *Foreign Affairs* 72, no. 3 (Summer 1993): 22–49, https://doi.org/10.2307/20045621; Charles Krauthammer, "The Unipolar Moment," *Foreign Affairs* 70, no. 1 (1990); and John J. Mearsheimer, "Back to the Future: Instability in Europe after the Cold War," *International Security* 15, no. 1 (Summer 1990): 5–56, https://doi.org/10.2307/253898.

13. James Addison Baker and Thomas M. DeFrank, *The Politics of Diplomacy: Revolution, War, and Peace, 1989–1992* (New York: G. P. Putnam's Sons, 1995); Hal Brands, *Making the Unipolar Moment: U.S. Foreign Policy and the Rise of the Post–Cold War Order* (Ithaca, NY: Cornell University Press, 2016); George H. W. Bush and Brent Scowcroft, *A World Transformed* (New York: Vintage Books, 1999); and Phillip Zelikow and Condoleezza Rice, *To Build a Better World: Choices to End the Cold War and Create a Global Commonwealth* (New York: Twelve, 2019).

14. Brands, *Making the Unipolar Moment*; and G. John Ikenberry, *Liberal Leviathan: The Origins, Crisis, and Transformation of the American World Order* (Princeton, NJ: Princeton University Press, 2011).

15. Adam Tooze, *Crashed: How a Decade of Financial Crises Changed the World* (New York: Viking Press, 2018).

16. Henry Kissinger, "The Coronavirus Pandemic Will Forever Alter the World Order," *Wall Street Journal,* April 3, 2020, https://www.wsj.com/articles/the-coronavirus-pandemic -will-forever-alter-the-world-order-11585953005.

17. Robert D. Kaplan, "A New Cold War Has Begun," *Foreign Policy,* January 7, 2019, https://foreignpolicy.com/2019/01/07/a-new-cold-war-has-begun/; "A New Kind of Cold War: How to Manage the Growing Rivalry between America and a Rising China," *The Economist,* May 16, 2019, https://www-economist-com.proxy1.library.jhu.edu/leaders/2019 /05/16/a-new-kind-of-cold-war; Kevin Rudd, "The Coming Post-COVID Anarchy: The Pandemic Bodes Ill for Both American and Chinese Power—and for the Global Order," *Foreign Affairs,* May 6, 2020, https://www.foreignaffairs.com/articles/united-states/2020-05 -06/coming-post-covid-anarchy; and "The New Scold War: The Pandemic Is Driving America and China Further Apart," *The Economist,* May 9, 2020, https://www-economist-com .proxy1.library.jhu.edu/leaders/2020/05/09/the-pandemic-is-driving-america-and-china -further-apart.

18. Richard Haass, "A Cold War with China Would Be a Mistake," *Wall Street Journal,* May 7, 2020, https://www.wsj.com/articles/dont-start-a-new-cold-war-with-china-11588860761; and Lawrence Summers, "Covid-19 Looks Like a Hinge in History," *Financial Times,* May 14, 2020, https://www.ft.com/content/de643ae8-9527-11ea-899a-f62a20d54625.

19. Tom McTague, "The Pandemic's Geopolitical Aftershocks Are Coming," *The Atlantic,* May 18, 2020, https://www.theatlantic.com/international/archive/2020/05/coronavirus -pandemic-second-wave-geopolitics-instability/611668/; and "China's 'Wolf Warrior' Diplomacy Gamble," *The Economist,* May 28, 2020, https://www.economist.com/china/2020 /05/28/chinas-wolf-warrior-diplomacy-gamble; and Minxin Pei, "China's Coming Upheaval," *Foreign Affairs,* May/June 2020, https://www.foreignaffairs.com/articles/united-states/2020 -04-03/chinas-coming-upheaval.

20. This is not to say that the US-China rivalry is the same as the Cold War, a debate that continues to play out at greater length in many other forums.

21. See Thomas Wright's and Elizabeth Economy's contributions to this volume (chapters 17 and 20, respectively).

22. In an interview in late January, US Commerce Secretary Wilbur Ross predicted the coronavirus would "help to accelerate the return of jobs to North America." Ana Swanson and Alan Rappeport, "Wilbur Ross Says Coronavirus Could Bring Jobs Back to the U.S." *New York Times,* January 30, 2020, https://www.nytimes.com/2020/01/30/business /economy/wilbur-ross-coronavirus-jobs.html.

23. Hal Brands, "Coronavirus Hasn't Killed the Global Balance of Power," *Bloomberg,* May 27, 2020, https://www.bloomberg.com/opinion/articles/2020-05-27/china-wants-co ronavirus-to-destroy-the-global-balance-of-power; and Hal Brands, "Cooperate with China on Coronavirus but Don't Trust It, *Bloomberg,* April 12, 2020, https://www.bloomberg.com /opinion/articles/2020-04-12/china-can-t-be-trusted-in-fight-against-coronavirus.

24. On the impact of disinformation campaigns on Western democracies, see Alina Polyakova and Spencer Phipps Boyer, *The Future of Political Warfare: Russia, the West, and the Coming Age of Global Digital Warfare,* Brookings Institution, March 2018, https://www .brookings.edu/research/the-future-of-political-warfare-russia-the-west-and-the-coming -age-of-global-digital-competition/. China has deployed facial recognition software on a

large scale in Xinjiang province to monitor the Uyghur population; see Paul Mozer, "One Month, 500,000 Face Scans: How China Is Using A.I. to Profile a Minority," *New York Times,* April 14, 2019, https://www.nytimes.com/2019/04/14/technology/china-surveillance -artificial-intelligence-racial-profiling.html.

25. Henry A. Kissinger, Eric Schmidt, and Daniel Huttenlocher, "The Metamorphosis," *The Atlantic,* August 2019, https://www.theatlantic.com/magazine/archive/2019/08 /henry-kissinger-the-metamorphosis-ai/592771/; and Henry A. Kissinger, "How the Enlightenment Ends," *The Atlantic,* June 2018, https://www.theatlantic.com/magazine/archive /2018/06/henry-kissinger-ai-could-mean-the-end-of-human-history/559124/.

26. The latest Freedom House report found that 2019 marked the 14th consecutive year of net decline in global freedom. Sarah Repucci, *Freedom in the World 2020: A Leaderless Struggle for Democracy* (Washington, DC: Freedom House, 2020), www.freedomhouse .org/report/freedom-world/2020/leaderless-struggle-democracy.

27. Derek Scissors, "Estimating the True Number of China's COVID-19 Cases," American Enterprise Institute, April 2020, https://www.aei.org/wp-content/uploads/2020/04 /Estimating-the-True-Number-of-Chinas-COVID-19-Cases.pdf; Emily Feng and Amy Chang, "Restrictions and Rewards: How China Is Locking Down Half a Billion Citizens," *NPR,* February 21, 2020, https://www.npr.org/sections/goatsandsoda/2020/02/21/806958341 /restrictions-and-rewards-how-china-is-locking-down-half-a-billion-citizens; and Lin Zhu et al., "China's Cities Lock Up Residents to Prevent Spread of Virus," *Bloomberg,* February 11, 2020, https://www.bloomberg.com/news/articles/2020-02-11/china-s-cities-lock-up -residents-to-prevent-spread-of-virus.

28. Former FDA commissioner Scott Gottlieb predicts the United States will have a better vaccine sooner than China. See "U.S. is Ahead of China in Vaccine Race, Former FDA Chief Says," *Politico,* May 24, 2020, https://www.politico.com/news/2020/05/24 /coronavirus-vaccine-china-gottlieb-276763. For a discussion of state and local government responses to COVID-19, see Rebecca L. Haffajee and Michelle M. Mello, "Thinking Globally, Acting Locally—the U.S. Response to Covid-19," *New England Journal of Medicine* 382, no. 22 (May 2020): e75, https://doi.org/10.1056/NEJMp2006740.%2010.1056/NEJ Mp2006740.

29. A Pew Research Center Coronavirus report, released in June 2020, reported 61% of Republicans felt the worst problems the country was facing from coronavirus were behind us, while 76% of Democrats felt that the worst was still to come. See "Republicans, Democrats Move Even Further Apart in Coronavirus Concerns," Pew Research Center, June 25, 2020, https://www.pewresearch.org/politics/2020/06/25/republicans-democrats -move-even-further-apart-in-coronavirus-concerns/; and Ronald Brownstein, "Red and Blue America Aren't Experiencing the Same Pandemic," *The Atlantic,* March 20, 2020. https://www.theatlantic.com/politics/archive/2020/03/how-republicans-and-democrats -think-about-coronavirus/608395/.

30. Matt Apuzzo and David D. Kirkpatrick, "Covid-19 Changed How the World Does Science, Together," *New York Times,* April 1, 2020, https://www.nytimes.com/2020/04/01 /world/europe/coronavirus-science-research-cooperation.html.

PART I / Applied History and Future Scenarios

Chapter One

Ends of Epidemics

Jeremy A. Greene and Dora Vargha

We know a good deal about beginnings: those first signal cases of pneumonia in Guangdong, influenza in Veracruz, and hemorrhagic fever in Guinea, respectively marking the origins of the SARS outbreak of 2002–4, the H1N1 influenza pandemic of 2008–9, and the Ebola pandemic of 2014–16. Recent history tells us a lot about how epidemics unfold, outbreaks spread, and how they are controlled before they spread too far. These stories only get us so far, however, in coming to terms with the global crisis of COVID-19. In the first few months of 2020 the coronavirus pandemic blew past most efforts at containment, snapped the reins of case-detection and surveillance across the world, and saturated all inhabited continents. To understand possible endings for this epidemic, we must look back much further indeed.

Historians have long been fascinated by epidemics, in part because they tend to form a similar sort of social choreography recognizable across vast reaches of time and space.[1] Even if the causative agents of the Plague of Athens in the 5th century BCE, the Plague of Justinian in the 6th century CE, the 14th-century Black Death, and the early 20th-century Manchurian Plague were almost certainly not the same

Jeremy A. Greene, MD, PhD, is the William H. Welch Professor of Medicine and the History of Medicine and director of the Institute of the History of Medicine at Johns Hopkins University. Dora Vargha, PhD, is a senior lecturer in medical humanities at the University of Exeter.

An earlier version of this essay was published in *Boston Review* under the title "How Epidemics End."

thing, biologically speaking, the epidemics themselves share common features that link past actors to our present-day experience. "As a social phenomenon," historian Charles Rosenberg argues, "an epidemic has a dramaturgic form. Epidemics start at a moment in time, proceed on a stage limited in space and duration, following a plot line of increasing and revelatory tension, move to a crisis of individual and collective character, then drift towards closure."[2] Rosenberg wrote these words a decade into the North American HIV/AIDS epidemic, a moment whose origin was assiduously, perhaps overzealously, being traced to a "Patient Zero," but whose end was, like the present condition, nowhere in sight.

As the coronavirus seeped further as an all-too-visible stain in the fabric of our society, we saw an initial fixation on origins give way to the more practical question of endings. In March, *The Atlantic* offered four possible "timelines for life returning to normal," all of which depended on the biological basis of a sufficient amount of the population developing immunity (perhaps 60%–80%) to curb further spread.[3] This confident assertion derived from models of infectious outbreaks formalized by epidemiologists such as W. H. Frost a century earlier.[4] If the world can be defined into those susceptible (S), infected (I), and resistant (R) to a disease, and a pathogen has a reproductive number R_0 describing how many susceptible people can be infected by a single infected person, the end of the epidemic begins when the proportion of susceptible people drops below $1/R_0$, meaning that one person would infect, on average, less than one other person with the disease.

These equations reassure us that a set of natural laws give order to the cadence of calamities. The curves they produce, which in better times belonged to the arcana of epidemiologists, are now common figures in the lives of billions of people learning to live with contractions of civil society promoted in the name of "bending," "flattening," or "squashing" them. At the same time, the smooth lines of these curves are far removed from jagged realities of the day-to-day experience of an epidemic. The textbook model of infectious disease modelling presents the epidemic as a quasi-biological function determined by a contagion parameter, R_0, inherent to the infectious agent in question: seasonal influenza has an R_0 of 1.3, Ebola has an R_0 of 2, where a more contagious disease like chikungunya has an R_0 greater than 4, and measles literally explodes through populations with an R_0 between 11 and 18.[5] Yet this only tells part of the story.

Epidemics are not merely biological phenomena. They are also always inevitably shaped by our social responses to them, from beginning to end. The question now being asked of scientists, clinicians, mayors, governors, prime ministers, and presidents around the world is not merely "when will the biological phenomenon of this epidemic resolve?" but rather "when (if ever) will the disruption to our so-cial life caused in the name of coronavirus come to an end?" As the peak inci-dence appears to have passed in some locations but looms larger in others, elected officials and think tanks from opposite ends of the political spectrum provide "road maps" and "frameworks" for how an epidemic that has shut down economic, civic, and social life in a manner not seen in at least a century might eventually recede and allow resumption of a "new normal."[6]

These two versions of an epidemic, the biological and the social, are closely in-tertwined but they are not the same. Yes, the biological processes that constitute the epidemic can shut down daily life by sickening and killing people. But the so-cial responses that constitute the epidemic also shut down daily life by overturn-ing basic premises of sociality, economics, governance, discourse, and interaction— while also killing people in the process. There is a risk, as we know from both the Spanish influenza of 1918–19 and the more recent swine flu of 2009–10, of relax-ing social responses before the biological threat has passed.[7] But there is also a risk in misjudging a biological threat based on faulty models and overresponding or disrupting social life in such a way that the restrictions can never properly be taken back.[8] We have seen in the case of coronavirus the two faces of the epidemic es-calating on local, national, and global levels in tandem. But the biological epidemic and the social epidemic don't necessarily recede on the same timeline.

History reminds us that the interconnections between the timing of the biologi-cal epidemic and the social epidemic are far from obvious. In some cases, when the epidemic disease itself is so clearly marked as abnormal, like the dramatic fea-tures of yellow fever or cholera in the 18th and 19th centuries or the classic pre-sentation of the Spanish influenza in the early 20th century, the end of the epi-demic may seem relatively clear. Like a bag of popcorn popping in the microwave, the tempo of visible case-events begins slowly, escalates to a frenetic peak, and then recedes, leaving a diminishing frequency of new cases which eventually are spaced far enough apart to be contained and then eliminated. In other cases, however—and here the polio epidemics of the 20th century are perhaps a more useful model than influenza or cholera—the disease process itself is hidden, threatens to come back, and ends not on a single day but at different timescales and in different ways for different people.

Campaigns against infectious diseases tend to be discussed in military terms and work with the assumption that both epidemics and wars must have a singu-lar endpoint. We approach the "peak" as if it were a decisive battle like Yorktown or Waterloo or Appomattox Court House, or a diplomatic arrangement like the Armistice at Compiègne in November 1918. Yet the chronology of a single, decisive ending is not always true even for military history. More than three months separated the end of the Second World War in Europe formalized by "V-E Day" from the end as experienced in the broader Pacific Theater as "V-J Day," let alone the end as experienced by Teruo Nakamura, the last Japanese soldier to lay down arms in 1974, after nearly 30 years of hiding in a remote island in the Philippines.[9] For occupied countries like Japan, Germany, and Austria, the end of the war had a different temporality as well. By the time Austria signed a World War II peace treaty in 1955, the Korean War's military operations had already ceased after a 1953 armistice, yet there is still no peace treaty between North and South Korea.

Just as the clear ending of a military war does not necessarily bring a close to the experience of war in everyday life, so too the containment of a biological agent does not immediately undo the social impacts of an epidemic. In the course of World War II, historians have calculated that sixty million people were displaced in Europe alone, among them Holocaust survivors, prisoners of war, refugees, and deportees.[10] Two years later, there were still close to a million people stranded in displaced persons camps, the last of which closed only in 1959. Returning to "normal" life for people in their home countries also took time: rationing food in Britain went on until 1954, nearly a decade after the last military battle.[11] So, too, were the social and economic effects of the 1918–19 pandemic felt long after the end of the third and putatively final wave of the virus—even if explicit conversations about the pandemic seem to have been swiftly "forgotten."[12] While the immediate economic effect on many local businesses caused by shutdowns appeared to have resolved in a matter of months, the effects of the epidemic on labor-wage relations were still visible in economic surveys in 1920, again in 1921, and in several areas of the economy as far out as 1930.[13] Some economic historians have argued that there was an even longer-term effect, detectable through generations: the Spanish flu's negative impact on social trust, which in turn influenced long-term economic development.[14]

Like the First World War with which its history was so closely intertwined, the influenza pandemic of 1918–19 appeared at first to have a singular ending. In individual cities, the epidemic often produced dramatic spikes and falls in equally rapid tempo. In Philadelphia, as John Barry notes in *The Great Influenza*, after an explosive and deadly rise in October 1919, which crested at a death rate of 4,597 people a week by the middle of the month, cases suddenly dropped so precipitously that by the end of the month the public gathering ban was lifted, and two weeks after that there were almost no new cases. Like any part of a materially determined universe, Barry describes, "the virus burned through available fuel, then it quickly faded away."[15]

And yet as Barry reminds us, scholars have since learned to differentiate at least three different sequences of epidemics within the broader pandemic. The first wave blazed through military installations in the spring of 1918, the second wave caused the devastating mortality spikes in the summer and fall of 1918, and the third wave began in December 1918 and lingered long through the summer of 1919. Some cities, like San Francisco, celebrated the success of their public health measures after passing through the first and second waves relatively unscathed only to be devastated by the third wave. Nor was it clear to those still alive in 1919 that the pandemic was over after the end of the third wave. In 1920 eleven thousand influenza related deaths took place in New York City and Chicago. Even as late as 1922, a bad flu season in Washington State merited a response from public health officials to be "dealt with the same as influenza . . . enforce absolute quarantine."[16] It is difficult, looking back, to say exactly when this prototypical pandemic of the twentieth century was really over.

Who can tell when a pandemic is over? Strictly speaking, only the World Health Organization (WHO) can. The Emergency Committee of the WHO is responsible for the global governance of health and international coordination of epidemic response. After the SARS coronavirus pandemic of 2002–4, this body was granted sole power to declare the beginnings and endings of Public Health Emergencies of International Concern (PHEICs). While SARS morbidity and mortality (roughly 8,000 cases and 800 deaths in 26 countries) is already dwarfed by the sheer scale of COVID-19, the pandemic's effect on national and global economies prompted revisions to the International Health Regulations in 2005, a body of international law that had remained unchanged since 1969.[17]

Perhaps the most fateful step implemented in the wake of SARS was the decision to expand the declarative powers given to the World Health Organization in the 2005 revisions to the International Health Regulations. This revision broadened the scope of coordinated global response from a handful of diseases to any public health event which the WHO deemed to be of international concern and shifted from a reactive mechanism to a proactive one based on real-time surveillance and from action at borders to detection and containment at the source.[18] Any time the WHO declares a public health event of international concern—and frequently when it chooses *not* to declare one—the event becomes a matter of front-page news. The World Health Organization has been criticized both for declaring a PHEIC too hastily (as in the case of the H1N1 pandemic) or too late (in the case of the Ebola pandemic).

The termination of a PHEIC is rarely subject to the same public scrutiny as its initiation. When an outbreak previously known as a PHEIC is no longer classified as an "extraordinary event" and no longer is seen to pose a risk of international spread, the PHEIC is simply considered unjustified, leading to a withdrawal of international coordination. In most of its day-to-day operation, the World Health Organization acts to support the actions of its constituent ministers of health, rather than perform any function like a supranational executive agency. Once countries can grapple with the disease within their own borders under their own national frameworks, it is presumed that international coordination is no longer needed, and the PHEIC is quietly de-escalated.

Yet as the response to the 2014–16 Ebola outbreak in West Africa has shown, the act of declaring the end of a pandemic can be just as powerful as the act of declaring its beginning, and a return to "normal" can indeed exist alongside the continuation of an emergency. When, in March 2016, WHO director-general Margaret Chan announced that the Ebola outbreak was no longer a public health event of international concern,[19] the pronouncement had significant consequences on international, national, and local levels. International donors no longer saw it justified to provide funds and care to the West African countries devastated by the outbreak, even as these struggling health systems continued to be stretched beyond their means by the needs of Ebola survivors. On a local level, for those struggling with physical and mental health consequences and for Ebola survivors and their families and communities traumatized by the epidemic, it was hardly over. The official ending of the epidemic also caused concern beyond the national contexts: international nongovernmental organizations feared that the end of an international emergency would hinder work and collaboration on vaccines, which were still under development at the time.[20]

Part of the reason that the role of the WHO in proclaiming and terminating the state of pandemic is subject to so much scrutiny is that it *can* be. Unlike other major global health funders, such as the Bill & Melinda Gates Foundation or the Wellcome Trust, who are accountable only to themselves, the WHO is the only international health agency that is accountable to every government in the world and contains the health ministers of every nation within its parliamentary body, the World Health Assembly. Since its foundation in 1948, the organization has been crucial in coordinating a response, making recommendations, and directing efforts in epidemic management. Its authority is not mainly based on its battered budget, but its access to epidemic intelligence and pool of select individuals, technical experts with vast experience in epidemic response. And yet, even though acknowledgement of this scientific and public health authority is key to its role in pandemic crises, ultimately the WHO's recommendations are carried out in very different ways and on very different timescales in different countries, provinces, states, counties, and cities.[21]

We can already see, tracking epidemic curves across the globe through our daily consumption of news, that the timeline of epidemics plays out in differing ways in various countries. One state might begin easing up restrictions to movement and industry, while another is about to enact more and more stringent measures, as case fatalities increase by the day. As international air travel has come to nearly a complete stop and global production and distribution networks have halted, or at least significantly reduced, the flow of goods, we are reminded daily by the lack of ties that connect us to the rest of the world that the end of an outbreak in one community, one nation, or one continent will not mean the end of the epidemic. While the cutoff may seem universal, the reconnection will show extraordinary local variance.

Many believe that the end of COVID-19 will simply arrive with the development of a vaccine. Yet a closer look at one of the central vaccine success stories of the 20th century shows that technological solutions rarely offer resolution to pandemics on their own. Contrary to our expectations, vaccines are not universal technologies. Vaccination practices and the infrastructures in place to deliver them are as diverse as the epidemic management strategies national governments follow. They are always deployed locally, with variable resources and commitments to scientific expertise.[22] This is nowhere more visible than in the management of polio epidemics that wreaked havoc across the globe in the 1950s.

The development of the polio vaccine is a relatively well-known story, usually told, as much of the history of polio, as an American one.[23] However, the 1950s saw polio epidemics sweep over the globe with no regard for borders, or even the Iron Curtain, and in many ways it united the politically divided Cold War world with a common goal. Locked in a conflict that would go on for decades, antagonistic superpowers were provided a safe haven by the disease in which they could meet and collaborate. A myriad of publications, scientists, and specimens crisscrossed the globe in an effort to share experiences and research in prevention and treatment. In a couple of years following the licensing of Jonas Salk's vaccine in the

United States, the use of the inactivated vaccine became widely used across the world. It did not work, however, in certain settings, or at least not as well as governments and scientists hoped.[24] This uncertainty with efficiency gave way to the mass testing of another live, oral vaccine developed by Albert Sabin, who collaborated in the final stages with Eastern European and Soviet colleagues, primarily Mikhail Chumakov. The successful Soviet polio vaccine trials became a rare landmark of Cold War cooperation, which prompted Basil O'Connor, speaking at the Second International Conference of Live Poliovirus Vaccines in 1960, to state that "in search for the truth that frees man from disease, there is no cold war."[25]

Yet the differential uptake of this vaccine retraced the divisions of Cold War geography. The Soviet Union, Hungary, and Czechoslovakia were the first countries in the world to begin nationwide immunization with the Sabin vaccine, soon followed by Cuba, the first country in the Western Hemisphere to eliminate the disease.[26] By the time the Sabin vaccine was licensed in the United States in 1963, much of Eastern Europe had done away with epidemics and was largely polio-free. The successful ending of this epidemic within the communist world was immediately held up as proof of the superiority of their political system.

Did the authoritarian nature of these regimes make them uniquely capable of ending polio epidemics? This question can be seen reflected in current debates over the heavy-handed interventions in Wuhan this year. Yet it was also being asked in 1948, in one of the first meetings of the freshly minted WHO.[27] After a devastating war with fascist dictatorships, and in the growing shadow of the Cold War, the invocation of authoritarian measures was uncomfortable, to say the least, but its necessity was widely acknowledged. Furthermore, it was the military-like organization of the Soviet health care system that Dorothy Horstman, Yale virologist and WHO envoy, emphasized in support of the validity of the Soviet vaccine trials.[28] Such a regime was well placed to organize and efficiently deliver the venture.

What united the Cold War East was not only authoritarianism and heavy hierarchies in state organization and society. It was also a shared belief in the integration of politics and health as a particular imagination of modernity, in a combination of a paternal state, biomedical approaches, and social and socialized medicine. Regardless of the availability of resources and how far the achievements of health care were from its goals, epidemic management in these countries combined an overall emphasis on disease prevention, relatively easily mobilized health workers, top-down organization of vaccinations, and the rhetoric of solidarity, all resting on a health care system that aimed to provide access to all citizens. However imperfect, vertical and technocratic interventions of vaccination met with horizontal infrastructures of health and social care.[29]

Authoritarian measures, then, are not sufficient, nor are they necessarily as beneficial as one might imagine. Alternative solutions, built on compassion and solidarity and coupled with adequate provisions, might ease and even remove tensions that often run high in epidemic contexts. Historian Samuel Cohn has examined the example of the cholera outbreak in Berlin in 1831, where authorities focused on assistance and negotiations instead of harsh clampdowns, establishing soup kitchens for the unemployed and care for the orphans of victims.[30] As a result, Berlin became unique in avoiding cholera uprisings, which swept across German cities and much of Europe at the time. There are other examples: in early modern Florence during a plague outbreak, its health board, the Sanitá, combined heavy-handed measures with punishment for whoever violated quarantine measures (for instance by dancing), and at the same time provided food and medicine to all inhabitants.[31] The assumption was that an insufficient diet, especially among the poor, would contribute to their vulnerability to the disease, therefore they received daily and weekly packages of bread, wine, sausages, cheese, and herbs. The overall death toll in Florence remained significantly lower than other Italian cities (around 12% as opposed to up to 61%) by the time the epidemic ended.

Still, authoritarianism as a catalyst for ending epidemics can be singled out and pursued with long-lasting consequences. Epidemics can be harbingers of significant political changes that go well beyond their ending, raising questions of what then becomes a new "normal" after the threat passes. Many Hungarians have watched with alarm the complete sidelining of parliament and the introduction of government by decree at the end of March 2020.[32] There was no date set for the termination of the emergency measures. The end of the epidemic, and thus the end of the need for the significantly increased power of Prime Minister Viktor Orbán, would be determined by Orbán himself. Likewise, many other states, urging the mobilization of new technologies as a solution to end epidemics, are opening the door to heightened state surveillance of their citizens. The apps and trackers now being designed to follow the movement and exposure of people in order to enable the end of epidemic lockdowns can collect data and establish mechanisms that reach well beyond the original intent. The digital afterlives of these practices raise new and unprecedented questions about when and how epidemics end.[33]

Although we want to believe that a single technological breakthrough will end the present crisis, the application of any global health technology is always locally determined. After its dramatic successes in managing polio epidemics in the late 1950s and early 1960s, the oral poliovirus vaccine became the tool of choice for the Global Polio Eradication Initiative in the 1980s, as it promised an end to "summer fears" globally.[34] But as vaccines are technologies of trust, the end of polio continues to be contingent upon maintaining trust in national and international structures through which it is delivered. Wherever that often-fragile trust is fractured or undermined, vaccination rates can drop to a critical level, giving way to vaccine-derived polio, which thrives in partially vaccinated populations.

In Kano, Nigeria, a ban on polio vaccination between 2000 and 2004 resulted in a new national polio epidemic that soon spread to neighboring countries.[35] As late as December 2019, polio outbreaks were still reported in fifteen African countries, including Angola and the Democratic Republic of the Congo.[36] Nor is it clear that polio can fully be regarded as an epidemic at this point: while polio epidemics are now a thing of the past for Hungary, the rest of Europe, the Americas, Australia, and East Asia as well, the disease itself is still endemic to parts of Africa and South Asia. A disease once universally epidemic is now locally endemic: this, too, is another way that epidemics end.

How do epidemics become endemic? Consider the global threat of HIV/AIDS. From a strictly biological perspective, the AIDS epidemic never ended. HIV/AIDS continues to spread devastation through the world, infecting 1.7 million people and claiming an estimated 770,000 lives in the year 2018 alone.[37] But HIV is not generally described these days with the same urgency and fear that accompanied the newly defined AIDS epidemic in the early 1980s. Like coronavirus today, AIDS at that time was a rapidly spreading and unknown emerging threat, splayed across newspaper headlines and magazine covers, claiming the lives of celebrities and ordinary citizens alike. Nearly forty years later, HIV/AIDS has largely become a chronic disease endemic, at least in the Global North. Like diabetes, which itself claimed an estimated 4.9 million lives in 2019, HIV/AIDS became a manageable condition—that is, if one had access to the right medications.[38]

We have a hard time continuing to attend to the urgency of an epidemic that has now been rolling on for nearly four decades. Even in the first decade of the epidemic, AIDS activists in the United States fought tooth and nail to make their suffering visible in the face of both the Reagan administration's dogged refusal to talk publicly about the AIDS crisis, and the indifference of the press who went on to cover other topics after the initial sensation of the new plague and the newly discovered virus had become common knowledge.[39] In this respect, the social epidemic does not necessarily end when biological transmission has ended, or even peaked, but rather when it no longer incites fear as a newsworthy topic compared to other potential headlines of environmental collapse, bioterrorism, a dirty bomb, instability in the Middle East, or another epidemic.

The ending of an epidemic is not much clearer even if there is eventually a successful vaccine in place. Polio has not been newsworthy for a while, even as thousands around the world still live with the disease with ever-decreasing access to care and support. Soon after the immediate threat of outbreaks passed, so did support for the people whose lives were still bound up in the disease. With the polio problem "solved," specialized hospitals closed, fundraising organizations found new causes, and poster children found themselves in an increasingly challenging world. Few medical professionals are trained today in the treatment of the disease. As intimate knowledge of polio and its treatment withered away with time, people living with polio became embodied repositories of lost knowledge. But people have all but disappeared from how we talk about the disease, despite the fact that hundreds of thousands continue to live with it and a number of people contract it each year as it remains a real threat—it has morphed from its clinical complexity to a virus, which is only ever discussed in the context of vaccines and endings. The social narrative of an epidemic ending, therefore, can impact hundreds of thousands of personal lives, especially those for whom the biological epidemic has not ended.

Our attention is more easily drawn to new diseases as they emerge. Well before AIDS drew the world's attention to the devastating potential of new epidemic diseases, a series of earlier outbreaks had already signaled the presence of emerging infectious agents. When hundreds of members of the American Legion fell ill with a mysterious new disease after their annual meeting in Philadelphia in 1976, the efforts of epidemiologists from the CDC to explain the spread of this virulent new epidemic disease and its newly discovered causative agent, *Legionella*, occupied front-page headlines.[40] In the years since, however, as the 1976 incident faded from memory, infections of Legionnaires' disease have become everyday objects of medical care, even though incidences in the United States have grown ninefold since 2000, tracing a line of exponential growth that looks a lot like COVID-19's on a longer timescale.[41] Yet few among us regularly pause in our daily lives to consider whether we are living through the slowly ascending limb of a Legionnaires' epidemic.

Likewise hepatitis C, the most common blood-borne infection in the United States, was also first described in the 1970s, after the rapid spread of a new and virulent form of hepatitis spreading among patients who tested negative for both hepatitis A and hepatitis B.[42] Because in hepatitis C, as in HIV, the causative virus can be carried without symptoms for decades, the CDC refers to hepatitis C as a "silent epidemic," noting a 150% increase in new cases in recent years even in the face of new curative agents, and there are at least 3.5 million cases currently in the United States alone.[43] Yet few among us regularly pause in our daily lives to consider we are living through the ascending limb of a hepatitis C epidemic.

Nor do most people living in the Global North stop to consider the ravages of tuberculosis as a pandemic, even though an estimated 10 million new cases of tuberculosis were reported around the globe in 2018 and an estimated 1.5 million people died from the disease.[44] Tuberculosis, the leading cause of death worldwide from a single infectious agent, is the target of concerted international disease control efforts, and occasionally eradication efforts, but the timescale of this affliction has been spread out so long—and so clearly demarcated in space as a problem of "other places"—that it is no longer part of the epidemic imagination of the Global North.[45]

DNA lineage studies of tuberculosis now show that the spread of the disease in sub-Saharan Africa and Latin America was initiated by European contact and conquest from the 15th century through the 19th century.[46] In the early decades of the 20th century, tuberculosis epidemics accelerated throughout sub-Saharan Africa, South Asia, and Southeast Asia due to the rapid urbanization and industrialization of European colonies.[47] Although the wave of decolonization that swept these regions between the 1940s and the 1980s established autonomy and sovereignty for newly postcolonial nations, this movement did not send tuberculosis back to Europe.

Like infectious agents on an agar plate, epidemics colonize our social lives and force us to learn to live with them, in one way or another, for the foreseeable future. There is no simple return to the way things were in the aftermath of an epidemic: whatever normal is built in the aftermath is a new normal. Just as the postcolonial period for most nations who lived under European empires is characterized by continuing structures established under colonial rule, so too are our post-epidemic futures indelibly inflected by each passing agent. Like "universal precautions" and blood-bank screening after HIV/AIDS,[48] or mask wearing in Asian societies after SARS, much of what we accept as everyday reality in the future will only be seen as different to those who look backward to find the subtle scars where the new normal was sutured onto the fabric of social life that came before.[49]

The uncertainty of the present does not stop countless modelers, politicians, and pundits from making predictions of what will come after the end of the epidemic. After the end of coronavirus, we are told, we will see the end of neoliberal austerity. After the end of coronavirus, we are told, we will see the folly of not investing in national health programs. After the end of coronavirus, we will divest fully from fossil fuels and embrace a green economy, we will see the consolidation of autocracy, we will see barbarism with a human face.

History does not predict what we will see when we see the end of the present epidemic. Like the world of scientific facts after the end of a critical experiment, the world that we find after the end of an epidemic crisis looks in many ways like the world that came before, but with new social truths established.[50] How these truths are established depends a great deal on current interactions among people, the instruments of social policy as well as medical and public health intervention with which we apply our efforts, and the underlying response of the material which we applied that apparatus against (in this case, the coronavirus strain SARS-CoV-2). While we cannot know now how the present epidemic will end, we can be confident that it in its wake it will leave different conceptions of normal in realms biological and social, national and international, economic and political.

Though we like to think that science itself, like a vaccine, can be a universal remedy to the pandemic, science is contingent upon local practices that are easily thrown over in an emergency and established conventions that do not always hold up in situations of urgency. Today, we see civic leaders claiming the availability of treatments, antibody screens, and vaccines well in advance of any scientific evidence,[51] while relatively straightforward attempts to estimate the true number of people affected by the disease spark firestorms over the credibility of medical knowledge.[52] Arduous work is often required to achieve scientific consensus, and when stakes are high, heterogeneous data give way to highly variable interpretations. As data move too quickly in some domains and too slowly in others, and urgent time pressures are placed on all investigations, the projected curve of the epidemic is transformed into an elaborate guessing game in which different states rely on different kinds of scientific claims to sketch out wildly different timetables for ending social restrictions.[53]

These varied endings of the epidemic across local and national settings will only be valid insofar as they are acknowledged as such by others—especially if any reopening of trade and travel is to be achieved. In this sense, the process of establishing a new normal will continue to be bound up in international consensus. What the new normal in global health governance will look like, however, is more uncertain than ever. Long accustomed to the role of international whipping boy, the WHO Secretariat seems doomed to either be accused of overreaching beyond its mandate, or not acting fast enough. Moreover, it can easily become a target of scapegoating, as the secessional posturing of Donald Trump demonstrates. Yet the American president's move is neither unprecedented nor unsurmountable. Although Trump's voting base might not wish to be grouped together with the other global power that seceded from the World Health Organization, after the Soviet Union's 1949 departure from the WHO it ultimately brought the Eastern Bloc back to task of international health leadership in 1956. Much as the return of the Soviets to the WHO resulted in the global eradication of smallpox—the only human disease so far to have been intentionally eradicated—it is possible that some future return of the United States to the project of global health governance might also result in a more hopeful post-pandemic future.[54]

As the historian of medicine and historian of time Anne Kveim Lie and Helge Jordheim have recently noted, in epidemic times "the present moves faster, the past seems further removed, and the future seems completely unpredictable."[55] How, then, are we to know when epidemics end? How does the act of looking back aid us in determining a way forward? Historians make poor futurologists, but we spend a lot of time thinking about time. And epidemics produce their own kinds of time, in both biological and social domains. Epidemics disrupt the social conventions with which we divide up a given week or day. They carry within them their own tempos and rhythms: the slow initial growth, the explosive upward limb of the outbreak, and the slowing of transmission that marks the peak, plateau, and the downward limb. This last part, the end of an epidemic, is perhaps always ever an asymptote, never disappearing but rather fading to the point where its signal is lost in the noise of the new normal, and even allowed, in some imaginable future, to be forgotten.

NOTES

1. David S. Jones, "History in a Crisis: Lessons for COVID-19," *New England Journal of Medicine*, 382 (2020): 1681–1683.

2. Charles E. Rosenberg, "What Is an Epidemic? AIDS in Historical Perspective," *Daedalus* 118, no. 2 (1989): 1–17.

3. Joe Pinsker, "The Four Possible Timelines for Life Returning to Normal," *The Atlantic*, March 26, 2020.

4. Alfredo Morabia, "Snippets from the Past: The Evolution of Wade Hampton Frost's Epidemiology as Viewed from the *American Journal of Hygiene/Epidemiology*," *American Journal of Epidemiology* 178, no. 7 (2013): 1013–1019.

5. Joseph Eisenberg, "R0: How Scientists Quantify the Intensity of an Outbreak like Coronavirus and Its Pandemic Potential," *The Conversation*, March 27, 2020.

6. Helen Branswell, "Two New Road Maps Lay Out Possible Paths to End Coronavirus Lockdowns," *STAT*, March 29, 2020.

7. John Barry, "The Single Most Important Lesson from the 1918 Influenza Epidemic," *New York Times*, March 17, 2020.

8. John P. A. Ioannidis, "A Fiasco in the Making? As the Coronavirus Pandemic Takes Hold, We Are Making Decisions without Reliable Data," *STAT*, March 17 2020, https://www.statnews.com/2020/03/17/a-fiasco-in-the-making-as-the-coronavirus-pandemic-takes-hold-we-are-making-decisions-without-reliable-data/.

9. Beatrice Trefalt, "The Straggler Returns: Onoda Hiro and Japanese Memories of the War," *War and Society* 17, no. 2 (1999).

10. Matthew Frank and Jessica Reinisch, "Introduction: Refugees and the Nation-State in Europe, 1919–59," *Journal of Contemporary History* 49, no. 3 (2014): 477–90.

11. "1954: Housewives Celebrate End of Rationing," On this Day 1950–2005, BBC, 2005, http://news.bbc.co.uk/onthisday/hi/dates/stories/july/4/newsid_3818000/3818563.stm.

12. Alfred Crosby, *America's Forgotten Pandemic: The Influenza of 1918* (Cambridge: Cambridge University Press, 1976).

13. Thomas A Garrett, "Economic Effects of the 1918 Influenza Pandemic: Implications for a Modern-Day Pandemic," research report (St. Louis, MO: Federal Reserve Bank of St. Louis, 2007), https://www.stlouisfed.org/~/media/files/pdfs/community-development/research-reports/pandemic_flu_report.pdf.

14. Le Moglie, M., F. Gandolfi, G. Alfani, and A. Aassve, "Epidemics and Trust: The Case of the Spanish Flu," IGIER Working Paper no. 661 (2020).

15. John Barry, *The Great Influenza: The Epic Story of the Deadliest Plague in History* (New York: Penguin, 2005), 371.

16. Barry, *The Great Influenza*, 391.

17. Andrew Lakoff, *Unprepared: Global Health in a Time of Emergency* (Oakland: University of California Press, 2017).

18. David A. Relman et al., *Infectious Disease Movement in a Borderless World: Workshop Summary* (Washington, DC: National Academies Press, 2010).

19. "Statement of the 9th meeting of the IHR Emergency Committee regarding the Ebola Outbreak in West Africa," World Health Organization, March 29, 2016, https://www.who.int/news-room/detail/29-03-2016-statement-on-the-9th-meeting-of-the-ihr-emergency-committee-regarding-the-ebola-outbreak-in-west-africa.

20. Samuel Kline Cohn, "Cholera Revolts: A Class Struggle We May Not Like," *Social History* 42, no. 2 (2017): 162–180.

21. Nitsan Chorev, *The World Health Organization between North and South* (Ithaca, NY: Cornell University Press, 2012); Marcos Cueto, Theodore M. Brown, and Elizabeth Fee, *The World Health Organization: A History*, Global Health Histories (Cambridge:

Cambridge University Press, 2019); Javed Siddiqi, *World Health and World Politic: The World Health Organization and the UN System* (Columbia: University of South Carolina Press, 1995).

22. Hannah Devlin and Sarah Boseley, "Scientists Criticise UK Government's 'Following the Science' Claim," *Guardian*, April 23 2020, https://www.theguardian.com/world/2020/apr/23/scientists-criticise-uk-government-over-following-the-science.

23. David M. Oshinsky, *Polio: An American Story* (New York: Oxford University Press, 2005).

24. Dóra Vargha, *Polio Across the Iron Curtain: Hungary's Cold War with an Epidemic*, Global Health Histories (New York: Cambridge University Press, 2018).

25. Dora Vargha, "'There is no Cold War': Global Networks in Polio Vaccine Research," Imperial and Global Forum, Centre for Imperial and Global History, University of Exeter, January 7, 2019, https://imperialglobalexeter.com/2019/01/07/there-is-no-cold-war-global-networks-in-polio-vaccine-research/.

26. Enrique Beldarraín, "Poliomyelitis and Its Elimination in Cuba: An Historical Overview," *MEDICC Rev* 15, no. 2 (2013): 30–36.

27. "After the End of Polio." In Vargha, *Polio Across the Iron Curtain*.

28. Dora Vargha, "Between East and West: Polio Vaccination across the Iron Curtain in Cold War Hungary," *Bulletin of the History of Medicine* 88, no. 2 (2014): 319–342.

29. Dora Vargha, "The Socialist World in Global Polio Eradication," *Revue d'études comparatives Est-Ouest* 1, no. 1 (2018): 71–94.

30. Cohn, "Cholera Revolts."

31. John Henderson, *Florence Under Siege: Surviving Plague in an Early Modern City* (New Haven, CT: Yale University Press, 2019); Shaun Walker and Jennifer Rankin, "Hungary Passes Law that Will Let Orbán Rule by Decree," *Guardian*, March 30, 2020, https://www.theguardian.com/world/2020/mar/30/hungary-jail-for-coronavirus-misinformation-viktor-orban.

32. Walker and Rankin, "Hungary Passes Law that Will Let Orbán Rule by Decree."

33. Stephen L. Roberts, "Tracking Covid-19 Using Big Data and Big Tech: A Digital Pandora's Box," *LSE British Politics and Policy, The London School of Economics and Political Science*, April 20, 2020, https://blogs.lse.ac.uk/politicsandpolicy/tracking-covid-19/.

34. "Global Polio Eradication Initiative," World Health Organization, http://polioeradication.org/.

35. Jefcoate O'Donnell, "Nigeria Just Won a Complex Victory over Polio," *Foreign Policy*, August 21, 2019, https://foreignpolicy.com/2019/08/21/nigeria-just-won-a-complex-victory-over-polio/.

36. "Polio in Africa," travel notices, Centers for Disease Control and Prevention, accessed June 23, 2020, https://wwwnc.cdc.gov/travel/notices/alert/polio-africa.

37. "Global HIV & AIDS Statistics—2019 Fact Sheet," UNAIDS, accessed June 23, 2020, http://afew.org/wp-content/uploads/2020/01/11.png.

38. "Diabetes Facts and Figures," International Diabetes Federation, February 12, 2020, https://www.idf.org/aboutdiabetes/what-is-diabetes/facts-figures.html.

39. Steven Epstein, *Impure Science: AIDS, Activism, and the Politics of Knowledge* (Berkeley: University of California Press, 1996).

40. Lawrence K. Altman, "In Philadelphia 30 Years ago, an Eruption of Illness and Fear," *New York Times*, August 1, 2006, https://www.nytimes.com/2006/08/01/health /01docs.html.

41. "Legionella (Legionnaires' Disease and Pontiac Fever): History, Burden, and Trends," Centers for Disease Control and Prevention, April 30, 2018, https://www.cdc.gov /legionella/about/history.html.

42. Leonard B. Seeff, "The History of the 'Natural History' of Hepatitis C (1968– 2009)," *Liver International: Official Journal of the International Association for the Study of the Liver* 29, suppl. 1, no. 1 (2009): 89–99.

43. "Hepatitis C: A Silent Epidemic," US Department of Health and Human Services, Centers for Disease Control and Prevention, 2020, https://www.cdc.gov/nchhstp/newsroom /docs/factsheets/Hepatitis-C-A-Silent-Epidemic-Infographic.pdf.

44. "Tuberculosis Fact Sheet," World Health Organization, March 24, 2020, https:// www.who.int/news-room/fact-sheets/detail/tuberculosis.

45. Paul Farmer, *Infections and Inequalities: The Modern Plagues* (Berkeley: University of California Press, 1999).

46. Natalie Jacewicz, "The Tuberculosis that Afflicts Much of the World Was Likely Spread by Europeans," *Goats and Soda*, NPR, October 19, 2018, https://www.npr.org /sections/goatsandsoda/2018/10/19/658797864/the-tb-that-afflicts-much-of-the-world -was-likely-spread-by-europeans?t=1592659437778.

47. Randall Packard, *White Plague, Black Labor: Tuberculosis and the Political Economy of Health and Disease in South Africa* (Berkeley: University of California Press, 1989).

48. "Perspectives in Disease Prevention and Health Promotion Update: Universal Precautions for Prevention of Transmission of Human Immunodeficiency Virus, Hepatitis B Virus, and Other Bloodborne Pathogens in Health-Care Settings," *MMWR Weekly* 37, no 24 (n.d.): 377–388.

49. Uri Friedman, "Face Masks Are In," *The Atlantic*, April 2, 2020, https://www .theatlantic.com/politics/archive/2020/04/america-asia-face-mask-coronavirus/609283/.

50. Peter Galison, *How Experiments End* (Chicago: University of Chicago Press, 1987).

51. Katie Thomas, "Trump Calls This Drug a 'Game Changer.' Doctors Aren't So Sure," *New York Times*, April 17, 2020, https://www.nytimes.com/2020/04/17/health/trump -hydroxychloroquine-coronavirus.html.

52. Erin McCormick, "Why Experts Are Questioning Two Hyped Antibody Studies in Coronavirus Hotspots," *Guardian*, April 23, 2020, https://www.theguardian.com/world /2020/apr/23/coronavirus-antibody-studies-california-stanford.

53. Quoctrung Bui et al., "What 5 Coronavirus Models Say the Next Month Will Look Like," *New York Times*, April 22, 2020, https://www.nytimes.com/interactive/2020/04/22 /upshot/coronavirus-models.html?action=click&module=News&pgtype=Homepage.

54. Robert Smith, "Did we Eradicate SARS? Lessons Learned and the Way Forward," *American Journal of Biomedical Science & Research* 6, no. 2 (2019): 152–155.

55. Helge Jordheim and Anne Kveim Lie, "Epidemic Times," *Somatosphere*, April 2, 2020, http://somatosphere.net/2020/epidemic-times.html/.

Chapter Two

The World after COVID

A Perspective from History

Margaret MacMillan

A mong the brilliant and flamboyant costumes they wear during Carnival in Venice, a sombre figure also stalks. It wears a white mask with dark spectacles and a long curving beak along with a black hat and gown. The "plague doctor" costume was once more than a diversion. It dates back to the middle of the 14th century when waves of the bubonic plague—the Black Death—hit the city, probably borne from further east by some of the many trading ships that had made Venice so rich. The authorities did what they could, setting up special burial grounds and quarantine stations throughout the city and eventually obliging newly arriving ships to isolate themselves for forty days on a remote island. The city also organized and paid for the plague doctors. The mask, with its spectacles and a beak stuffed with special herbs, would, it was hoped, ward off the noxious vapors suspected of carrying the disease. The great trading city of Genoa on the other side of Italy endured its own outbreak around the same time and the plague spread outwards throughout Europe, carrying off a third or more of all its inhabitants.

It was a different world of course with very different values, institutions, and science and technology. Yet the reactions of Europeans and their governments then— fear, denial, resignation, hope, blind optimism, experimentation—are not so different from ours today. Moralists and theologians blamed the pandemic on the decline

Margaret MacMillan specializes in the international history of the late 19th and 20th centuries.

in public morality; in one of the stranger responses, wandering bands of flagellants whipped themselves raw to atone for their sins. Conspiracy theorists preferred to single out minorities, at that time Jews. Governments floundered; some virtually collapsed while others did their best to cope and to contain the disease, clearing out garbage because it produced supposedly dangerous odors, locking up the sick in their houses or forcing them out into the countryside to die there. And, as many are doing today, the rich fled the cities to their country estates while the poor remained where they were, jammed into slums and at the mercy of the disease.

There was a desperate search for prophylactics and cures just as there is today: nosegays perhaps, like the herbs in the plague doctors' masks, might keep the evil vapors away. Pilgrims flocked to holy relics, particularly those of St. Sebastian who, it was held, protected worshippers against the plague. While there were many instances of selfishness and indifference to the suffering of others, there were also great acts of altruism, with local groups springing up to nurse the sick and bury the dead. What made the times even more difficult and troubling is that the Black Death was not the only crisis in Europe. Across the continent, conflicts—the Hundred Years' War between England and France, for example—carried on despite the pandemic. More, the Great Schism in the Church of Rome shook public faith in the institution itself and in morality.[1] Shocks, as we are discovering with COVID-19, do not always come at convenient times, and when they intersect with other crises, as happened in 2020, their impact is amplified.

Historians disagree on how much change the Black Death brought.[2] Governments did not fall as a result of that first great outbreak, and the Church eventually regained much of its authority, at least until its next crisis during the Reformation. Because there were fewer people to work, wages in some areas went up and workers were often somewhat better treated. It is possible that the need to deal with the repeated waves of the plague encouraged the move to stronger centralized states, but war was already doing that. The plague, if anything, reinforced a lesson Europeans already knew well—that life is uncertain and unfair, and death can come quickly. And it was going to take another five and a half centuries after those first outbreaks in the late 1340s for scientists to finally work out how the Black Death was transmitted, and it took longer still for the development of the antibiotics which could treat it.

It will be harder for us to come to terms with the prospect that we may not find a cure or treatment for COVID-19 soon. For we have got used to a world where science and technology forge ahead, eliminating what were once ordinary diseases, prolonging life, and producing consumer goods and innovations on a scale and with a rapidity our ancestors could only dream of. We have come to expect what the British government fetishized in 2020, that science and our institutions will solve our problems and keep us safe. The impact of our pandemic may, paradoxically, be greater than that of the even more deadly Black Death precisely because we are unaccustomed to dealing with uncertainty. The COVID-19 crisis is often compared to the Spanish influenza at the end of the First World War, which may have killed as many as fifty million people around the globe. Certainly there are similarities: the virus spread quickly in a globalized world and governments varied their responses, from ignoring its spread to imposing curfews, with the result that mortality rates varied widely from place to place. Yet in other ways the reactions to the influenza were closer to those of the 14th century. Medical science did not yet have the tools to fully understand the influenza's transmission and impact or to develop ways of treating it quickly. People at the time also lived in an uncertain world where life could be cut short at any time by a whole host of diseases which have now virtually disappeared, such as smallpox, or that can be managed and treated, such as cholera or typhoid. There is so little comment about the influenza in the memoirs and novels of the time that perhaps the millions of dead in the war had further habituated the world to sudden death.

The COVID-19 pandemic has shaken even strong societies. It has brought into sharp relief flaws that were already starting to emerge in our globalized world: growing social and economic inequalities, for example, or the dangerous fragility of international supply lines. And it has exacerbated existing international tensions, between the United States and China for example, as governments blame each other for the spread of the virus. Just as 14th-century Europe suffered from a convergence of different crises, so too today problems and issues that had been developing on parallel paths are increasingly intersecting. The higher death rate among ethnic and racial minorities in several countries, including the United States and the United Kingdom, has heightened existing concerns and resentment over racism. Resistance to globalization or at least to this current form of it has been given new force by the rapid international spread of COVID-19. The public's disillusionment of the past decades with their own elites and institutions has been further fueled by the incoherent and often ineffective responses of their governments.

A debate has started about what we did wrong and what we did right in confronting the pandemic, but it is already developing into a broader discussion of what is wrong with our societies and what we need to do in order to cope better with the next great challenge, whether it is economic, medical, or environmental. We will need to examine and debate our own assumptions about how to prepare for sudden large-scale crises, about the proper role of government, or about how to build stable and effective domestic and international societies. As we start to take stock of the costs and impact of the COVID-19 pandemic and prepare to deal with an uncertain future, history, I suggest, can help us answer crucial questions. Most importantly, why are we repeatedly surprised by catastrophes? While there are what Nassim Taleb has called "black swan" events—rare and hard or impossible to predict—most cataclysmic events have warning signs beforehand, if only people care to notice. If we can get a better understanding of why we and, crucially, those in positions of power fail to do so, we may be able to guard against that complacency in the future. Then there is the question, once the crisis is upon us, why do some leaders and some societies cope better than others? And, then, how do we deal with the consequences and pick up the pieces? When have societies learned from catastrophes and put in place needed reforms and measures for the ones yet to come? By looking at history, we can gain a better idea of the role played in crises by values and ideas, the strengths or weaknesses of institutions, and leadership.

History can help as we raise questions and look for answers, but we must not expect clear lessons or convenient blueprints for the future. We must understand and acknowledge differences over time and in societies, whether in institutions, capabilities, or values. The United States is often compared to the Roman Empire, but the two are far apart in both time and character. American presidents may have an imperial style, but they do not sacrifice to the gods or indeed believe that they are gods themselves. And the order in which events unfold matters. The military planners and strategists going into the Second World War were influenced by their experience of the first. The French thought the defense would still be stronger than the offensive, and so they built the Maginot Line and waited to shatter German attacks. The Allied leaders who planned the post-1945 world were conscious of what had gone wrong in the 1920s and 1930s and hoped to set up institutions to avert those political and economic failures.

The study of the past offers instructive examples, showing what has worked in the face of challenges and what has not. In the financial crisis of 2008, the chair of the Federal Reserve, Ben Bernanke, and Timothy Geithner, chair of the Federal Reserve Bank of New York, were helped in their decision making by their knowledge of previous crashes and depressions, particularly the Great Depression of the

1930s. Indeed, Bernanke had researched and written about the subject in his academic career. History also warns of unintended consequences and shows what the price of failure might be. The Tsarist regime in Russia went to war in 1914 assuming that the conflict would be short and hoping that a common cause might pull a badly fractured society together. The opposite happened and large numbers of Russians, including, critically, much of the military, simply withdrew their support. The first revolution, of February 1917, toppled what was a hollow shell, and the second, in October, brought the tiny Bolshevik Party into power with lasting consequences for Russia and the world. Finally, examples of similar situations—such as depressions, war, revolutions—allow us to ask what we might do ourselves. Knowing what questions to ask is the first step to getting good answers.

Using analogies to analyze situations and determine what policies and actions might work has to be done with care of course, and we must always guard against getting locked into just one analogy. Think of the ways in which the Munich analogy has been misused both in the initial assessments and expectations. Anthony Eden was persuaded that Gamal Abdel Nasser of Egypt was a dictator like Benito Mussolini or Adolf Hitler, whom Eden had dealt with in the 1930s, and that he must be confronted early on while he still was consolidating his regime and not yet militarily strong. And so Britain, in league with France and Israel, embarked on the disastrous Suez adventure. In reality Nasser was an Arab nationalist who was bent not on war and conquest but on situating Egypt at the center of the Arab world. Unlike Hitler and Mussolini he could have been managed with a combination of skilful diplomacy and containment.

In a few months many of us have gone from assuming that pandemics were only in the past to living with an unaccustomed degree of uncertainty. We still do not understand completely how COVID-19 spreads, why it affects some demographic groups more than others, or how best to contain and treat it. Although we have made considerable progress, the effective vaccine may be a long way off—or not come at all. The pandemic has shaken our faith in science, in our leaders, and in our societies.

Yet COVID-19 should not have come as such a shock. Epidemiologists and other scientific experts have been warning for years that we faced increasing risks from viruses that jump from other living creatures, such as birds or swine, to human beings. As populations increased and pressed into hitherto wild natural areas, the chances of that grew greater. More, the ease and extent of travel around the globe made it likely that new viruses would spread rapidly. There have been warnings from past influenza pandemics: the Asian flu, 1957–8; the Hong Kong flu, 1968–9; the swine flu, 2009–10; and of course, long before those, the Spanish flu, 1917–20, which may have killed as many as fifty million people worldwide. And coronaviruses such as MERS, Middle East Respiratory Syndrome, and SARS, Severe Acute Respiratory Syndrome, gave warnings of other strains of potentially lethal disease occurring on a large scale.

There are, alas, many examples in the past of people ignoring evidence, or when that became impossible, explaining it away. Often it is a consequence of being preoccupied with other problems which seem more immediate. In January 2020 scattered reports that a strange new virus had appeared in Wuhan were overshadowed by the sharp rise in tensions between the United States and Iran or, in the United States itself, the Democratic primaries. In addition, as psychologists have pointed out, we tend to suffer from a confirmation bias. We fit what we observe into an existing system of beliefs and assumptions. That is reinforced increasingly today by media "echo chambers" which keep out contrary views. There were signs before the Wall Street Crash of 1929 that the stock market was dangerously overheating and that levels of debt were too high, but the ever-growing pool of investors wanted to believe in their chances of making great profits. Indeed, they often resented those who tried to issue warnings as only interested in keeping the wealth for themselves. In 1998 the investment firm Long-Term Capital, which prided itself on having taken risk out of finance, suddenly imploded when the capital markets did not behave as the computer models had predicted. Its failure threatened the stability of the whole American system, and it had to be salvaged and then quietly wound up when the Federal Reserve Bank of New York organized a bailout by major financial institutions.[3] Yet for all the postmortems and recommendations for greater regulation, very little was done and the derivatives market continued to grow. The belief among those investors who were making extravagant profits thanks to increasingly arcane instruments was, as the title of Carmen Reinhart and Kenneth Rogoff's study of centuries of financial folly says, "this time is different." As those who have written about what went wrong in 2008, including Reinhart and Rogan, Gillian Tett, Andrew Ross Sorkin, and Michael Short, have all pointed out, the warnings, from academics, government officials, and businesspeople, were simply brushed aside.[4]

The First World War was a turning point in the 20th century, and its outbreak provides a vivid example of how decision making can enter a narrow tunnel and how those making the decisions fail to account for potential and unintended consequences. Without that long and costly struggle which put the societies in-volved under such strain, Europe might well have been spared the violent milita-rized politics of the 1920s and 1930s. We can never know, but it is possible that Austria-Hungary and the Ottoman Empire might have evolved into multinational states. Russia in 1914 had survived an earlier revolution and was moving by fits and starts towards constitutional and representative government. More, its econ-omy and society were modernizing rapidly. The war cut short that promise and, by bringing about the destruction of the old regime, made possible the Bolshevik coup d'état of October 1917. The spread of the Bolsheviks' revolutionary ideol-ogy and the growth of anti-democratic communist parties increasingly under the direction of Moscow, as well as the establishment of new states based on ethnic-ity, made European domestic and interstate politics dangerously polarized and overheated. The First World War did not lead directly to the Second but it made it possible. If they could have seen the future or even imagined a part of it, would Europe's leaders have acted otherwise than they did in the final crisis of July 1914? That failure of imagination is a case study in why we are shocked by events that, especially in hindsight, had been threatening.[5]

In the summer of 1914 Europeans were, for the most part, stunned by the speed—just over a month—with which the continent went from peace to a gen-eral war. Thousands of people who had gone on holidays as usual in July found themselves scrambling to get home as borders snapped shut and trains were di-verted for troops. The long century of peace in Europe after the Napoleonic Wars had persuaded many Europeans that their civilization had moved beyond the need for nations to settle disputes by violence. And the political and military leaders, who had thought they could still use war as an instrument of policy, had been banking on a short decisive war. As a consequence, they had made no plans either to stockpile large amounts of war matériel or convert a peacetime economy into a war one, and they were surprised and appalled at how quickly mass industrial war consumed resources. Within a month the French used up half the ammuni-tion they had on hand and German artillery had fired all the shells available by the end of six weeks. And, as the two sides settled into their trenches in the late autumn of 1914, it became clear that a war planned as one of movement was on its way to becoming a stalemate.[6]

The war should not have come as such a surprise. After all, the military and diplomatic establishments of the great powers had been thinking and planning for potential war since the end of the 19th century. And the first decade of the 20th century had shown that peace in Europe was resting on increasingly shaky foundations. Heightened nationalisms, aided by the spread of literacy, the mass media, and the extension of the voting franchise, put governments under pressure to defend national honor and interests, if necessary, through war. And governments and lobby groups were in turn prepared to use public sentiments to promote activist foreign policies or get more funds for the military. Before 1914 an arms race gripped the major powers which further heightened tensions among them. Added to that was the influence of social Darwinism which encouraged a belief that a struggle for survival was inevitable among nations. For some Europeans war was seen as desirable, a way of demonstrating the nation's virility and determination to succeed. Any war, it was assumed, would necessarily be short because after about six months, empty treasuries and bankrupt economies would force the powers to negotiate.

European planners should not have been surprised at the nature of the war or by the inability of either side to overcome the other. They certainly had enough evidence by 1914 to make an informed guess about how a major European war might unfold. The military had closely studied recent conflicts around the world. It was increasingly clear that advances in technology had given an advantage to a well-dug-in defense. Yet evidence from wars such as the American Civil War or colonial wars was dismissed on the grounds that, as one European general put it, "Those savage encounters do not deserve the name of war." Perhaps because they remained uneasy about the evident power the new weapons gave defenders, the military took refuge in calculations of how many attackers would be needed to overcome one defender or magical thinking about imbuing all their soldiers with a longing to sacrifice their lives.

Europeans had ample warning that a major war would be hard to control and perhaps unwinnable by either side. Their strategists and political leaders should have been able to envisage the possibility of a stalemate, for the balance of power was so evenly divided by 1914. Ivan Bloch, a highly successful entrepreneur in Russia, devoted much of the last part of his life to a massive study of war in which he argued that Europe's own economic strength could be turned inwards to tear it apart and that any conflict was likely to produce years of deadlock rather than the weeks and months of swift battles the generals imagined. The French politician Jean Jaurès made a study of war and came to a similar conclusion. Because both were civilians and the former a Jewish businessman and the latter a socialist, they were ignored by the experts.

The road to the First World War also shows how dangerous the division of responsibilities can be. The politicians tended to leave military affairs to their experts—much as some governments in the COVID-19 crisis have claimed to be following the science when in reality the decisions that must be made are broad political ones. In the major European powers, civilian control over the military, even in Britain and France, which had stronger traditions in that area than Germany or Austria-Hungary, was inadequate or nearly nonexistent. So the military made plans, which they did not always share with the civilian leadership, to fight offensively or only on two fronts. Too often the civilians were content to remain in the dark only to find that, as the war approached, the choices before them had been dangerously narrowed. In the final days before the First World War started, the Kaiser in Germany and the Tsar in Russia tried to limit the coming conflict by fighting on a single front only to be told by their generals that was impossible.

Of course there were those, including political leaders such as Jaurès or Sir Edward Grey, the British foreign secretary, who worried about growing tensions and careless talk about how a good war would clear the air, but an important psychological barrier had been crossed and war had become thinkable. In the years before 1914 a series of crises—the annexation of the Ottoman territory by Austria-Hungary in 1908, the Italian seizure of Libya from the Ottoman Empire in 1911, and the Balkan Wars of 1912 and 1913—brought talk of war and threatening moves such as military mobilizations. The powers muddled through but each crisis left both lingering resentments and a fatal complacency, similar to the one at the start of the COVID-19 pandemic, that all such challenges could be successfully dealt with. The brinkmanship served further to weaken what was already a fragile European order and increased the temptation for preventive wars. As mutual suspicions grew, what was intended as deterrence on one side was read in other capitals as a threat. In 1914, Russia's decision to mobilize some forces as "a precaution" was read in Berlin as preparation for an attack, and the high command pressured the government to order the German armies into action before it was too late.

In the final days before a general war, Europe's leaders let it down. The British government and the media were not paying attention to the confrontation developing in the Balkans after the assassination of the Archduke because of the Irish question that was threatening to tear apart British society, while the French were focused on the sensational trial of the wife of a leading politician who had shot a critic of her husband. In Berlin the Kaiser recklessly promised his "blank check" of support to Austria-Hungary as it moved to destroy Serbia and his government meekly backed him up. When they realized that they were about to unleash a general war, the Kaiser and his cousin Tsar Nicholas II of Russia both hesitated to sign the fatal mobilization orders, yet both gave way to their own military.

How then can societies and their governments avoid being taken by surprise and prepare themselves better to make decisions when great events occur? When we look at previous crises and the COVID-19 pandemic, certain tendencies stand out that must be guarded against. Complacency: the faith that we have muddled through before, avoiding a war or finding a cure, and we can do so again. Tunnel vision: those in positions of power and authority fall into the trap of speaking and listening only to those who reinforce what they already believe, and competing viewpoints are belittled or ignored and awkward pieces of evidence explained away. And finally, an unwillingness to learn from experience: the temptation after a crisis has been dealt with to relax and go back to business as usual, yet that is precisely the moment society should be resolving to do better and to set in place insurance, whether that be better banking regulations or stockpiles of crucial medical goods.

In the COVID-19 pandemic, democratic states, especially those with a history of moderate politics where parties tend to seek the middle ground, were able to successfully appeal to their citizens to think of a common good without needing coercion. In Germany, South Korea, and New Zealand, which were among the more successful countries in managing the pandemic, governments did not have to order people to wear masks or do social distancing. As the two world wars demonstrated, patriotism or ideologies of other sorts bring people together. Accepting sacrifices and mobilizing resources, especially in a long struggle, cannot be imposed merely by fiat. Soviet citizens in the Second World War had little choice over their leaders, but they trusted them as Russians had not in the First World War. Soviet men and women volunteered to fight the German invaders, organized partisan groups behind the lines, and endured long years of hardship. They did so, it is clear, not for communism but for Mother Russia, and official propaganda came to reflect that. Britain was able to maintain its war effort because its citizens agreed on the common cause of surviving and defeating the Axis powers. Labour politicians joined a Conservative government led by Winston Churchill. In France, by contrast, the divisions over what sort of society France should be, over values such as religion, and over whether Nazi Germany or Soviet Russia was the greatest enemy had already threatened to tear the country apart in the 1930s. When the war came, neither French society nor its leaders were united in their values or goals and that contributed to the defeat and capitulation of 1940.[7]

Success in coping also depends on existing institutions, which include effective governing bodies and civil services, well-resourced education and research, and strong industrial and economic organizations. Britain endured and prevailed in two world wars, in part, because it mobilized its economy and society more efficiently and thoroughly than its enemies. The government persuaded unions and employers, on the whole successfully, to work together to sink their differences for the war effort, and it persuaded the public to accept a high degree of control over their lives.[8] Russia held together for a surprising length of time in the First World War thanks largely to the patriotism of its people, but by 1917 its institutions, never strong to begin with, were buckling under the strain. Soldiers at the front were so short of equipment that they had to share rifles and could only fire a handful of bullets a day. The railways were clogged and chaotic and the cities were slowly starving because crops could not be brought in from the country. The Tsar's government was incapable of providing leadership, and rumors of corruption, even treason, undermined its few remaining shreds of authority.[9]

As the experience of Russia in the First World War shows, leadership counts too. The countries that have done well in the 2020 pandemic tend to be those with leaders who are both responsive to their publics and are not afraid to make difficult decisions. Angela Merkel in Germany and Jacinda Ardern in New Zealand had the benefit of leading strong and cohesive societies before the pandemic, and their decisions and style have only enhanced that fact rather than undermined it. Both have addressed their peoples bluntly and have not attempted to minimize the severity of the crisis or the challenges in managing it. Nor have they been afraid to make decisions. By contrast, the British government has sent out a series of conflicting messages and irritated the public by telling transparent untruths about, for example, the availability of testing. In the United States, the federal government has been largely absent in managing the crises and, when it has intervened, has often issued dangerous or misleading advice. Leadership there has devolved largely to the state and municipal level with understandably mixed results. In more authoritarian societies, the response, as so often has been the case, has depended too much on the leader. Brazil's president Jair Bolsonaro made light of the threat of COVID-19—a "mere case of the sniffles," he said—and quarrelled with his own bureaucrats, the medical establishment, and state governors. In Russia, President Vladimir Putin denied the existence of cases for far too long even as he secluded himself in a special hygienic bunker. China has been more successful, but that may be less a consequence of Xi Jinping's leadership—after all, he largely absented himself in the early stages of the pandemic—and more on the size and strength of the Communist Party and a society which values cohesiveness and conformity to social norms.

Good leaders also have a willingness to draw on advice and support from whatever quarter. Just as President Abraham Lincoln had assembled a cabinet full of talented individuals, President Franklin Delano Roosevelt in the 1930s brought into government Republicans, businesspeople, university professors, and, in the case of Frances Perkins in the Department of Labor, a strong social activist. During the Second World War the governments of both the United States and Canada had the "dollar-a-year men," successful businessmen who volunteered their services. In Britain Winston Churchill pioneered the use of scientific advisors, and the famous code-breaking center at Bletchley Park raided the universities for their most talented students. It is said that when Churchill paid a visit to Bletchley he remarked to the director that, while he had urged that no stone be unturned to find the brightest minds, he had not expected to be taken literally. In addition, leaders such as Lincoln, Roosevelt, and Churchill can be firm in purpose and confident of the rightness of their long-term goals but still willing to listen to contradictory views. Indeed, that helped them to think through their decisions. During the Cuban Missile Crisis, President Kennedy assembled an Executive Committee, ExComm, of his most important officials and advisers and had them thrash out the merits and demerits of possible responses to the Soviet provocations.

In that crisis Kennedy also showed that he had learned from the failure of the Bay of Pigs the year before not to believe everything the military told him or the assurances they gave. That brings me to the last issue I wish to raise. How can individuals or groups of individuals such as nations best learn from major crises? That we can and must learn seems obvious. In the past century democratic governments have fallen into the habit of setting up official inquiries to probe what went wrong and to offer recommendations. After both world wars a number of governments commissioned official histories whose purpose was not merely to create a record of events but to analyze and probe what had worked and what had not. How much governments heed such conclusions is another matter. The American military and many in the foreign policy establishment concluded after the United States' failure in Vietnam that it should never again fight a counterinsurgency war. So, strategies and tactics that had been learned through painful experience were not studied at military colleges and the best book on counterinsurgency was allowed to go out of print. With the invasion of Afghanistan and then the invasion and occupation of Iraq at the start of this century, many of those lessons had to be relearned. As a counterexample, certain young army officers, among them Charles de Gaulle and Heinz Guderian, learned from their experiences in the First World War to respect the offensive potential of the tank, and they were able put their ideas into practice in their own armies. The British post-1945 Labour government and other European governments took in the lessons of the 1930s, when the Great Depression caused massive economic misery and opened up dangerous rifts in society. The welfare state and similar social-democratic measures across Europe were the result and have contributed greatly to Europe's well-being and stability.

In the 17th century the prolonged miseries of the Thirty Years' War, when the powers meddled in each other's internal affairs, finally persuaded European leaders to accept the principle of sovereignty which was enshrined in the peace settlement of Westphalia. In the next century the European powers clung to the notion of a balance of power in a zero-sum game despite the high costs, but the French Revolution and the rise to power of a hegemonic France under Napoleon made them think again. As Paul Schroeder has argued, the statesmen who met at Vienna in 1814 and 1815 had the goal not of a balance but an "equilibrium," based on a respect for laws and borders and aimed at creating stability.[10] During the Second World War, the leaders of the Grand Alliance took note of the failures of the Paris Peace Conference at the end of the First World War and the more recent ones of the 1930s, when appeasement and a lack of support for the League of Nations only emboldened the dictators who were bent on revising the international order.[11] This time the United States not only took the lead in building new institutions of which the centerpiece was the United Nations but Roosevelt ensured that the United States would become a member. At the same time, Allied leaders, with the experience of the Great Depression and the collapse of world trade as nations scrambled to erect tariff barriers, came together, again under the leadership of the United States, to create the Bretton Woods institutions of the World Bank, the International Monetary Fund, and the General Agreement on Tariffs and Trade to keep the world's economy stable and encourage the spread of trade, investment, and prosperity. In Western Europe, forward-looking leaders, mindful of the corrosive national rivalries of the 1930s that had led to the outbreak of war in 1939, laid the foundations of the European Union. In the postwar years the United States took on the responsibilities of being a superpower and both encouraged European states to cooperate with each other and aided recovery directly through the Marshall Plan. The trouble is that memories fade and lessons lose their force as those who learned them firsthand depart from the scene. Perhaps the COVID-19 crisis will remind us yet again of the benefits of international cooperation.

While it is too soon to draw firm conclusions or formulate lessons, some things are already becoming clear. COVID-19 has brought to prominence the failings in our societies, such as growing social and economic inequality, the dangerous lack of medical provision in certain countries, and the downsides of globalization, such as long and easily disrupted supply lines. On a more positive note, a major crisis can also bring changes and advances that in normal times were not thought possible. Producing penicillin on a large scale was not economically feasible in the 1930s. In the Second World War, Allied governments deemed it essential for their troops and so worked with major drug companies to produce it on a large scale. The response to COVID-19 has shown, contrary to what has been assumed in conservative circles, that governments can intervene to considerable effect in society and can spend on a large scale without going bankrupt. We now have a renewed appreciation of the power of government to take and, where necessary, enforce measures for the good of society. We have also seen that governments can trust their citizens, their judgment, and their resilience, more than they sometimes do. In the 1930s successive British governments and their advisers took for granted that the first experience of aerial bombing would so demoralize the British public that they would be overcome with panic, behave irrationally, and as a result, society would collapse. As the experience of the war showed, the British were able to endure repeated bombing attacks and, if anything, British society grew stronger in the face of a shared threat. In early March 2020, as the number of infections was mounting, the British government hesitated to impose a lockdown because it feared people would not understand or obey it. In fact, large numbers of the British were already going into self-isolation.

The war metaphor may be overdone, but dealing with a major challenge such as COVID-19 demands increased authority and arbitrary measures which in more ordinary times we would shrink from. And, as in a war, social values and assumptions can shift. In the past, women were not held to be capable of doing certain jobs; total war and the need for their labor exploded that belief. Today, as the former governor of the Bank of England Mark Carney has argued, we may be starting to detach value from price and think of other measures.

Let us hope that he and others are right and that some good will come from the pandemic. Let us try and follow the examples of those societies that study and learn from their mistakes. And let us guard against the sort of tunnel thinking and complacency which leaves us unwilling or unable to contemplate and prepare for great shocks. Key to that will be accepting that we are entering a period of great uncertainty. The post-1945 and post-1989 arrangements are falling apart and a new world order has yet to emerge; the economy faces a long struggle to recover; it is almost certain that COVID-19 will be followed by other pandemics; and climate change, the greatest challenge of all to humanity, is speeding up. As in major wars, we are going to need to see the problems and possible solutions properly explored and debated and the necessary resources made available. We should harness the knowledge of the scientific experts but also those whose work it is to understand how societies function—among them, behavioral psychologists, sociologists, anthropologists, political philosophers, and, yes, historians too.

NOTES

1. For the impact of disease on society, see Jared Diamond, *Guns, Germs, and Steel: The Fates of Human Societies* (New York: W. W. Norton, 1999); and William H. McNeill, *Plagues and People* (New York: Doubleday, 1976). For the Black Death in Europe, see Rosemary Horron, *The Black Death* (Manchester, UK: Manchester University Press, 2013).

2. See, for example, Samuel K. Cohn, "The Black Death: End of a Paradigm," *American Historical Review* 107, no. 3 (June 2002): 703–738; and part V of Walter Scheidel, *The Great Leveler: Violence and the History of Inequality from the Stone Age to the Twenty-First Century* (Princeton, NJ: Princeton University Press, 2017).

3. See chapter 5 in Gillian Tett, *Fool's Gold: How the Bold Dream of a Small Tribe at J.P. Morgan Was Corrupted by Wall Street Greed and Unleashed a Catastrophe* (New York: Free Press, 2009).

4. Michael Lewis, *The Big Short: Inside the Doomsday Machine* (New York: W. W. Norton, 2009); Carmen M. Reinhart and Kenneth S. Rogoff, *This Time Is Different: Eight Centuries of Financial Folly* (Princeton, NJ: Princeton University Press, 2009); Andrew Ross Sorkin, *Too Big to Fail: The Inside Story of How Wall Street and Washington Fought to Save the Financial System from Crisis—and Themselves* (New York: Viking, 2009); Tett, *Fool's Gold*.

5. For an exploration of the counterfactual and the slide of Europe to war, see Richard Ned Lebow, "Franz Ferdinand Found Alive: World War I Unnecessary," in *Forbidden Fruit: Counterfactuals and International Relations* (Princeton, NJ: Princeton University Press, 2010): 69–102.

6. For recent works on the causes of the war, see Christopher M. Clark, *The Sleepwalkers: How Europe Went to War in 1914* (New York: Harper Perennial, 2013); Margaret MacMillan, *The War That Ended Peace: The Road to 1914* (New York: Random House, 2013); Thomas G. Otte, *July Crisis: The World's Descent into War, Summer 1914* (Cambridge: Cambridge University Press, 2014).

7. Julian Jackson, *The Fall of France: The Nazi Invasion of 1940* (New York: Oxford University Press, 2003); Daniel Todman, *Britain's War: Into Battle, 1937–1941* (New York: Oxford University Press, 2016).

8. David Edgerton, *Britain's War Machine: Weapons, Resources, and Experts in the Second World War* (London: Allen Lane, 2011); Arthur Marwick, *Britain in the Century of Total War: War, Peace and Social Change, 1900–1967* (Boston: Atlantic Monthly / Little Brown, 1968).

9. For a discussion of leadership, see Daniel Byman and Kenneth Pollack, "Let Us Now Praise Great Men," *International Security* 25, no. 4 (Spring 2001): 107–146; and the clas-

sic 1919 lecture by Max Weber, "Politics as a Vocation," in H. H. Gerth and C. Wright Mills, *From Max Weber: Essays in Sociology* (New York: Oxford University Press, 1946). For the Russian Revolution, see Orlando Figes, *A People's Tragedy: A History of the Russian Revolution* (New York: Viking, 1997).

10. Paul W. Schroeder, "Did the Vienna Settlement Rest on a Balance of Power?" in *Systems, Stability, and Statecraft: Essays on the International History of Modern Europe* (New York: Palgrave Macmillan, 2004); Paul W. Schroeder, *The Transformation of European Politics, 1763–1848* (New York: Oxford University Press, 1994).

11. Mark Mazower, *Governing the World: The History of an Idea, 1815 to the Present* (New York: Penguin Books, 2012).

Future Scenarios

"We are all failed states, now"

Philip Bobbitt

> all things stedfastnes doe hate
> And changed be: yet being rightly wayd,
> They are not changed from their first estate;
> But by their change their being doe dilate:
> And turning to themselues at length againe,
> Doe worke their owne perfection so by fate:
> Then ouer them Change doth not rule and raigne;
> But they raigne ouer change, and doe their states mantaine.
>
> EDMUND SPENSER,
> "TWO CANTOS OF MUTABILITIE"

A s I write this, the constitutional environment of the United States is experiencing its greatest stresses since the American Civil War. A viral pandemic has engulfed the world and especially stricken the United States; as of this writing more than 3 million coronavirus cases have been reported in the United States, more than in any other country. Although the United States has about 4.2% of the global population, it has suffered 25% of the deaths worldwide—more than 132,000 Americans have died from the COVID-19 virus. Partly as a consequence of this viral apocalypse, US unemployment is experiencing levels approaching 20%[1]—numbers not seen since the Great Depression, and US gross domestic product is expected to contract by 7% in a single year.[2] The chairman of the Federal Reserve has predicted a steep recession of uncertain length[3] and the federal debt has climbed to levels unseen outside of wartime.

Philip Bobbitt is the Herbert Wechsler Professor of Federal Jurisprudence and Director of the Center for National Security at Columbia Law School.

Coincidentally, a mass interracial movement has been ignited by instances of police brutality toward African Americans, made indelible by smartphone cameras that have seared into the memory of a horrified world the death throes of unarmed persons in police custody. Not so coincidentally, the White House is occupied by a president who has an attitude of inflamed contempt for US constitutional norms and an incompetence at foreign policy that has prompted concern even from America's adversaries. Respect for the deadlocked Congress and for public officials is approaching historic lows.[4] The public is sharply divided against itself; members of both parties at record levels would not wish to see their children marry outside the faith. The commitment to democracy itself has sharply decreased among its heirs, the generation born in the 21st century.[5] Opinion polls taken abroad confirm that America's global image has plummeted[6] and the nonproliferation initiatives of the US administration toward North Korea[7] and Iran[8] have collapsed. In this fraught summer, it has hardly captured the headlines that temperatures in Siberia have soared to levels unseen in a hundred thousand years.[9] To say that the world, and especially its leading power the United States, is facing a series of crises hardly needs to be said.

But, imagine, for a moment, that the United States—or for that matter all developed states—did not face a public health crisis caused by a pandemic. Or a crisis in the fragility of their financial systems. Or a democracy crisis in those states that are liberal democracies and in those countries that aspire to have democratic systems. Or a critical infrastructure vulnerability crisis. Or a climate change crisis. Or face the looming security crisis caused by the proliferation of weapons of mass destruction. Or a crisis in race relations and growing economic inequality.

What we do face, however, is a crisis of change.[10] Or, more precisely, a crisis of managing change brought about by a historic shift in the constitutional order of the state. This shift has delegitimated the constitutional order of industrial nation-states as they strive, unsuccessfully, to cope with the various problems besetting them that, unlike previous challenges, actually thrive in a global environment dominated by industrial nation-states. As a result, the most profound change of all is coming to world order as the constitutional order of its constituent states is transformed. It is this crisis that underlies all the others because it is converting those other challenges into existential crises for governance. It is this change in the constitutional order that must be managed before these crises can be dealt with successfully.

The extraordinary failure of the United States to deal with the COVID-19 pandemic has its roots not in previous failures but in previous historic successes.

Indeed, it was these successes that enabled the United States to shape a world order in its own image. Its current epic failure will inevitably have an impact on its ability to shape the architecture and character of the 21st-century international order.

The crisis in the current constitutional order of industrial nation-states is the legacy of the greatest triumph of that order, the defeat of fascism and communism and the ascendancy of market-based, liberal democracy. A half dozen critical innovations brought about that victory. Now each of these innovations has spawned threats for which the current constitutional order (and the international order) is not designed and cannot cope.

The development of weapons of mass destruction discredited the fascist regime in Japan without ever actually having to defeat its vast land armies; further developments of these weapons technologies kept communist regimes at bay until they too could be discredited in the eyes of their own populations. US extended deterrence not only protected the populations of its allies; it also gave the United States the paramount voice in the global affairs of the anti-Soviet coalition that it organized. But now those very technologies and the means of their delivery have become so much cheaper that we are entering a period when impoverished and otherwise weak states like Pakistan and North Korea can threaten nuclear attacks and even small groups without state backing will be able to marshal biological weapons, undoing the deterrence theories that spared humankind another experience of mass destruction on the scale of Hiroshima and Nagasaki. There is universal doubt in the epidemiological community that COVID-19 originated in a bioweapons lab in Wuhan, China, though there is little doubt that the lab has worked with deadly coronaviruses. Given the world's experience with COVID-19—a virus whose latency makes it especially potent as a weapon, and whose close genetic relationship to familiar coronaviruses means that it might be engineered from commonly available and well-known genetic materials—it may turn out that the long-term importance of the pandemic will be manifested in new weapons in the hands of relatively unsophisticated operators. A state that cannot protect its own citizens is unlikely to persuade other states that it can protect theirs.

The development of an international system of trade, transport, financing, and labor has brought unprecedented wealth not only to its authors in the developed world but to the mass of impoverished persons in South and East Asia. Although Bernie Sanders and Jeremy Corbyn may not have gotten the news, this surge in global wealth has removed socialism as a viable alternative to market-based economies. This vast increase in wealth, however, has come at a price: markets have grown more fragile as they have grown more interdependent, and inequality in the wealthiest states has soared, creating a reservoir of resentment among the 90% at least as keenly felt as are the anxieties of the richest 10%. The system of transport that has expanded manufacturing centers and their markets is now bearing a deadly virus by the same efficient means that carried businesspeople to foreign meetings.

A global network of electronic communications that penetrates every society provided the basis for disillusionment within totalitarian countries and kept ever-present in the minds of persons everywhere the atrocities of the Holocaust, the Maoist depredations, and the true nature of Western societies that had been portrayed as impoverished political and social plantations. If there is a silver lining to the COVID-19 cloud, it is the astonishing international cooperation in research, the sharing of data, and vaccine research and potential manufacture that has occurred. This electronic connectivity, however, has empowered global networks of terror and brought the critical sectors of all advanced economies—the sectors of energy, banking, information, commerce, health, and defense—new vulnerabilities to penetration and paralysis.

The web of international organizations—including alliances like NATO, economic backstops like the International Monetary Fund and the World Bank, political forums like the United Nations, and juridical bodies including the International Court of Justice and the International Criminal Court—linked the well-being of the United States to that of other countries and thus enabled an unprecedented period of collective growth and security. Whether we say that these postwar international institutions were once capable but have become deadlocked, or that they were never designed to deal with the transnational complexities of an interconnected world, the result is the same:[11] the COVID-19 pandemic has exposed these institutions as useless in coping with global threats that pit states against each other. Their successes brought into being the very interdependent world that made pandemics inevitable. Yet the UN Security Council has not had one meeting on the subject of COVID-19.

Doctrines of human rights exposed totalitarian governments by changing our expectations of sovereignty but eventually disabled states from dealing with migration that was in part a consequence of Western interventions to protect human rights. What will the states of the developed world do when the next pandemic drives millions of refugees to their borders?

The individuation of political and social cultures enabled by the World Wide Web made possible the flourishing of many nations—Scotland, Lombardy,

Catalonia—that did not have their own states and many non-elite groups that had been subordinated to a dominant political and social archetype. But this individuation also empowered demands for isolationism, the wounding of the European Union through the defection of Britain, populist neonationalism in the United States and many other countries, and finally widespread and entrenched disagreement on facts and truth itself. A poll out this morning, the 24th of June, 2020, discloses that if Donald Trump loses his campaign for reelection, most Republican voters say they will believe the election was rigged,[12] and one wonders what reported facts could possibly disabuse them of this notion.[13] It cannot be a coincidence that the virus is currently raging to its highest infectious level by its spread to those states whose governors cast doubt on the danger of the threat itself.

The prologue to the industrial nation-state's inept confrontation with the COVID-19 pandemic—the interface between a rapidly decaying constitutional order and the precise sort of challenge it would have profound trouble handling—has led to a further loss of legitimacy that makes civil cooperation even more difficult, which leads to an ever further loss of legitimacy. This has affected all states, but the United States has done uniquely badly.

A political scientist might not have predicted this, especially in the case of the American form of the prevailing constitutional order. One key pillar of that unusual form is the US system of federalism. At the framing of the US Constitution, different responsibilities were assigned to the national government and to the states (counties, municipalities, townships, and the like have no independent constitutional status). This ought to have meant that the United States would be better able to control the virus. As Professor Danielle Allen argued in *Foreign Affairs,*

> Viruses spread through social networks. Efforts to control them that take into account existing social structures perform better than those that do not. . . . The lesson for the United States is that authority for key public health decisions should be lodged with state and local authorities. After all, they are the ones who best understand the dynamics of community spread. . . . In the context of the coronavirus, this system of federalism should be an asset, not a liability. It provides flexibility and the ability to tailor responses to the context—just what the United States needed. Rural areas with no COVID-19 cases did not require the same response as cities with thousands.[14]

Professor Allen thinks the federal system failed us because the president did not set the broad guidelines for states to follow and did not educate the public from his "bully pulpit." There is something to this; it's hard to imagine how a president could have done a worse job. But the guidelines the president should have determined for the states were no secret, and despite his unspeakable efforts to rouse mobs to defy state-ordered sheltering, he did not organize those mobs. They are in fact a feature of federalism as it is refracted through the broken legitimacy of the current constitutional order. It is not a coincidence that the states where hostility to preventative measures was highest were states that supported Trump.

The national government can enforce very limited mandates on the states when they refuse to act in accordance with national law: President Dwight D. Eisenhower sent the 101st Airborne Division into Little Rock on just such an occasion when Arkansas authorities refused to accept court-ordered mandates to desegregate the public schools. But it is idle to think that that sort of coercion could have made millions of persons wear masks or refrain from gathering in social groups of more than six. That kind of cohesion comes from a federalism that, in the words of the Great Seal, is founded on solidarity: *E Pluribus Unum*—out of many, one— the motto of the US federal system. Federalism in a collapsing constitutional order operates in exactly the opposite direction. Its motto might be: *Ex Uno Pluribum*, out of one, many.

Just as the system of federalism ought to have been an advantage for the United States in dealing with the COVID-19 pandemic, it can be a positive structure in the transition away from the constitutional order of industrial nation-states to an order of informational market-states. The opportunity for variation, for experimentation (Louis Brandeis famously observed that states were the laboratories of democracy),[15] and the ability to move more nimbly could give the United States an advantage in this transition. But that depends, as all political life ultimately depends in a democracy, on the awareness of its citizens as to what is at stake.

When the state goes from the reliance on regulation and legal institutions so characteristic of the nation-state to deregulating not only industries but, far more importantly, women's reproduction; when the state moves from conscription to an all-volunteer force to raise armies, as all the most powerful NATO states have done; when the state ends policies of tuition-free higher education in favor of some combination of fees and merit-based scholarships in order to cope with the rising costs that are themselves the result of the demands of students who see themselves as customers; when the state transitions from administering direct cash transfers like the dole and workers' compensation schemes to providing job training and teaching the skills necessary to enter a changed labor market; when state-owned enterprises are replaced by sovereign wealth funds; when regimes of market democracy like referenda, recall votes and voter initiatives that circumvent parliamentary practices and traditional systems of representation become widespread; when these developments occur, we are seeing the stirring of a nascent constitutional order, the informational market-state.

One of the salient features of this new order is that it treats citizens as consumers—and this is true across all classes, races, and political parties. It has been said that "the only valid purpose of the State is to create the citizen," which means—if the citizen is simply a "consumer"—adding value to the lives of those persons who are both the subject and the sovereign of the democratic state. Because the state has a monopoly on law, value can be created by constitutional innovation, like varying the states in a federal system to offer what individuals and groups want. For national groups that have historically faced legal and social barriers to equality, this might be a welcome development; paradoxically, the same might be true for other groups that wish to exclude them. This constitutional evolution is closer than we think; indeed, I fear that we are racing toward a constitutional environment in the United States that would abandon the commitment to uniform guarantees of human rights throughout the Union. It may well be that the greatest political threat to the United States today—to which the COVID-19 pandemic has given further momentum—lies in a fissioning of American constitutional rights, a chain reaction set off within the very structure of federalism that was designed to protect the state against such a collapse.

That threat looks like this. With one dramatic exception, constitutional rights in the United States are normalized across the various constituent states. This was not an achievement of our founding constitutional order, which I have characterized as that of an "imperial state nation," and the relationship it ordained between the central government and the states. On the contrary, it is the result of the constitutional order created by Lincoln and his contemporaries, that of the industrial nation-state, and it took more than a century before the Johnson administration and the Warren Court brought the guarantees of human rights to a consistent application across all states. Today, if you are arrested for shoplifting in Detroit, you are read the same Miranda warnings a shoplifter gets in Miami; if a local district attorney tries to strike jurors on account of their race, she must obey the same rules in Birmingham that her counterpart does in Los Angeles; and so on for all the guarantees of the Bill of Rights that have been incorporated into the 14th amendment against the states. The one exception—unique in the developed world—is capital punishment, which is now a matter of local constitutional option.

Since the end of the Cold War, Americans have been sorting themselves into ever-more homogeneous communities. As a political matter, this increases the ideological polarization it in part reflects, but the key constitutional question is how this demographic sorting will play out in conjunction with US federalism. Imagine that, partly owing to demographic sorting, more issues—abortion rights,[16] narcotics regulation, affirmative action, even sanctuaries that defy the enforcement of federal immigration laws—will become subjects for local option in the same way that capital punishment is today. Some states might mandate that a certain percentage of their legislature must be composed of women or members of particular ethnic groups, and some would doubtless defy such measures. Some states would allow prayers in the schools, others would forbid them.

This development would have the effect of reducing the uniformity of human rights guarantees among the states as a whole, resulting in a more diverse state with less diverse constituent states. It would be a replay of the historic move west that led to Frederick Jackson Turner's and Walter Prescott Webb's Frontier thesis, only this time the migration would be for constitutional culture rather than farmland.

If you think the courts and the Constitution would never permit such variations in how constitutional guarantees are applied, reflect on this fact: the US constitutional structure provides that the ratification of constitutional amendments and, more importantly, the calling of a constitutional convention depend upon a count of the states in which all are equal. Article V thus provides, "On the application of the Legislatures of two thirds of the several States, [the Congress] shall call a Convention for proposing Amendments, which . . . shall be valid to all Intents and Purposes, as Part of this Constitution, when ratified by the Legislatures of three fourths of the several States."

At present, twenty-nine state legislatures are controlled by the Republican Party; the votes of thirty-four would be required to call a constitutional convention. The difficulty for the future of the United States comes with the continued sorting of the population by which more and more persons live on the coasts and the non-coastal states are hollowed out. By far the greatest number of states will be those with lesser populations. Picture a map of the United States showing a group of states, like the Trump coalition of states that lost the popular vote in 2016 but won the electoral college, painted red.[17]

If such trends continue, it is not hard to imagine thirty-four states with only a third of the population of the country calling a constitutional convention, proposing amendments by a majority of the states at the convention, and even ratifying those amendments not by three-quarters of the population but by three-quarters of the states with far less than half the national population. Thus, a number far less than two-thirds of the population could call a convention, proposing amendments that far less than three-quarters of the population of the United States ratified. One might conclude that the most urgent order of business for those who want to preserve the American liberal tradition of judicial independence, uniform human rights norms, the primacy of the Constitution over state and federal laws, and federal supremacy is to prevent a new constitutional convention from coming into being.

It's not that the United States has done especially badly at coping with the pandemic because its federal structure impedes needed reforms or inhibits a transition to a market-state. It's rather that a federal structure is easily infected by the movement to such a new constitutional order, like a virus taking over the nucleus of a living cell. So it isn't that federalism accounts for the poor performance of the United States' response to the pandemic any more than that it has been an enabler for a decentralized and thus more effective response. It's that the political divisions in American society are turning this transition away from one that preserves liberal democratic values to one that fractionates the state. That will have profound effects on the ability of the United States to shape world order.

Now let us consider a description of the impact of COVID-19 by one of our most distinguished and sophisticated political analysts,[18] operating without the benefit of the thesis about a change in the constitutional order, indeed, whose analysis depends upon what one might call the "Westphalian Fallacy." This is the assumption that the constitutional order of states has not changed since 1648 and is unlikely to do so now.

This analysis begins, as so many do, with three events: the 9/11 attacks, the financial crises of 2008, and the coronavirus pandemic of 2019–20. Major crises have major consequences, but no connection is drawn *among* these crises that might tell us the nature of the predicted consequences. Instead we are told that success or failure in confronting the pandemic cannot be a matter of regimes. "Some democracies have performed well, but others have not and the same is true for autocracies," for that is the only way most analysts can distinguish regimes. Once the state itself has been put to one side, the factors on which success or failure depend are competent state apparatus, trust by citizens, and leadership. A dysfunctional state, a polarized society, and poor leadership are bound to lead to failure.

Looking ahead to what may be a lingering epidemic, job losses, recession, and mounting debt are bound to produce a political backlash, "but against whom is as yet unclear." Once again, it appears inconceivable that the backlash will be against the state itself whatever its political system. In fact, the industrial nation-state is not equipped to handle completely predictable crises like 9/11, the 2008 financial breakdown, and the present pandemic, and its poor responses to these crises undermine its capabilities even further. We should be asking ourselves, "What are other predictable crises? Can we infer certain challenges will become crises by the fact that they play on the weakness of the prevailing constitutional order?"

It is suggested that the global distribution of power "will continue to shift eastward, since East Asia has done better at managing the [COVID-19] situation than Europe or the United States." Presumably this is because these societies have a more competent state apparatus, the trust of the citizens, and better leaders, but is this true? Some East Asian states like the Philippines have been a notable failure; Iceland, a notable success. Is it possible that those states who have responded most effectively to the pandemic are those who have moved the furthest towards the new constitutional order of the informational market-state? Singapore comes to mind, as do Germany, New Zealand, and South Korea.

To see the difference in these approaches, consider the claim that in the United States, "its current highly polarized society and incompetent leader blocked the State from functioning effectively." Without disputing this assertion, one is moved to ask *why* these particular characteristics have disabled the state. How did we become so polarized? Why did we choose such a manifestly divisive and media-obsessed celebrity to lead us? And if one is persuaded that these phenomena are the result of the declining legitimacy of the state, one may be moved to ask what is the basis for the legitimacy of a state—the compact with its society on which a particular constitutional order relies—and why it has declined. It's certainly not impossible that highly polarized societies and incompetent leaders have successfully managed health crises in the past and that it's the management of crises that has gotten so much harder. Even if this were not the case, how helpful is the advice "Don't be so polarized!"? Don't stoke division rather than promote unity, don't politicize the distribution of aid, don't cast responsibility onto governors for making key decisions while encouraging protests against them, and don't attack international institutions rather than galvanizing them!

Such advice is unlikely to affect the actions of a neonationalist political leader whose greatest gifts have to do with manipulating the media by capturing the attention of a citizenry that thinks of itself as a collection of customers—in other words, the sort of leader who can be successful at gaining power in an informational market-state. In the situation of the US citizenry, polarization, politicization, inflammatory rhetoric, division, and especially attacks on international institutions might be just the ticket to achieve power (if not enhancing the chances of success in managing a crisis). That perspective can help us understand what we must do better other than simply replacing the president.

Of course, scenarios can be generated from the kind of analysis I am criticizing. The question is, how helpful are these scenarios? For example, it has been posited that two outcomes of the COVID-19 debacle might be "Rising Fascism" or a "Rebirth of Liberal Democracy."[19] These sound like scenarios but don't have much to do with scenario planning.

To see why, consider the analytic gaps in these two descriptions. The "Rising Fascism" future posits continuing increases in nationalism, isolationism, xenophobia, and attacks on the liberal world order. These are indeed characteristic of fascism, but they are not confined to fascism, which was a widespread movement in the first half of the 20th century as fascist, communist, and parliamentary industrial nation-states sought dominance for their form of that constitutional order. Only if one ignores the evolution of that order and the resolution of that long struggle for the sole legitimate paradigm could one see fascism as a realistic option. Thus is the Westphalian Fallacy at work. Note that this scenario assumes that international security will remain stable.[20] If that is right, it is because the threat posed to liberal democracy comes from a neonationalism which forsakes the militarism and foreign adventures that are an integral part of fascism. Neonationalism—like neoliberalism and neoconservatism—is a reaction to the emergence of the informational market-state. Ignoring the historic shift in the constitutional order results in a sort of category mistake, such that the competing scenario ("Rebirth of Liberal Democracy") is a different story but not an alternative possible world to the rise of fascism, and it might be tightly linked to the very events that have tempted some to think that fascism is imminent. Indeed, in the case of the Weimar Republic, the one might well prompt the other. More importantly, such scenarios throw away the identification of the fundamental drivers that are common to all possibilities in scenario planning. They therefore sacrifice those alerts that might help decision makers determine what exactly is happening.

Instead, these sorts of scenarios sketch out how a state of affairs might arise in the aftermath of the pandemic: "polls suggest that a large majority of Americans trust the advice of government medical experts in dealing with the crisis; this could increase support for government interventions to address other major social problems."[21] That makes them turn on the likelihood of events, which is to say they lose completely the power of scenario planning to assist the decider.

Scenario planning is not about pinpointing the future. In some ways, it's not even about the future. It is about the present and therefore much of its benefit lies in the doing, preparing us to appreciate the uncertainties that lie before us, guiding us to the most flexible and robust plans, and sensitizing us to possible futures as they unfold.

In 1985 the Kennedy School at Harvard sponsored a conference to discuss the future of international conflict at the turn of the 21st century. A group of academics, journalists, strategists from think tanks, and distinguished public servants speculated on the international environment to come and the risks of warfare that would accompany it. According to one participant who was present as a young graduate student and who later became an accomplished policy maker in his own right,

> No one dared speculate about an end to the Cold War or the demise of a narrow, bipolar alignment in global affairs. There was, however, considerable conversation about the prospects of major military clashes . . . centered on a still divided Europe [arising from] inadvertent or intentional conflict there. . . . In short, the experience was a classic example of the limits of linear thinking.[22]

Fifteen years later, after the card of the century's calendar had flipped, apparently anticlimactically, on Y2K, the Bush administration also became notable for having been surprised by events. These events included not only the September 11 atrocities but also the escape of the Al Qaeda and Taliban leadership from Afghanistan, French intransigence at the United Nations toward the Iraq War, Turkey's refusal of timely cooperation before that invasion, the coordinated murder and sabotage campaign led by Baath Party remnants and Al Qaeda elements in Iraq, and the widespread mood of truculent Iraqi impatience with the American presence there culminating in a deadly insurgency. These events were so predictable, critics say, that someone, surely, was thinking about them before they occurred, yet the White House was forced to improvise hasty responses.

The question was asked: Was the US administration blindsided by the poor work of its intelligence community, or was the problem poor coordination by the National Security Council that is supposed to integrate the work of the various intelligence, diplomatic, and defense agencies?

Actually, the answer is that none of these events were really surprises. Everything that appeared to catch the White House off guard had been anticipated in various reports, some by the National Security Council itself. The problem wasn't foresight but forethought: the Bush administration, like the Clinton White House before it, had yet to come up with an effective process to marshal judgment on the events it did foresee.

The COVID-19 pandemic, or something like it, was a certainty. It would come when it would come. What could not have been predicted was the utter foolhardiness of the responses of countries, including those that might have been expected to do better precisely because they had the enormous state capacity, scientific expertise, and educated populace to have fielded the state apparatus, social trust, and leadership necessary to prevail in this sort of crisis. Unless we appreciate the deep changes underway in the legitimacy of the constitutional order, we will be surprised again when a not-very-surprising catastrophe overtakes us, which it most assuredly will.

In the longer run, those crises will usher in a new constitutional order, the informational market-state. Our task, like Lincoln's (and Washington's), will be to ensure that a new constitutional order is created that is a "more perfect union" because it better serves the values of the Declaration of Independence in a new context of threats and opportunities.

What does all this have to do with "Future Scenarios"? Why isn't the title of this chapter, "Constitutional Law Professor Thinks Biggest Problem for the United States and World Order Is a Constitutional Law Problem"? Because the real failure thus far in preparing for and guiding our country through this transition has been a failure of imagination. Unlike strategic planning, the creation of scenarios can prepare a society and its leaders for multiple potential futures and thus for otherwise paralyzing and destabilizing change.

In this chapter, I have offered an interpretation of the COVID-19 crisis that connects domestic politics to the global order. The pandemic that is increasing its grip as I write these pages was quite predictable; it wasn't that we didn't know this challenge was coming. It's that we were politically and institutionally paralyzed because the nature of the threat fit so well the vulnerabilities of the contemporary constitutional order. In the case of the United States, one feature of that order—US federalism—greatly heightened the damage done by the pandemic and, by discrediting the United States, also did damage to the shaping of an international order that would protect and promote our values of liberal and humane governance. This needn't have been the case. Federalism could have been a valuable asset in overcoming the pandemic because it is well adapted to the emerging constitutional order. Instead, it may lead to a version of that order that cripples the United States as an international leader.

We may think of "applied history" as using past patterns to predict present ones, and this is sometimes true, as Graham Allison's chapter shows. But more often, history helps us to see the differences with the past—what is really new. That is why scenario construction is so valuable a tool for decision makers. That is why recognizing the historic shift in the nature of the constitutional order is an imperative.

NOTES

1. Nelson D. Schwartz, Ben Casselman, and Ella Koeze, "How Bad is Unemployment? 'Literally Off the Charts,'" *New York Times*, May 8, 2020, https://www.nytimes.com /interactive/2020/05/08/business/economy/april-jobs-report.html.

2. "The Conference Board Economic Forecast for the US Economy," The Conference Board, last modified July 8, 2020, https://www.conference-board.org/research/us-forecast.

3. Martin Crutsinger, "Fed Chairman Jerome Powell Warns U.S. Economy Faces Deep Downturn With 'Significant Uncertainty,'" *Time,* June 16, 2020.

4. "Congress and the Public," *Gallup*, accessed June 2020, https://news.gallup.com/poll /1600/congress-public.aspx.

5. Ian Bremmer, "Is Democracy Essential? Millennials Increasingly Aren't Sure—and That Should Concern Us All," Think, *NBC News*, February 13, 2018, https://www.nbcnews .com/think/opinion/democracy-essential-millennials-increasingly-aren-t-sure-should -concern-us-ncna847476.

6. Richard Wike, Bruce Stokes, Jacob Poushter, Laura Silver, Janell Fetterolf, and Kat Delvin, "Trump's International Ratings Remain Low, Especially Among Key Allies," *Pew Research Center,* October 1, 2018, https://www.pewresearch.org/global/2018/10/01/trumps -international-ratings-remain-low-especially-among-key-allies/.

7. Kelsey Davenport, "Chronology of U.S.-North Korean Nuclear and Missile Diplomacy," *Arms Control Association,* last modified May 2020, https://www.armscontrol.org /factsheets/dprkchron.

8. David E. Sanger and Lara Jakes, "Iran Is Accused of Hiding Suspected Nuclear Activity," *New York Times,* July 2, 2020, https://www.nytimes.com/2020/06/19/us/politics /iran-nuclear-iaea.html.

9. Anton Troianovski, "A Historic Heat Wave Roasts Siberia," *New York Times,* June 25, 2020, https://www.nytimes.com/2020/06/25/world/europe/siberia-heat-wave-climate -change.html.

10. David Judson, review of *Realistic Hope—Facing Global Challenges*, ed. Angela Wilkinson and Betty Sue Flowers, *World Futures* 76, no. 2 (January 2020): 118–131, https:// www.tandfonline.com/doi/abs/10.1080/02604027.2019.1698236?af=R&journalCode =gwof20.

11. Judson, review of *Realistic Hope*.

12. Bruce Anderson, "What Americans Don't Know . . . Should Worry Us," *Maclean's*, June 22, 2020, https://www.macleans.ca/politics/washington/what-americans-dont-know-should-worry-us/.

13. "As many Americans think Russia is America's best friend as think France, Italy or Germany is. . . . Right now, with racial divides widening (half see a serious chance of a civil war), America feuding with most of its allies, an economy stumbling, a deficit at unprecedented levels, and a pandemic that has killed 120,000 and remains out of control in many areas . . . 80 per cent of Republicans think Trump has made America greater." Bruce Anderson, "What Americans Don't Know."

14. Danielle Allen, "A More Resilient Union: How Federalism Can Protect Democracy from Pandemics," *Foreign Affairs* 99, no. 4 (July/August 2020), https://www.foreignaffairs.com/articles/united-states/2020-06-01/more-resilient-union.

15. In New State Ice Co. v. Liebmann, 285 U.S. 262, 272 (1932), Justice Louis Brandeis wrote that "it is one of the happy incidents of the federal system that a single courageous state may, if its citizens choose, serve as a laboratory and try novel social and economic experiments without risk to the rest of the country."

16. One enraged member of the pro-life/anti-abortion movement recently wrote in reaction to the Supreme Court's decision in *June Medical Services v. Russo*,

> Why are the Supreme Court and a nearly half-century-old ruling that you consider illegitimate the be-all end-all anyway? You know already that at the state level there are decent men and women far more committed to the cause than the national Republican Party. Why not borrow a lesson from sanctuary cities or, if you support it, as one suspects an increasing number of you do, the legalization of marijuana in various states? The Nine say that abortion is legal; let them enforce it, or rather, let the president who claims to be on your side do so, and make his real feelings known one way or the other. Urge your governors and state senators and representatives to ban abortion tomorrow. Empower state police to close down facilities. Will Trump really send in the National Guard? Will the next Democratic president do so, in 2021 or 2025 or whenever the White House again comes under the control of the party whose resolve on cultural questions has not been tested thanks to the high court's willingness to implement its agenda by fiat?

See Matthew Walther, "The Ashes of the Pro-Life Movement," *The Week*, June 30, 2020, https://theweek.com/articles/922717/ashes-prolife-movement.

17. At present, twenty-eight states have adopted resolutions calling for a convention to discuss a balanced budget amendment. Four states that Donald Trump carried in 2016 have yet to call for a balanced budget convention (Montana, Idaho, South Carolina, Kentucky). Five states have adopted calls for a campaign finance amendment and none of these five are among the thirty-two that have either adopted a resolution calling for a convention or were carried by Trump. That means that a call that bundled campaign finance reform with a balanced budget could be only one state away from bringing a new constitutional convention into being.

18. See Francis Fukuyama, "The Pandemic and Political Order," *Foreign Affairs* 99, no. 4 (July/August 2020), https://www.foreignaffairs.com/articles/world/2020-06-09/pandemic-and-political-order.

19. Fukuyama, "The Pandemic and Political Order."

20. "Given the continued stabilizing force of nuclear weapons and the common challenges facing all major players, international turbulence is less likely than domestic turbulence." Fukuyama, "The Pandemic and Political Order."

21. Fukuyama, "The Pandemic and Political Order."

22. Kurt Campbell, "Possibilities of War: The Confluence of Persistent Contemporary Flashpoints and Worrisome New Trouble Spots," paper for Changing Nature of Warfare (a conference sponsored by the National Intelligence Council's 2020 Project) (Washington, DC: May 25, 2004): 13–15, https://www.cna.org/CNA_files/PDF/D0011005.A1.pdf.

PART II / Global Public Health
and Mitigation Strategies

Chapter Four

Make Pandemics Lose Their Power

Tom Inglesby

C OVID-19 has had the power to do what few other international shocks could have done. It has sickened millions around the world in a matter of months, killed hundreds of thousands, and created a global economic crisis unprecedented in modern times. People around the world have been directed to stay at home for months to avoid catching the disease or contributing to its rapid spread. Massive job losses and economic ruin have occurred globally. Most schools around the world closed for a prolonged period, or they are still out. At least one national leader appears to have died from COVID-19,[1] and other national leaders who are either older or have certain underlying medical conditions run the risk of having a severe outcome should they become ill. Travel around the world has diminished to a fraction of what it was. While the disease has unified some countries in their collective effort to pursue a vaccine and to assist lower-income countries, it has deepened international fissures between others. It has underscored the importance and limits of international organizations in this kind of crisis. In the big picture, COVID-19 has shown the extraordinary power of pandemics to do harm.

Pandemics are in a small category of events that have destructive power on a global scale, posing risks that have been called global catastrophic risks.[2] The risks

Tom Inglesby is the director of the Center for Health Security of the Johns Hopkins Bloomberg School of Public Health and a professor in the Department of Environmental Health and Engineering in the Johns Hopkins Bloomberg School of Public Health, with a joint appointment in the Johns Hopkins School of Medicine.

of future pandemics and biological threats are going to continue to grow. The next one could arise without warning or lead time at any point, just as SARS-CoV-2 appeared with no notice at the end of 2019. Even as the world continues its struggle to cope with this pandemic, it is critical to consider how to prevent something like this from happening again. Doing so will require a major re-envisioning of our effort to prevent and prepare for biological threats. Given its capabilities in science, medicine, health, technology, and manufacturing, the United States must be a central part of all these efforts. In US foreign policy, there has been a long-standing debate about US unilateralism versus multilateralism and the benefits and risks of those paths. The effort to drastically diminish the impact and consequence of pandemics in the future will require a strong combination of the two.

In the time ahead, the project for the United States will be to do what it can to prevent a new pandemic threat from emerging, to prepare a strong national program to respond to the next event, and to be a driver of international partnerships needed to solve critical global problems that emerge in this kind of crisis. If we can accomplish the necessary work within the United States and in partnerships internationally, we can give ourselves more warning about new outbreaks, diminish the risk that science will create new pandemics, accelerate the development of vaccines and therapies, and prepare our national and international systems for rapid, strong, and effective response that would limit illness and economic impact. This is how the United States can make pandemics lose their power.

Anticipate Biological Threats on the Horizon

There has been a series of acute infectious disease crises in the last twenty years, including the anthrax mailed letters in 2001, SARS in 2002–4, H5N1 bird flu in 2005, H1N1 influenza pandemic, MERS, Zika, and Ebola in West Africa and in the Democratic Republic of the Congo, to name just some. If you go back to the 20th century there were three major influenza pandemics, the most serious of which by far was in 1918. National and global systems for preparing and responding to these crises have evolved and improved over time, though progress waxes and then wanes as time passes after these events occur. The World Health Organization (WHO) has helped lead an effort to improve nations' capacity to prepare and respond to regionally serious epidemics and pandemics by measuring national capabilities to respond to infectious disease crises using an assessment tool called the Joint External Evaluation. The majority of countries in the world have voluntarily engaged in that transparent evaluation process, and scores from the assessment have helped drive government and philanthropic funding to improve preparedness.

It might be imagined that the COVID-19 pandemic is a once-in-a-century event, and that since it has now happened, we are safe from another such event until far off into the future. Some might also believe that the severity of this virus, with its ability to sicken and kill so many, cannot be matched or exceeded by future pandemics. Neither of these notions is true. There are no natural waiting periods after a pandemic, and no certain limits to how lethal a future pandemic might be. Future pandemics could have higher lethality and/or a greater capacity to spread. One of the few comparatively silver linings of COVID-19 has been that it has caused substantially less serious illness in children compared to adults. Tragically it has caused death in some children but at a rate that is orders of magnitude less than older adults or those with certain underlying conditions. Future pandemics may not follow that pattern, however. If children were to get sick and die at rates similar to adults, that would create major global shocks beyond even the ones we are experiencing now as countries would consider drastic actions to protect young people.

At the high end, future natural, accidental, or deliberately initiated pandemics could lead to global catastrophe on the scale we are suffering now or even worse. At the highest end, these risks have been called global catastrophic biological risks, defined in this way: "Global Catastrophic Biological Risks are those events in which biological agents—whether naturally emerging or reemerging, deliberately created and released, or laboratory engineered and escaped—could lead to sudden, extraordinary, widespread disaster beyond the collective capability of national and international governments and the private sector to control. If unchecked, GCBRs would lead to great suffering, loss of life, and sustained damage to national governments, international relationships, economies, societal stability, or global security."[3]

In addition to severe naturally occurring pandemics, there are other kinds of biological risks that need to be considered. The deliberate or accidental release of smallpox from its known global repositories could result in a smallpox pandemic in a world with very little immunity and enough vaccine to cover only a small minority of the world's population.[4] The scientific manipulation of a bird flu virus to turn it into a more transmissible variant could start a pandemic with high lethality in the event of laboratory accident or misuse. Science may also develop the capability of creating organisms using artificial genetic code that would be harmful to humanity on a large scale.[5]

Countries will need to improve the way they consider and plan for these kinds of risks. Special efforts will need to be made to prevent these kinds of events from occurring, but governments have not been particularly attentive to these kinds of potential harmful consequences of life science research or technological developments. If efforts to prevent pandemics or other global catastrophic biological risks fail, then there will need to be extraordinary national and global action in response. Preparing those systems will take a United States that is far more capable of responding, combined with an international pandemic response effort that is far stronger than what exists now.

Scale Up the Efforts to Prevent New Pandemics

Efforts to prevent pandemic threats from emerging will take a combination of surveillance and early-warning systems, better governance of science that could create new pandemic risks, and strong international diplomatic effort and agreement.

New viruses emerge from nature on a regular basis, with the jump from animals to humans being the most common way that novel epidemics appears.[6] Existing viruses may also evolve new properties and so change in ways that make them more transmissible, lethal, or resistant to existing therapies. There are many conditions that are increasing the risks of big epidemics or pandemics.[7] Humans are continuing to encroach on animal ecosystems that were previously undisturbed. Megacities continue to grow with people living more densely, in some places without access to good sanitation. The climate is warming, increasing the range of the animal vectors that carry diseases. Rising numbers of large, concentrated livestock operations around the world provide conditions for the rapid spread and amplification of pathogens within animal populations that could increase the risks of contraction for the humans working with and around them. People can travel around the world rapidly, incubating and spreading the disease, a means of spread that contributed to the rapid global spread of COVID-19.

Prevention efforts around natural pandemics should include improving early disease surveillance, both in the animals that are a frequent source of disease spread, but also in humans hospitalized with serious febrile illness, a substantial portion of whom are never definitively diagnosed. To build our understanding of the global baseline of human viral infections causing serious illness, we should increase the effort to identify specific viral causes of serious human illness.[8] Science now provides the tools for that, but cost concerns and widespread access to technologies has limited their use. On the animal side, we need to build the science around animal virus discovery, geographic range, and rate of evolution, with a special focus on viral families that have already caused serious outbreaks in humans. Other key capacities related to the prevention of natural epidemics are a country's ability to make rapid laboratory diagnoses and to mobilize public health and communicate with doctors and nurses at the earliest signs of a new outbreak. We should build these rapid systems aimed at the earliest possible recognition of a new outbreak so that we can move to contain it before it spreads.

Prevention efforts also need to be focused on preventing the misuse of science. Biotechnology, and the life sciences more broadly, while they do bring enormous benefits to the world, could also be misused in ways that increase the risk of accidentally or deliberately starting a new pandemic. Scientific tools and approaches now exist that allow scientists to increase the lethality or transmissibility of a pathogen, creating a novel strain not before seen in nature. If laboratory accidents were to occur while working on a novel pathogen that is highly transmissible and lethal—either through engineering failures, administrative mistakes, human errors, or subversion of safety systems—then that strain could start spreading in a community with the possibility of generating a large outbreak, even a pandemic.[9] Similarly, if scientists with the skills to create these kinds of novel strains decided to create and release them deliberately into the world, they could themselves start an outbreak, perhaps leading to a pandemic. Such scientists could conceivably be working with a country's biological weapons program, a terrorist organization, a cult, or even be working by themselves or with small numbers of others.

Governments should have strong policies in place for the governance and funding of biotechnology and life science research that could generate novel pathogens that are transmissible and injurious,[10] but most countries do not at this point. Any work that could result in pathogens with these characteristics should require very clear justification, senior government approval, public transparency, and with benefits determined to exceed the serious risks. If work is to be permitted to create such pathogens, then the highest possible biosafety and biosecurity systems should be in place to prevent possible accidental escape or deliberate dispersion from the laboratory. Viruses with pandemic potential that are no longer circulating, most notably SARS-CoV-1 and smallpox, should also be handled with the highest possible level of global biosafety and biosecurity. The current plan to hold all smallpox reserves and allow research in only two places in the world, and only after WHO approval, is one strong global model for noncirculating viruses with pandemic potential. Now that viruses can be created de novo, it is also possible to synthesize viruses from nonliving parts. Efforts need to be made to improve screening and impose interdiction for those trying to order, without authorization, the parts of those viruses with epidemic and pandemic potential from DNA synthesis companies.

Given that biological weapons could be created that had the capacity to start epidemic or pandemic disease, the United States and other countries should also be fully committed to the terms of the Biological Weapons Convention (BWC),[11] the only treaty that bans an entire class of weapons. Most countries of the world have signed the convention, but there are no practical verification measures that are in place. It is critical to build confidence and assurance that countries are in compliance with the treaty in order to preserve the norm against biological weapons, with particular importance given to stopping the development, trade, and use of biological weapons that could start epidemics or pandemics. If a country is proven to be out of compliance with the BWC, the United States should work closely with the signatories of the BWC to impose sanctions, with particularly serious consequences for a country that has developed, acquired, or used a biological weapon with the capacity to cause serious and highly transmissible human illness.

Transform US Preparedness for Future Pandemics

To consider what the United States needs to build in order to stop future pandemics, it is important to consider our current response to COVID-19. While some parts of the world have had success in their efforts to control this disease, including New Zealand, Thailand, Taiwan, Iceland, the Czech Republic, and Australia, the United States has not done well. The United States was slow to transition diagnostic testing to public health labs, hospitals, and private-sector diagnostic companies. It also placed confidence in a strategy of trying to keep the disease entirely out of the country by focusing initially on banning incoming flights from China. The result was a delayed recognition that the United States was confronting pandemic spread of the disease, a delayed start to testing around the country, and the discovery of an extraordinary amount of COVID-19 infections in places around the country in March 2020. The United States also has had far too little personal protective equipment to safeguard its health care workers, essential businesses, or the public. Other countries provided medical masks for the general public,[12] but the United States did not even have enough for its own health care workers.[13] The US Centers for Disease Control and Prevention (CDC), usually a highly visible pillar of public health response during infectious disease emergencies in the country, was restricted in its communications with the American public.[14] New York City was one of the hardest hit cities in the world, with as many as one in four hundred New Yorkers dying from this disease in the first three months of the pandemic there.[15] Widespread state-level imposition of social distancing, public mask use, and expanded diagnostic testing worked to flatten the epidemic curve and slow the spread nationally. However, many states continued to have daily rises in the rate of new infections through at least June, at the time of writing this commentary. Communication from the top of government was confused, inconsistent, and too infrequent to continue broadcasting the message throughout the country. So, even as other developed countries have had major improvements in their epidemics, the United States continues to struggle.

The reasons for these mistakes are many. There seemed to be a political decision to minimize the virus at the start of the pandemic so as to avoid economic setbacks. There were also decisions to reopen economies in states around the country too quickly and fully, even for some of the higher-risk activities. In addition, in the years leading up to the pandemic, there has been waxing and waning support in the presidential administration and in Congress for pandemic-preparedness activities. In the setting of an acute infectious disease shock, there would, for a time, be a period of activity and funding. As time moved on, though, the attention paid to the threat would diminish.

Strong preparation for a future pandemic will require that the United States become highly capable on its own. The country will need to have the ability to rapidly develop and mass-manufacture vaccines. It should have the ability to manufacture personal protective equipment and ventilators on a large scale, sufficient for all the needs of the health care system, the public, and the many organizations that require or want this equipment for their operations. It will need the capacity to scale up diagnostic testing right from the start of a major new epidemic or pandemic. It also will require changes to medical and public health systems to make them much better prepared, as well as a plan to deal with long-standing racial inequities that have deepened the impact of this crisis.

Preparedness for a naturally occurring pandemic would resemble in most ways preparedness for one deliberately started by a biological weapon capable of pandemic spread, or accidentally initiated by a laboratory accident with a pathogen that was both lethal and highly transmissible. All of these would appear as an epidemic requiring early detection, rapid surveillance to understand the extent of disease, analysis of risk factors, health care for the sick, and development of medical countermeasures. And all of these parts of the response would require basically the same workforce.

If it were deliberate biological weapon use, there would be the additional concerns related to national security, law enforcement, and government intelligence, which would require their own careful response. But the public health and medical response for all would be similar. It should be said that efforts to prevent biological weapons development or use would be quite distinct from efforts to prevent a natural pandemic from emerging. Preventing deliberate efforts requires strong diplomatic initiative, strong law enforcement coordination, and interdiction work. It would also require good governance of the life sciences to avoid funding and supporting research that could be used to create novel pathogens capable of causing a pandemic.

Faster Development and Manufacturing of Vaccines, Therapeutics, and Diagnostics

With an extraordinary number of COVID-19 vaccine projects under way,[16] this is the biggest and fastest vaccine development project in history. The major lines of effort are being funded by the United States, China, and an international collaboration run by the Coalition for Epidemic Preparedness Innovations in a partnership with WHO—all working in partnership with biotech or leading global vaccine companies. Some leading vaccine experts have said there is the possibility of having a safe and effective COVID-19 vaccine approved by the US Food and Drug Administration (FDA) by the end of 2020, with production starting at the end of this year or the beginning of next year.[17] If so, that would be faster development by far than ever before for a new vaccine. Other leading experts believe it will take much longer to develop and produce on large scale a safe and effective vaccine. In any event, it is not fast enough to head off incredible sickness, death, and economic catastrophe around the world.

The United States will need to invest much more in preparing to make vaccines for unknown threats that emerge without warning. Given that there is no private-sector market for such investment between crises, readiness will require a dedicated government effort aimed at preparing for the emergency development of a vaccine for the next pandemic.[18] That kind of program would fund the development and optimization of new vaccine platforms and technologies, as well as acceleration and optimization of proven vaccine development approaches. It would have the necessary contractual mechanisms in place for speed. It would have agreements with leading vaccine companies to initiate development at the earliest indication of an emerging pandemic. It would prepare for new manufacturing operations that could rapidly produce vaccine on a great scale, and it would have worked through as many regulatory issues and as was feasible with the FDA in advance to identify the most efficient path to approval. We should resolve to do what it takes never to be in the position of waiting twelve to eighteen months, or possibly much longer, to have a vaccine to fight a new pandemic.

The rapid development and manufacture of a safe and effective vaccine should be the highest-order goal. A vaccine would change almost everything related to the response for the better. But because it will remain uncertain whether even a substantial new effort to prepare to make vaccine for unknown emerging infections will succeed, we also need to press forward with the capability to accelerate therapeutic development for the next pandemic. In the earliest days of a new therapeutic, there needs to be a rapid effort to assess whether existing medications can be repurposed with any effectiveness. These medications are already approved for other purposes, so they do not need to be developed. The case of hydroxychloroquine has shown us again that randomized clinical trials are crucial before therapies are recommended by leaders. Even if a medication seems to have promise in early treatment efforts, a randomized trial can show it causes more harm than good, as a series of trials have now shown for hydroxychloroquine.

New antiviral medications, monoclonal antibodies, and immune system modulators are all being developed now for COVID-19. Given the way trials work for these products, it may be possible to develop and demonstrate the safety and efficacy of these medications faster than is possible for a new vaccine. The United States and other countries have been moving along at a good pace with many of these trials, helped in part by an emerging infectious disease clinical trial network developed in the aftermath of the Ebola outbreaks in Africa. But this process could get faster and produce more information that could help with the approval process and decisions around use, and we should work to streamline and accelerate these clinical trial efforts. The large and fast-moving UK trial called Randomised Evaluation of COVID-19 Therapy recently announced the results of a study showing that a commonly used medical steroid reduced mortality in the sickest COVID-19 patients.[19] This is an example of what we should aspire to do in the United States. That is the kind of speed and scale for a trial that is needed in pandemic conditions.

Diagnostics have been critical in this pandemic for identifying people infected with COVID-19 and for getting them isolated and properly treated as needed. Diagnostics will be crucial in future pandemics as well. They are key in monitoring disease control efforts within a state or country, and they are critical to assessing the overall course of an outbreak. In the COVID-19 response in the United States, the process of transitioning the initially developed diagnostic test into a widely available one was seriously delayed by technical challenges and policy decisions. We need to be prepared in future pandemics to bring in the full diagnostic power of the leading US companies in clinical diagnostics and the health care system laboratories of the United States at the earliest sign of pandemic spread. Earlier widespread diagnostic testing could have limited the early spread of the disease and diminished the impact of COVID-19 in the United States.

Greater Supply of Personal Protective Equipment and Ventilators

When epidemics are local or regional in one part of the world, the emergency supply chain can pivot toward helping that region. But in a pandemic, all countries need the same critical materials at the same time. The United States had woefully too few N95 masks, too few surgical masks, too few gowns, and inadequate eye protection and face shields to cope with the COVID-19 pandemic. All countries were dependent on the same small number of global suppliers, some located in the United States but a substantial portion of them overseas. If we do not change that situation, we will again see in a future pandemic our doctors and nurses having to care for patients without the right protective equipment, high numbers of infections for health care workers, and too small a supply to give to businesses and organizations that need them. The United States needs to create the right incentives to develop its own robust manufacturing base for the personal protective equipment it will need. Some emergency supply should be stockpiled for immediate need in a crisis, but in addition we need the capability to emergently ramp up through increased US industrial supply. In the Strategic National Stockpile, a similar kind of arrangement is called keeping a warm base. If a supplier makes X number of masks in a year, the US government should establish a contract to pay the supplier to scale up rapidly to perhaps five times X or ten times X above their usual annual capacity in a time of national emergency. We need to build in this kind of surge capacity.

Another concern in the early months of the COVID-19 pandemic was the potential for ventilator shortages around the country. While social distancing measures and stay-at-home orders diminished the rate of new hospitalized cases in New York City in time to avert ventilator shortages overall, there were some hospitals in the city that reported having come extremely close to running out of ventilators given the rapid peak in COVID-19 patients. Future pandemic planning will need to plan appropriately both for the number of ventilators that should be stockpiled and for rapid ramping up of production of low-cost ventilators should our national stockpile of ventilators not be sufficient.

Strengthen US Health Care and the Public Health Response and End Racial Health Inequities

Health care workers and hospitals will need to be better prepared for future pandemic events. A big part of that preparation relates to having the right protective equipment and material assets. COVID-19 has shown that many health care workers were not trained to manage these kinds of events. Many hospitals had not sufficiently prepared staff or acquired the needed facilities. Health care workers around the country stepped up to provide outstanding care for COVID-19 patients, despite the uncertainties. In the aftermath of this pandemic, it will be critical to go back to identify how some health care systems were able to succeed whereas other systems struggled to cope.

Public health agencies have been critical to state and local responses to COVID-19. They have a central role in advising political leaders, communicating with the public, running their state laboratories, identifying the highest risks and sources of transmission, establishing diagnostic strategies, and running contact tracing and quarantine efforts, among other key responsibilities. They are chronically underfunded in between times of epidemic crisis, and this needs to change. Our public health system should be built to rival any in the world, but it is clear that public health agencies such as those in Hong Kong, Singapore, Taiwan, New Zealand, and Iceland, to name a few, have capabilities that exceed ours in important ways. There are public health data management systems, outbreak investigation capabilities, crisis communication, and contact tracing efforts that are far stronger in countries around the world than they are in the United States. We should learn from others by emulating them and turning our public health systems into ones that can cope with the challenge of future pandemics.

Federal health agencies are also an important part of our health care and public health systems. The CDC provides some of the best technical advice in the world, both to the public and to local health agencies, and that has for the most part been true during the COVID-19 pandemic. The CDC has expertise across a range of disciplines that are key to pandemic preparedness and response. In major infectious disease crises of the past, the CDC was allowed to explain and guide the public and medical and public health leaders. Unfortunately, the CDC has not been allowed to serve in that role for COVID-19; the CDC has been permitted to make relatively few public announcements as the pandemic progressed. That should change. The country needs the CDC to regain its advisory role.

The Department of Health and Human Services also has the Office of the Assistant Secretary for Preparedness and Response (ASPR), which is responsible for preparing hospital systems for crises. The hospital preparedness effort needs to be substantially expanded from where it stood before the pandemic. The ASPR should also be prepared to take on major responsibility for logistics in future pandemics, centrally coordinating the distribution of scarce resources to states and hospitals as needed. The ASPR has control of the Strategic National Stockpile and so can deploy those resources,[20] but it also must be ready to contract with companies to make products or assets that are in short supply or that might not have been anticipated. If the ASPR is unable to fill that kind of national logistics role, then the Department of Defense or the Federal Emergency Management Agency could also serve in that role, or do it jointly with the ASPR, as came to happen over time in the US response to COVID-19.

One more priority in building the nation's response is to correct gross inequities in the health care and public health response that has resulted in people of color being disproportionately sickened and killed by COVID-19.[21] This population of people is more likely to have jobs categorized as essential and so would be unable to telecommute, which puts this population at higher risk of catching the disease on the job. People in essential jobs need to be better protected, with masks, spacing, and changes to work operations that decrease their risks. People of color also have less access to health care and more difficulty overall in getting a diagnostic test in many parts of the country. Those things would need to be addressed with urgency at the start of a future pandemic. It is also known that people of color have more underlying medical conditions that place them at a higher risk of having severe outcomes with COVID-19, and these medical conditions themselves are often determined by social factors including less access to healthy food and good outpatient care, higher environmental risks to health, and other challenges. Those are the kinds of issues that should be dealt with and changed now as part of improving the quality of and access to health care in the United States, well in advance of any future pandemic.

One particularly important task for strengthening US preparedness for pandemics is to rebuild public trust in public health and the interventions we will need to rely on in the future. Substantial portions of the public have concerns about vaccines or will refuse to get them. During the COVID-19 response, a sizable portion of the national population has resisted wearing masks, social distancing, or otherwise changing their lives to slow down the spread of the virus. That kind of reaction has been rare elsewhere in the world. For the United States to develop a strong preparedness program, we have much work to do to understand the root causes of public mistrust of these public health tools and recommendations. We will need the public to be strong and full partners in efforts to prepare the country for infectious disease crises of the future.

Strengthen the Multilateral System of Response

Even while the United States is doing all that it can to build up its own capacities to respond vigorously and successfully to future pandemics, it also needs to prepare and plan effectively and intensely with other governments, international organizations, and the private sector. Together with these partners around the world, the United States needs to anticipate and address problems that can only be solved through multinational efforts, public-private partnerships, and international approaches. Even if the United States should become largely able to solve its own challenges in a future pandemic, it will be in the country's clear interest to help the international community get through a global pandemic crisis as quickly as it can, whether that is a pandemic with the severity of COVID-19 or something even worse. Not only would it be the morally right approach for a strong United States to help the rest of the world cope with and recover from a future pandemic, it would also be in the national and economic interest of the United States to do so. There are some who may say that preparing for and responding to a pandemic is a zero-sum game that requires us to go our own path and compete with other countries over scarce resources. And, in fact, that is to some extent how the United States has operated in response to COVID-19. Not having developed its own manufacturing infrastructure for masks, for example, the United States has tried to muscle its way past others to get scarce resources. However, in the future, were the United States to operate with a longer-term strategy and seek synergy with partners around the world, pandemic planning would then not be a zero-sum matter. We do better when other countries do better. If much of the rest of the world remains badly disrupted, economically failing, fragmented in its trade efforts, overwhelmed with sickness and mortality—and perhaps unstable politically, unable to fulfill international obligations, and no longer capable of sending its students abroad or having its businesspeople and travelers come to the United States—then the United States will suffer.

The United States should be helping to build systems to manufacture and provide on vast scale what the United States will need to be making for itself: vaccines and therapeutics, personal protective equipment, and necessary medical equipment. For example, vaccines will need to be manufactured quickly at sites around the world. A global system of distribution that relies on international organizations and private-sector distributors will be needed. How this is all accomplished could produce greater solidarity or long-term fissures between countries.

While some countries in the world can and will increase their domestic manufacturing base for these products, there are many that will not be able to, either financially or technically or both. The United States, working with other governments, international organizations, and the private sector, should increase the stockpile of vaccines, therapeutics, diagnostics, and personal protective equipment at WHO. There are important products for known infectious diseases (e.g., yellow fever, Ebola, influenza) that can be stored now for anticipated emergencies, and this will help create the logistics and decision-making processes needed when new vaccines and therapeutics for previously unknown pandemics are created and require a process of global dissemination. In the COVID-19 pandemic, the process of distributing vaccine, when one becomes available, will likely rely in part on the WHO stockpile system as it exists now. We should learn from this process and strengthen and expand it going forward.

Governments should incentivize major biopharmaceutical companies to invest in distributed-manufacturing approaches so that the same critical vaccine and therapeutic products can be made in many parts of the world concurrently. This will require navigating legal and regulatory issues ahead of time. Without a widely distributed manufacturing process, lifesaving products may become restricted to the countries where they are created or to their close allies. We need to create a system that does not lead to that.

Global business should be a strong part of these efforts. It is very clear now what the economic toll of pandemics may be in the future. So global businesses should be fighting for much more robust national planning efforts, stronger international organizations, and better preparedness within their own organizations. COVID-19 has shown that a severe pandemic greatly interferes with workforce health, business operations, and the movement of goods and services, with potentially long-lasting effects on whole industries and national and global economies. It has also become clear that economies will not be able to fully recover without strong COVID-19 disease control efforts. The public is unlikely to go out and engage with the economy, buy things in the way they used to, go to entertainment venues, or travel, until they feel safe doing those things.

Governments and the private sector should also focus on establishing better processes for sharing scientifically and medically correct and useful information with the public and better coping with misinformation in the setting of a pandemic. Governments rely on traditional and social media companies to communicate with the public. Establishing partnerships in advance of future pandemics will help increase the spread of information that is reliable and scientifically valid, amid a flood of stories that are inadvertently or deliberately incorrect. The more that people get reliable and accurate information, the better societies will do at making good decisions and taking wise action.

To cope effectively with future pandemics will require strong international organizations that have the political and financial support of countries around the world. Of these organizations, WHO is particularly vital. In this pandemic, WHO sounded an early warning about COVID-19 at the start of January and started sending out technical reports from that time forward. It has been criticized for moving too slowly because of political interference. But if one looks at the timeline of WHO's actions and decisions in early January, it is clear that it was quickly communicating what it was learning to the public, and it was rapidly developing and publishing guidance. It is true that WHO did not declare a public health emergency of international concern until the end of January, and many in the public health community were arguing that a declaration should have happened sooner. WHO later said it had worried that declaring a public health emergency too soon might lead China to let up on its containment efforts. As a point of comparison in terms of timing, at the end of February, President Donald J. Trump was still saying that the virus was going to disappear and was under good control in the United States.

WHO has been providing guidance to countries around the world since the pandemic began, and it has sent technical assistance teams and medical assets to places with the greatest need.[22] WHO got a public health assessment team into China early on, when other countries could not on their own. It helped rally the world around a new approach to vaccine and therapeutic trial design that should accelerate results. It helped create a coalition of countries from around the world to donate to vaccine development efforts. The United States should be doing all that it can to strengthen WHO by enabling it to provide more technical and material assistance to countries that need it.

Instead of doing that, however, the United States is currently in the process of withdrawing from the organization. When the COVID-19 crisis subsides in the world, there should be an assessment of the overall WHO response to COVID-19, with an aim of strengthening its response in advance of the next global pandemic crisis. No doubt there are things that it can do to improve its response, decisions that it may have made differently given what we know now. But in the midst of this crisis, WHO needs to be strongly supported. It is a critical international institution and has the confidence of most countries around the world on technical and health matters. We should help work to strengthen it. In a substantial portion of the US public, though, there is an antipathy to international organizations, including WHO. This public antipathy has been fostered by a number of political leaders over the years. It will require strong leadership to counter that narrative going forward. It will require that presidential administrations and Congressional leaders make the case for international engagement, particularly for WHO engagement. In the case of WHO, it will be important to convey what the world would look like without WHO in a pandemic. It will also be key to offer a vision of how US leaders want WHO to evolve. Effective leadership can and should make the case for WHO's high value and paint a picture of how the United States will support it and help it move forward with strong multilateral partnerships to be better prepared for future pandemics.

Pandemic Resilience

COVID-19 has established that pandemics are a terrible source of global upheaval and destruction, a form of catastrophe that has to be clearly reckoned with in humanity's future. Unlike some other potential global catastrophic risks, the path to take for averting or mitigating pandemics is relatively clear, even if it is not easy or fast to carry out. The United States needs to understand the risks of natural and manmade epidemics and pandemics. It needs to plan for and invest in large-scale innovations, technologies, programs, and strategies that will transform its national ability to prevent and prepare for pandemics in the future. At the same time, it needs to be a strong partner with other countries in the world, working to create a post-COVID-19 system that is far more capable of anticipating and responding to future pandemics. International organizations, especially WHO, as well as the private sector will need to be key partners in that global effort. If and when we do all these things, we will strengthen our medical and public health systems in ways that make the United States more resilient to infectious disease threats. We will also diminish the power of pandemics to wreak havoc on the world.

NOTES

1. Jason Burke, "Burundi President Dies of Illness Suspected to Be Coronavirus," *Guardian*, June 9, 2020, https://www.theguardian.com/world/2020/jun/09/burundi-president-dies-illness-suspected-coronavirus-pierre-nkurunziz.

2. Nick Bostrom and Milan M. Ćirković, eds., *Global Catastrophic Risks* (Oxford: Oxford University Press, 2011).

3. Monica Schoch-Spana et al., "Global Catastrophic Biological Risks: Toward a Working Definition," *Health Security* 15, no. 4 (2017): 323–28, doi.org/10.1089/hs.2017.0038.

4. D. A. Henderson et al., "Smallpox as a Biological Weapon: Medical and Public Health Management," *JAMA* 281, no. 22 (1999): 2127–37, doi:10.1001/jama.281.22.2127.

5. John D. Loike and Robert Pollack, "Opinion: Ethical Boundaries Needed on the Uses of Synthetic DNA," *Scientist*, March 1, 2019, https://www.the-scientist.com/news-opinion/opinion--ethical-boundaries-needed-on-the-uses-of-synthetic-dna-65549.

6. Louise H. Taylor, Sophia M. Latham, and Mark E. J. Woolhouse, "Risk Factors for Human Disease Emergence," *Philosophical Transactions of the Royal Society of London B* 356, no. 1411 (2001): 983–89, https://royalsocietypublishing.org/doi/abs/10.1098/rstb.2001.0888.

7. World Health Organization, *A World at Risk: Annual Report on Global Preparedness for Health Emergencies* (Geneva: World Health Organization, 2019).

8. Amesh A. Adalja, Matthew Watson, Eric S. Toner, Anita Cicero, and Thomas V. Inglesby, "Characteristics of Microbes Most Likely to Cause Pandemics and Global Catastrophes," *Global Catastrophic Biological Risks* 424 (2019): 1–20, doi:10.1007/82_2019_176.

9. Mark Lipsitch and Thomas V. Inglesby, "Moratorium on Research Intended to Create Novel Potential Pandemic Pathogens," *mBio* 5, no. 6 (2014): e02366-14.

10. Thomas V. Inglesby and Mark Lipsitch, "Proposed Changes to U.S. Policy on Potential Pandemic Pathogen Oversight and Implementation," *mSphere* 5, no. 1 (2020): e00990-19.

11. "The Biological Weapons Convention: Convention on the Prohibition of the Development, Production and Stockpiling of Bacteriological (Biological) and Toxin Weapons and on Their Destruction," United Nations Office for Disarmament Affairs, accessed June 25, 2020, https://www.un.org/disarmament/wmd/bio/.

12. E. Tammy Kim, "How South Korea Solved Its Face Mask Shortage," *New York Times*, April 1, 2020, https://www.nytimes.com/2020/04/01/opinion/covid-face-mask-shortage.html.

13. Lois Parshley, "The Mask Shortage Is Forcing Health Workers to Disregard Basic Coronavirus Infection Control," *Vox*, April 3, 2020, https://www.vox.com/2020/4/3/21206726/coronavirus-masks-n95-hospitals-health-care-doctors-ppe-shortage.

14. Robert Kuznia, Curt Devin, and Nick Valencia, "'We've Been Muzzled': CDC Sources Say White House Putting Politics ahead of Science," *CNN*, May 20, 2020, https://www.cnn.com/2020/05/20/politics/coronavirus-travel-alert-cdc-white-house-tensions-invs/index.html.

15. "Coronavirus Resource Center," Johns Hopkins University and School of Medicine, https://coronavirus.jhu.edu/us-map.

16. Derek Lowe, "Coronavirus Vaccine Update, June 11," *In the Pipeline* (blog), *Science Translational Medicine*, June 11, 2020, https://blogs.sciencemag.org/pipeline/archives/2020/06/11/coronavirus-vaccine-update-june-11.

17. Jen Christensen, "US Should Have a 'Couple Hundred Million' Doses of a Covid-19 Vaccine by the Start of 2021, Fauci Says," *CNN*, June 3, 2020, https://www.cnn.com/2020/06/03/health/fauci-coronavirus-vaccine-2021/index.html.

18. Amesh Adalja, *Expediting Development of Medical Countermeasures for Unknown Viral Threats: Proposal for a "Virus 201" Program in the United States* (Baltimore: Johns Hopkins Center for Health Security, 2020).

19. "Low-Cost Dexamethasone Reduces Death by Up to One Third in Hospitalised Patients with Severe Respiratory Complications of COVID-19," RECOVERY (clinical trial), June 16, 2020, https://www.recoverytrial.net/news/low-cost-dexamethasone-reduces-death-by-up-to-one-third-in-hospitalised-patients-with-severe-respiratory-complications-of-covid-19.

20. "About the Strategic National Stockpile," US Department of Health and Human Services, accessed June 25, 2020, https://www.phe.gov/about/sns/Pages/about.aspx.

21. David R. Williams and Lisa A. Cooper, "COVID-19 and Health Equity—a New Kind of 'Herd Immunity,'" *JAMA* 323, no. 24 (2020), 2478–80, doi:10.1001/jama.2020.8051.

22. "COVID-19 Virtual Press Conference—20 April 2020," World Health Organization, accessed June 25, 2020, https://www.who.int/docs/default-source/coronaviruse/transcripts/who-audio-emergencies-coronavirus-press-conference-20apr2020.pdf?sfvrsn=b5656a70_2.

Chapter Five

Origins of the COVID-19 Pandemic and the Path Forward

A Global Public Health Policy Perspective

Lainie Rutkow

Although the world has experienced pandemics before, including several in the last fifteen years,[1] the COVID-19 pandemic has caused an unprecedented global public health crisis. The synergy among multiple factors—including the relative ease of transmission of SARS-CoV-2, the failure to identify and contain early outbreaks of COVID-19, and the at times fraught relationship between political and public health priorities—has fundamentally jolted the world order. What began as a local outbreak in Wuhan, China, rapidly expanded to impact private and public sectors throughout the world, including governments at every level, across a host of domains. The phrase "COVID-19 crisis" has evolved to become shorthand for challenges to health care systems, labor markets, supply chains, and even geopolitics.

In the coming months and years, as countries shift from the COVID-19 emergency response to the recovery process, the world must reconsider, and perhaps fundamentally shift, its approach to protecting and promoting the health of populations. Without such a change, global recovery from the COVID-19 crisis will remain tenuous, with fragile intra- and inter-country public health systems serving as the only shield against a future pandemic. The precise path forward may not be clear, but an immediate and intense focus on global public health policy is

Lainie Rutkow is a professor of health policy and management at the Johns Hopkins Bloomberg School of Public Health.

imperative. With that lens, this essay considers two questions: (1) How should we understand the origins and consequences of the COVID-19 crisis? (2) What should be our vision to craft a better world order for the future?

This essay argues that, from the perspective of global public health policy, multiple factors converged and contributed to the rapid spread of the novel coronavirus. These include the traditionally less prominent role of public health within international affairs, the inconsistent patchwork of laws and policies that governs public health preparedness within and among countries, and structural limitations relative to pandemic preparedness and response experienced by the World Health Organization (WHO). After exploring these factors, the essay pivots to identifying opportunities to promote a more effective world order. From a global health policy standpoint, these include anticipating and avoiding societal complacency once the pandemic abates; promoting wide-ranging collaborations that span countries, sectors, and disciplines to protect the public's health; and re-envisioning WHO based on lessons learned from current and prior pandemic responses.

Origins of the COVID-19 Pandemic

The origins of the COVID-19 pandemic are complex and multifaceted, with several key themes emerging. First, despite the primacy of public health to the survival of humankind, public health is often an invisible discipline within international affairs. Individuals typically become briefly aware of public health in times of crisis and tend to ignore it during periods of relative salubrity. As a result, public health systems are chronically underappreciated and underfunded. Second, the laws and policies that have been created within and among countries to secure public health are a sundry and inconsistent patchwork. This patchwork effect is exacerbated by an overlay of diverse emergency preparedness and response policies. As a result, intra- and inter-country public health emergency preparedness varies greatly. Finally, the primary body charged with protecting global public health, WHO, may deploy policy tools but has limited authority over their implementation and enforcement. In addition, WHO's funding model is subject to political whims, often leaving this global body on precarious footing.

Public Health Is a Largely Invisible Discipline

Public health is a broad field focused on protecting and promoting the health of populations. The US Centers for Disease Control and Prevention defines public health as "the science of protecting and improving the health of people and their communities . . . by promoting healthy lifestyles, researching disease and injury prevention, and detecting, preventing, and responding to infectious diseases."[2] Epidemiology, the scientific discipline underlying public health, is the study of the distribution and determinants of health and related events within populations.[3] This may include environmental exposures, outbreaks of foodborne illness or infectious diseases, violence in a community, incidence and prevalence of chronic conditions, and natural and human-made disasters. While public health is often conflated with health care, it is distinct. Public health practitioners and researchers consider population health at the local, regional, national, or global level. In contrast, the field of health care tends to involve individual-level encounters, typically between a health care provider and a patient.

For most people, the provision of health care has one or more faces associated with it: individuals may know their health care providers relatively well and value these relationships. Because public health work occurs at the population level, however, this type of personal relationship is absent. If asked who their public health provider is, people may mention, at most, their local health department. And even though a local health department's purview may be quite broad—including chronic disease prevention, emergency preparedness and response, environmental health, infectious disease prevention, maternal and child health, mental and behavioral health, and violence prevention[4]—the actual work feels abstract to the general public. As a result, during noncrisis periods, public health is a largely invisible discipline, particularly within international affairs.

The exception to public health's invisibility within international affairs occurs during periods of emergency or disaster. When individuals' lives and societal norms are disrupted, the cause of this disorder comes to the fore. For example, during and shortly after a major tropical cyclone, such as Hurricane Katrina in 2005 or Typhoon Haiyan in 2013, communities may experience displacement, lack of access to potable water, exacerbation of chronic health conditions, and infectious disease outbreaks.[5] During a pandemic, such as H1N1 in 2009, Zika in 2016, or COVID-19 in 2020, societies across the globe become intensely focused on disease detection, treatment, containment, and mitigation. For some period of days, weeks, or even months, public health metrics, tools, and vocabulary populate the news cycle and daily conversations. In 2020, as countries throughout the world experienced the COVID-19 pandemic, terms familiar to any public health practitioner—terms such as *social distancing*, *self-quarantine*, and *mortality rate*—joined our shared lexicon.

During a widespread or high-profile emergency, when public health, emergency preparedness, and response command the focus of policy makers, the increase in attention is often accompanied by an increase in funding. For example, in the United States, after the terrorist attacks of September 11, 2001, and the dissemination of anthrax via mail, the federal government appropriated nearly $1 billion for state and local public health preparedness efforts, which are typically tied to public health departments.[6] Over nearly two decades, that funding decreased by 30%, leaving a chronically underfunded public health system in its wake.[7] While this may be an extreme example, it is not unusual: as societies move out of a disaster's response phase and begin the recovery process, public health's visibility fades along with perceptions about its importance within the global policy agenda. Once a feeling of "return to normal" sets in—especially for those who did not experience the disaster's most acute impacts—policy makers and the public turn their attention to quotidian concerns.

This may suggest a degree of societal resilience, but it fails to account for the life course of a public health disaster, which is cyclical and not linear.[8] The highly visible response phase, when the public and private sectors may not be able to carry out their normal functions, is followed by the recovery phase. During recovery, a disaster may fade from public view, once, for example, hospitals are no longer overwhelmed with COVID-19 patients. Governments and communities rebuild systems, replace depleted resources, and attempt to implement lessons learned that may reduce vulnerability in the future. The recovery phase then transitions into the mitigation phase, which focuses on prevention or lessening the impacts of disasters. In this phase, researchers may develop new disease surveillance systems or strengthen efforts to limit disease transmission from animals to humans. Because new disasters are inevitable, mitigation transitions into the preparedness phase. At this point, preparation occurs for aspects of a disaster that cannot be mitigated, which includes planning and training for health care and public health responses to a future pandemic. The recovery, mitigation, and preparedness phases may be less visible, but they encompass critical public health activities that, ideally, lengthen the periods between disasters. These efforts are as important to protecting the public's health as those that occur in the response phase.

Public Health Laws and Policies Are a Patchwork

One of the oldest roles of government, which remains a core function today, is protecting and promoting individuals' health. The earliest known use of quarantine—the public health practice of breaking the chain of disease transmission by separating individuals exposed to a disease from those not exposed—can be traced to 14th-century Venice. Ships that arrived in Venice from locations with known cases of plague were required to anchor in the port for forty days before making landfall.[9] The Italian words that described this forty-day practice evolved over centuries into today's *quarantine*. In addition to revealing the origin of a public health tool, this example demonstrates that implementation of public health laws and policies has traditionally rested with subnational jurisdictions.

In the United States, the foundational case for public health law concerns a local government's attempt to keep its residents safe during a smallpox epidemic. In 1905, the US Supreme Court issued its opinion in *Jacobson v. Massachusetts*, which considered whether a local government could enact a compulsory vaccination law. In 1902, facing an outbreak of smallpox, Cambridge, Massachusetts, adopted a law requiring individuals over 21 years old to receive a smallpox vaccination. Henning Jacobson declined to be vaccinated, and he refused to pay the required fine. In essence, he argued that the Cambridge law compromised his autonomy in violation of several provisions of the US Constitution. In its decision the court found for the local government: "in every well ordered society charged with the duty of conserving the safety of its members the rights of the individual in respect of his liberty may at times, under the pressure of great dangers, be subjected to such restraint, to be enforced by reasonable regulations, as the safety of the general public may demand."[10]

With this, the US Supreme Court established a balancing test that persists today, with reasonable governmental action to protect public health and safety on one side and respect for individuals' liberty on the other. In practice, this has meant that, whenever possible, the least restrictive means of accomplishing a public health goal is preferable.[11]

These two elements—the key role of subnational governments in the implementation of public health law and policy and efforts to balance government action with preservation of individuals' rights—help explain the patchwork nature of public health law. Because public health challenges almost always originate locally, subnational jurisdictions traditionally serve as the front line for policy responses.[12] And the response selected by one local, regional, state, or territorial government may differ from other subnational governments' responses to the same public health issue. This variation may be attributed to multiple factors including the availability of resources, previous experiences with disasters, prioritization of government action over individuals' autonomy or vice versa, actions of neighboring jurisdictions, and incentives or disincentives provided by a higher level of government.

The patchwork effect of public health law also appears within public health emergency preparedness and response policies. For example, in recognition of outmoded or absent subnational public health preparedness laws in the United States, the Centers for Disease Control and Prevention commissioned the Model State Emergency Health Powers Act (MSEHPA) shortly after the 9/11 terrorist attacks and anthrax scare.[13] As a model law, MSEHPA carried no legal force on its own, but it provided a useful road map for subnational governments seeking language to update all or part of their public health preparedness laws and policies. More than two-thirds of US states ultimately adopted at least part of MSEHPA. However, because subnational governments selected which, if any, parts of MSEHPA to incorporate into their public health preparedness laws, the patchwork effect persisted. This, coupled with the ongoing funding challenges mentioned earlier, may impair the development of strong, cohesive public health and emergency response systems.

Today, intra- and inter-country public health preparedness and response laws and policies vary greatly. The Global Health Security Index, the first comprehensive assessment of health security capabilities in 195 countries, found vast differences across a host of categories, including disease detection and reporting, health system preparedness, and the ability to rapidly mitigate an epidemic.[14] As witnessed by the range of responses to the COVID-19 pandemic, both within and among countries, variation in law and policy can impede a swift, coordinated, and effective response.

WHO Has Limited Power to Protect the Public's Health

Among the United Nations agencies and public-private partnerships that interface with global public health, WHO is arguably the most prominent. Established in 1948, WHO is the United Nations agency responsible for "the attainment by all peoples of the highest possible level of health" and serves as the "co-ordinating authority on international health work."[15] Today, WHO's seven thousand employees hail from over 150 countries and carry out WHO's mission in country and regional offices as well as WHO's headquarters in Geneva. WHO's governing body is the World Health Assembly, with delegations from WHO's member countries. The World Health Assembly determines WHO's policies and approves the organization's budget on an annual basis.

WHO describes itself as protecting the public's health through several focus areas: (1) promoting universal health coverage through improved access to primary care, workforce training, and sustainable financing; (2) supporting populations' health and well-being by fostering collaborations across sectors and championing a health-in-all-policies approach; and (3) preparing for and responding to public health emergencies through early detection of risks, development of outbreak response tools, and provision of essential health services in locations with fragile health care and public health systems.[16]

In each of these areas, WHO serves as a centralized body for collecting, developing, and disseminating information and for devising recommendations. For example, WHO produces the *International Classification of Diseases*, which gives countries a standardized approach for identifying and reporting diseases, health conditions, and related trends.[17] WHO also works within countries to implement its recommendations and provide technical assistance. These efforts range from support for in-country vaccination programs to implementation of global health campaigns to reduce the prevalence of noncommunicable diseases. WHO's work has secured global public health, perhaps most prominently through the Smallpox Eradication Program, which led to the first global eradication of a disease in 1980.[18]

Given the breadth of its mission, the precarious nature of WHO's funding structure may appear surprising. WHO is funded through contributions from its member countries as well as voluntary contributions. Member country dues, officially referred to as "assessed contributions," are a percentage of a member country's gross domestic product set by the United Nations General Assembly and approved by the World Health Assembly.[19] Assessed contributions account for approximately 20% of WHO's budget, and WHO can determine how to use these funds. The remaining 80% of WHO's budget comes from voluntary contributions from member countries, philanthropic organizations, the private sector, and other entities. More than 90% of voluntary contributions are designated for particular uses: for instance, a particular programmatic area, geographic location, or time frame. During 2018–19, with assessed and voluntary contributions aggregated, WHO's top three donors were the United States ($851.6 million), the United Kingdom ($463.4 million), and the Bill & Melinda Gates Foundation ($455.3 million).[20]

As a result of its funding structure, WHO is often implementing work of greatest priority to its voluntary contributors, which does not necessarily align with the most objectively urgent global public health challenges. WHO has called for a more stable and flexible funding structure so that it can become increasingly nimble as it executes strategic priorities and pivots to address emerging health threats. Presently, WHO's budget is divided among seven areas, with the largest percentages allocated to universal health coverage (23%), country support (19%), emergency operations and appeals (17%), and health emergencies (15%).[21] WHO typically cannot shift funds among these areas, although there is some flexibility with the emergency operations and appeals category, which can be critical during a pandemic response.

During a public health emergency, such as the COVID-19 pandemic, WHO has a key role in coordinating the global response. The International Health Regulations (IHRs) establish the framework for this coordination. Updated in 2005, the IHRs create binding obligations for WHO member countries regarding disease surveillance, information reporting, and emergency response, with an overall goal of preventing and mitigating pandemics while limiting "interference with international traffic and trade."[22] While WHO provides assistance and guidance, including dissemination of relevant information and data and updates to the IHRs and related documents, it ultimately depends on its member countries to implement the IHRs at the country level. This is a critical distinction—despite its broad mission, WHO lacks enforcement authority and, thus, does not have a legal means to require countries to act. Instead, it serves as a coordinating body to assist sovereign nations in implementing their own policy responses.

Given this dynamic, one of WHO's greatest strengths is the ability to put the world on notice when an infectious disease outbreak—particularly involving a novel, or not previously known, disease—occurs. The IHRs delineate the process by which WHO may declare a Public Health Emergency of International Concern (PHEIC), defined as "an extraordinary event which is determined to constitute a public health risk to other States through the international spread of disease and to potentially require a coordinated international response."[23] WHO's director-general weighs various factors when deciding whether to issue a PHEIC declaration, including information provided by the country experiencing the outbreak, advice from a WHO-appointed Emergency Committee, scientific evidence, and an assessment of the risk of disease spread across countries and the risks to human health.[24] Since the creation of PHEIC in a 2005 revision to the IHRs, WHO has made six declarations: H1N1 in 2009, polio in 2014, Ebola in 2014, Zika in 2016, Ebola in 2019, and COVID-19 in 2020.

A PHEIC declaration has several potential effects, including heightening global awareness of an emerging disease risk, putting countries on notice to initiate infectious disease response efforts, and potentially driving donations to WHO or other organizations focused on mitigating any outbreaks. Importantly, as noted above, WHO does not have the ability to enforce any aspect of a PHEIC declaration. This means that WHO must rely on its position as the coordinating body for global public health to convey the severity of a threat and then wait for countries to act in accordance with its recommendations. WHO may use persuasion, data, and information to catalyze countries' responses to a PHEIC declaration, but it does not have any formal enforcement tools.

Crafting a More Effective World Order

Several systemic changes are needed to secure global public health. First, societies must overcome the cycle of intense interest and commitment during a public health emergency that is followed by widespread complacency. Future pandemics are inevitable. Bold action must occur now—while the COVID-19 pandemic continues to rage—before the crisis fades from memory and is replaced with a feeling of returning to normal. Second, because jurisdictional boundaries are not recognized by infectious diseases, newly invigorated multinational coalitions should facilitate wide-ranging collaboration as the world moves into the recovery, planning, and preparedness phases of the disaster cycle. By capitalizing on the periods between disasters, governments can work together to establish systems that facilitate a more nimble response to future disasters. Finally, lessons learned from COVID-19 and prior pandemics can inform a re-envisioned WHO. The greatest chance of success for this institution, and for robust oversight of the global public health response, rests on an orientation that favors science over politics.

ANTICIPATE SOCIETAL COMPLACENCY ABOUT
PUBLIC HEALTH DISASTERS

Individual and societal memories can be short. Everyone is naturally drawn in by events that impact them or their loved ones directly, and cataclysmic events—like the Indian Ocean tsunami of 2004 or the terrorist attacks of 9/11—capture the world's attention for some period of time. This can be attributed to a variety of factors, including hyper-attentiveness by the news media, the vast and sometimes incomprehensible scope of a disaster, disruptions to everyday life, and fear that encompasses imminent and potential longer-term impacts. Over weeks or months, the period of intensity fades, and slowly a feeling of returning to normal seeps in. This typically coincides with a societal sigh of relief as individuals and policy makers determine that the disaster is over and they can move on to the next pressing thing. The impulse makes sense—within the individual, community, and policy-making spheres, there will always be something new and urgent to address.

As COVID-19 roars across the globe, reactions have been aligned with what one might expect during the response phase for a public health disaster of this magnitude. The period of intense interest and fear has brought unprecedented policy responses with implementation of social distancing measures, closures of workplaces and schools, and allocation of government funds. While the response phase to COVID-19 will persist for the foreseeable future, governments are taking steps to reopen, and individuals are experiencing the fatigue that accompanies an enduring disaster response. Because future and potentially worse pandemics are inevitable,[25] it would be irresponsible if governments were to fail to capitalize on the COVID-19 response to secure the long-term investment needed for the full disaster cycle of mitigation, preparedness, response, and recovery. While the pandemic continues and its impacts are felt on a daily basis, policy makers should use their political capital to establish a well-resourced infrastructure for the full public health disaster cycle. Many activities within this infrastructure—such as disease surveillance, innovation relative to personal protective equipment, and development of new therapeutics—will be largely invisible to the general public between disasters. Yet this type of work is critical to ensuring greater societal readiness and resilience for future pandemics.

The type of policy change described above is not inevitable. It would be naïve to assume that the magnitude of the COVID-19 pandemic and its rippling impacts will overcome the societal complacency likely to descend once the pandemic wanes. Incremental change characterizes public policy, with stasis being the norm.[26] When viewed retrospectively, most disasters do not produce significant policy change, but some do. The political science theory of punctuated equilibrium offers helpful insights for understanding the factors that may coalesce to bring about meaningful departures from previous policy approaches.[27] According to punctuated equilibrium theory, the greater societal context for policy making leads to one of two paths: reinforcement of current approaches or questioning of these approaches. When current approaches are reinforced—which happens most of the time, as the policy process ultimately tends to favor the status quo[28]—only incremental change occurs because there is little motivation to consider alternatives. On the other hand, when a single issue dominates the political agenda and commands the attention of a broad cross-section of policy makers for a sustained period, change becomes possible.

The COVID-19 pandemic has caused a sustained impact that touches on all aspects of society, leaving no one apathetic to the disaster's consequences. This has brought the pandemic into clear focus for policy makers. While a public health disaster is traditionally viewed as touching health care and public health systems, the current pandemic has expanded well beyond that to disrupt the world economy, leaving rampant unemployment and systemic uncertainty in its wake. These society-wide impacts have led to massive political pressure for change, making it difficult for governments *not* to respond. For example, the US Congress—often slowed by extreme partisan gridlock—has passed multiple pieces of legislation, including the Coronavirus Aid, Relief, and Economic Security Act. This includes direct payments to individuals and families, emergency loans for small businesses, expansion of unemployment benefits, and funds to support health care system infrastructure.[29] The window for major policy change is open, but it will quickly close as COVID-19 fatigue sets in and attention shifts to other concerns. Before this happens, policy makers at every level of government should capitalize on this moment to strengthen public health infrastructure and secure funding to support public health preparedness, response, and recovery.

While the window for significant policy action may soon close, the opportunity to raise the profile of public health as a discipline will not. The exigency of a pandemic may have brought public health to the fore, but there are multiple opportunities to reimagine public health's place in society. Prior to the COVID-19 pandemic, public health was often viewed as a domestic policy concern, meaning that it was tied to the stability of a country's health care system and infrastructure. The pandemic has clearly demonstrated the fallacy of limiting public health domestically; instead, it should be framed as intimately tied to international affairs. COVID-19 has demonstrated that public health challenges, particularly biothreats, can rapidly scale up. In other words, public health does not simply keep populations healthy—it also keeps them safe. It should thus receive the same respect, implementation support, and continuous investment given to other aspects of international affairs.

Finally, although local governments are on the front lines of public health policy and implementation, public health should not operate only within the purview of local government. Localities typically have a broad grant of authority to act in ways that protect and promote the public's health, and their work is essential. However, local public health work inevitably impacts higher levels of government. For example, throughout the world, vaccinations are typically provided by a local public health workforce. The COVID-19 pandemic has already destabilized vaccination schedules in many parts of the world, raising the potential for outbreaks of diseases like measles and diphtheria.[30] These secondary public health impacts of the pandemic are first experienced locally, but they can quickly transcend local borders to become regional, country-level, and even global health challenges. In developed and developing countries, societal complacency may be overcome by elevating public health's place beyond the local government and reimagining its role within both foreign and domestic planning and policy.

Promote Wide-Ranging Collaboration to Protect Public Health

Pandemics have long proven that infectious diseases do not respect jurisdictional boundaries, and the COVID-19 pandemic has reinforced this point. Over the course of several months, COVID-19 cases were reported on every continent except Antarctica and in virtually all of the world's countries.[31] On a daily basis, COVID-19 incidence and prevalence were tracked and communities watched with a combination of awe and horror as the disease progressively populated global maps. Importantly, while there may be some genomic variation among the strains of COVID-19 in circulation,[32] the fundamental biology of the virus is not affected by geography. The traditional public health tools of isolation, quarantine, social distancing, testing, and surveillance are used consistently in efforts to mitigate COVID-19, regardless of the society in which it appears.

What does change, depending on the country in which the virus surfaces, are political responses and the activation of intra- and inter-country efforts to limit transmission and address the virus's health effects. In addition to in-country variation, countries' overall political environments do not necessarily remain predictable from one pandemic to the next. A change in leadership can dramatically alter a country's priorities and its role relative to global public health. The United States provides an illustrative case study over several presidential administrations. In his 2003 State of the Union address, President George W. Bush, a Republican, announced plans to establish the President's Emergency Plan for AIDS Relief, which received bipartisan support and has become the largest single-country funding commitment dedicated to one disease.[33] During the Ebola pandemic of 2014, under President Barack Obama, a Democrat, the United States played a major role in coordinating a global response and sent thousands of health officials to West Africa to focus on disease containment.[34] The administration viewed the Ebola response as both a public health and health security priority. In contrast, under President Donald J. Trump's America First approach, the United States has retreated from global public health leadership during the COVID-19 pandemic, focusing instead on an isolationist response.[35]

In an era when some leaders around the world have embraced nationalism and populism, the traditional ways of conceptualizing global public health security may no longer apply. The global coordinating body for pandemic response, WHO, must account for donor-driven rather than public health priorities. The United States has backed away from a position of global leadership relative to public health, and many leaders have lost enthusiasm for inter-country efforts in general. While political whims may change, effective public health approaches will not: global public health challenges will continue to necessitate a collaborative approach that spans the developed and developing worlds. COVID-19 has temporarily slowed our increasingly interconnected world, but the same pathways that allowed COVID-19 to spread so quickly will eventually reemerge. And the pandemics of the last fifteen years, culminating in COVID-19, have repeatedly demonstrated that an isolationist stance does not yield positive public health outcomes.

While effective collaboration may arise spontaneously during a pandemic, the strongest collaborations will be built and nurtured during inter-pandemic periods, when governments, organizations, and individuals can focus on structure and goals, rather than the exigency of response. The recovery and mitigation phases of the disaster lifecycle—which are inherently less chaotic than the response phase—offer an ideal time to learn from the strengths and failures of collaborative responses to prior pandemics. As the global community shifts from the most acute COVID-19 response into longer-term planning for a lingering pandemic, lessons can be learned from responses to prior coronavirus pandemics, particularly SARS in 2002–4.

SARS was a coronavirus disease, but it differed from COVID-19 in important ways. COVID-19 is easier to transmit than SARS, but its case fatality rate is lower, meaning that it is less deadly for those who contract it.[36] This means that COVID-19 is unlikely to fade away like SARS. Despite these differences, the SARS response offers important lessons about collaboration at individual and societal levels. In some countries that experienced SARS, especially those in eastern Asia, individuals implemented public health measures like mask wearing, handwashing, and social distancing to facilitate a collective response. Some have theorized that these societies retained their collective memory of population-level compliance from the SARS response, making them early adopters of public health practices during the COVID-19 pandemic.[37] Importantly, this type of collective response may emerge more predictably in countries that tend toward centralized governance or more widely shared norms. In a country like the United States—with a long tradition of decentralized governance and local or regional norms—public health practices may be embraced inconsistently.

The SARS response also put the world on notice about the need for country-spanning collaborations to ensure timely disease surveillance and outbreak response.[38] A National Academy of Sciences review of the SARS response noted that key collaborations related to linking laboratory research to epidemic response partners had been established years before SARS emerged.[39] In addition, diagnosis, treatment, and mitigation were supported because SARS appeared primarily in countries with stronger health care and public health systems. This realization should have alerted the global community to the potentially devastating effects of a pandemic throughout the developing world, where containment or mitigation would depend on international assistance. As the COVID-19 response has shown, while the world made some strides to improve surveillance capabilities and strengthen global outbreak alert systems, countries did not fully internalize critical lessons from SARS.

The question then becomes, What might a future approach to global public health preparedness look like? It will depend on effective collaborations within and between countries, grounded in a shared recognition that jurisdictional boundaries are irrelevant to infectious diseases. Regardless of the patchwork effect in public health law and policy, governments at every level must embrace a shared, nonpartisan goal of protecting the health of their populations, with pandemics viewed as public health, health security, and existential threats. Because no country can mitigate a global threat on its own, public health systems should be viewed as interconnected entities, both within countries and across international borders. While these systems, of course, will vary greatly in terms of resources, technology, and longevity, the success of the whole—defined as effective mitigation, preparedness, response, and recovery from pandemics—depends on the functioning of each part.

Rather than challenge national sovereignty, this orientation seeks to ensure that populations continue to thrive under the leadership of their respective governments. But it also recognizes the fundamental limitation of stand-alone public health efforts in an interconnected world. Critically, effective global public health preparedness must recognize the essential role of nongovernmental or quasi-governmental institutions. For example, over two decades, Gavi, the Vaccine Alliance, has demonstrated the power of public-private partnerships to tackle seemingly intractable challenges such as global vaccine access.[40] By bringing together diverse, multidisciplinary collaborators, these types of institutions can foster the innovation needed to supplement governments' public health work and can fill global health policy gaps not addressed by WHO.

Apply Lessons Learned from the COVID-19 Response to WHO

During recent pandemics, two observations about WHO have gained traction: (1) the organization plays a key role in pandemic response, as the international co-ordinating body for this work; and (2) WHO's effectiveness is curbed by structural limitations. To understand WHO's strengths and weaknesses—and the potential for change moving forward—the timeline of its engagement relative to COVID-19 proves instructive.[41] On December 31, 2019, WHO received a report of a cluster of pneumonia cases from the Wuhan Municipal Health Commission in China. On January 4, 2020, WHO shared this information with the world via a tweet and noted, "Investigations are underway to identify the cause of this illness."[42] The next day, WHO published information in its *Disease Outbreak News* about "cases of pneumonia of unknown etiology" in Wuhan, China,[43] followed by technical guidance later that week. On January 12, WHO confirmed that China had shared the disease's genetic sequence, and on January 14, a WHO official noted the possibility of human-to-human transmission. On January 20–21, a team of WHO officials visited Wuhan and, the next day, issued a statement confirming human-to-human transmission.

On January 22–23, Dr. Tedros Adhanom Ghebreyesus, WHO's director-general, convened an Emergency Committee, in keeping with the process established by the IHRs. The committee, composed of independent experts from throughout the world, failed to reach a consensus about whether available information supported a PHEIC declaration. On January 28, Dr. Tedros led a WHO delegation to China to confer with Chinese leaders about their response to the novel coronavirus. Two days later, the Emergency Committee was reconvened, leading to a recommendation for a declaration of PHEIC. Dr. Tedros issued the official declaration on January 30.[44] Significantly, WHO did not refer to the COVID-19 outbreak as a "pandemic" until March 11, 2020.[45]

As these events demonstrate, WHO must rely on information provided by its member countries when making determinations about a disease outbreak. In the case of COVID-19, immense concerns have arisen about the timing and accuracy of information provided by the Chinese government. And, because the pandemic began in the Wuhan region of China, any delays, omissions, or flaws attributed to China had wide-ranging implications for the rest of the world. For example, while doctors in China raised concerns about human-to-human transmission of the novel coronavirus,[46] the Chinese government hedged, and the mode of disease transmission was not confirmed for weeks by WHO.[47] Even without a WHO declaration of PHEIC, confirmation of human-to-human transmission would likely have led to much greater concern and swifter action by countries throughout the world. Instead, countries delayed their own responses—in many cases until late January or early February, after the PHEIC declaration. In addition, by not using the word *pandemic* until mid-March, WHO potentially gave a false sense of security to countries that had not yet identified COVID-19 cases within their borders.

In an ideal world, countries would report accurate, timely information to WHO, but varied reasons may constrain this. A country's government may not want its own residents, let alone the entire world, to know that it failed to identify and contain a novel disease outbreak, especially if it arises at a politically inconvenient time. In China, Lunar New Year celebrations, in which individuals travel and spend time with family and friends, coincided with the emergence of the novel coronavirus. Countries may also fear that disclosing a novel disease outbreak may compromise their global standing, perpetuate stigma and stereotypes, or impact tourism and trade. This last concern resonates strongly with countries where tourism is a major economic driver. These concerns have been validated by prior pandemics, which is why the IHRs state that their purpose is "to prevent, protect against, control and provide a public health response to the international spread of disease in ways that are commensurate with and restricted to public health risks, and which avoid unnecessary interference with international traffic and trade."[48] Yet, despite this, pandemics are routinely accompanied by country-specific decisions that do not reflect tenets of the IHRs. As a result, a country may have multifaceted reasons for withholding or limiting the information it shares with WHO while it attempts to contain a novel disease outbreak.

WHO's COVID-19 response raises a second structural limitation, related to its funding mechanisms. Because approximately 80% of WHO's funding comes from earmarked donor contributions, WHO must routinely view its member countries as both constituents and funders. Concern has arisen that this duality explains WHO's actions during the initial weeks of the COVID-19 outbreak. China is among WHO's largest contributors,[49] which suggests that WHO is particularly attuned to that government's preferences. This dynamic may have led WHO to resist declaring a PHEIC for a disease that had clearly originated in China, or at least postponed the declaration while it engaged with the Chinese government throughout the month of January.

If the timing of the PHEIC was a political decision, it certainly had public health consequences—countries throughout the world delayed their own responses, including country-level emergency declarations, until WHO had acted. During these several weeks of wait-and-see, individuals carrying the novel coronavirus traveled and hastened its spread throughout the world. WHO's actions may have also strengthened its ties to China: in the first half of 2020, China emerged as one of the leading donors to WHO's COVID-19 response, with $50 million pledged.[50] At the same time, WHO faces potentially catastrophic ramifications from recent US threats to withhold future funding;[51] in addition to affecting the global response to the COVID-19 pandemic, other WHO efforts—to control infectious diseases, mitigate noncommunicable diseases, and prevent injuries—would suffer. Because the United States is WHO's largest single funder, it remains unclear what country or organization might fill the void, raise its own profile in global health, and potentially reorient WHO's donor-driven priorities. This suggests that, for WHO, politics and public health are inexorably intertwined. And, within the current funding model, advocates of good global health governance must enlist well-resourced partners to effectively compete for influence within the organization.

Despite this, it would be a mistake to forsake WHO and its critical coordinating role. No country can tackle a pandemic on its own, which means global health security depends on an entity that can facilitate inter-country mitigation, preparedness, response, and recovery. After SARS, the IHRs were revisited to strengthen WHO's functions,[52] and that will need to happen again to account for the lessons of COVID-19. As part of this process, member countries could consider the One Health perspective, to ensure that pandemic response is situated within the broader context of connections among people, animals, plants, and the environment.

WHO is unlikely to gain enforcement authority, given the geopolitical implications that would accompany such a shift, so WHO's member countries must together develop processes that will yield compliance and timely, accurate information. Ultimately, all countries benefit from such an approach, as infectious diseases will continue to ignore jurisdictional boundaries and all populations remain susceptible to novel diseases that emerge. And these same member countries must determine their comfort level with a funding structure that forces WHO to constantly navigate the interface of politics and public health. A largely donor-driven agenda places global public health in peril if WHO is driven too heavily by politics rather than science. On the other hand, the door remains open for new funders to emerge—potentially even partnerships or funding consortiums that transcend country-level politics and span governments, civil society, and the private sector—to provide capital that allows WHO to address the world's most pressing global public health priorities.

Conclusion

The COVID-19 pandemic will bring fundamental changes to the conceptualization of global health security, but it is much too early to understand any long-term impacts. After the world experienced SARS in the early 2000s, some believed that a new world order relative to public health was imminent. Populations became skilled at implementing public health practices, such as wearing face coverings and social distancing, and WHO's IHRs were revised. While some global systems were strengthened, the COVID-19 pandemic has proven that the world's reaction to SARS was not nearly strong enough. After SARS, governments failed to fully internalize the lesson that public health is not merely a domestic policy issue—it must join governments' foreign policy agendas.

While society is in the midst of the current pandemic, heightened interest in public health preparedness and response must be channeled by policy makers. A window has opened in which leaders can address at least some of the factors that contributed to the origins of the COVID-19 pandemic, but this opportunity is fleeting. Leaders should use this period to look beyond the high-profile response and toward the next pandemic. Now is the time to ensure that all stages of the disaster cycle are accounted for, in terms of planning, resources, and infrastructure. Unless public health preparedness systems throughout the world are strengthened, any given country is at risk; infectious disease outbreaks require much more than lines on a map for containment.

As the world moves forward and envisions a post-COVID-19 era, science and politics will inevitably intermingle. Public health is inherently political for many reasons, including the frequent tension between government action to protect the health of a population and respect for the autonomy of individuals. It would be too simplistic to suggest that governments are now ready to view global public health through a purely technocratic lens. But it would also be incorrect to assume that politics alone will determine whether the world will be better prepared for the next pandemic. To surmount today's geopolitical and ideological fractures, new collaborations, coalitions, and networks—perhaps some that cannot yet be fully imagined—will be needed. Such innovative partnerships may hold the key to spanning the political divide, fortifying WHO, and contributing to a world order that recognizes and responds effectively to infectious disease threats.

NOTES

1. "Disease Outbreaks by Year," World Health Organization, accessed June 22, 2020, https://www.who.int/csr/don/archive/year/en/.

2. "What Is Public Health?," CDC Foundation, accessed June 22, 2020, https://www.cdcfoundation.org/what-public-health.

3. David D. Celentano and Moyses Szklo, *Gordis Epidemiology* (Philadelphia: Elsevier, 2019), 2–5.

4. "National Profile of Local Health Departments," National Association of County and City Health Officials, accessed June 22, 2020, http://nacchoprofilestudy.org/wp-content/uploads/2017/10/Summary_Report_Oct2017_Final.pdf.

5. James M. Shultz and Sandro Galea, "Mitigating the Mental and Physical Health Consequences of Hurricane Harvey," *JAMA* 318, no. 15 (2017): 1437–38.

6. Megan McHugh, Andrea B. Staiti, and Laurie E. Felland, "How Prepared Are Americans for Public Health Emergencies? Twelve Communities Weigh In," *Health Affairs* 23, no. 3 (2004): 201–9.

7. Crystal R. Watson, Matthew Watson, and Tara Kirk Sell, "Public Health Preparedness Funding: Key Programs and Trends from 2001 to 2017," *American Journal of Public Health* 107, no. S2 (2017): S165–67.

8. Daniel A. Farber, "International Law and the Disaster Cycle," in *The International Law of Disaster Relief*, ed. David D. Caron, Michael J. Kelly, and Anastasia Telesetsky (Cambridge: Cambridge University Press, 2014), 9–10.

9. "History of Quarantine," Centers for Disease Control and Prevention, accessed June 22, 2020, https://www.cdc.gov/quarantine/historyquarantine.html.

10. Jacobson v. Massachusetts, 197 U.S. 11 (1905).

11. Lawrence O. Gostin, Eric A. Friedman, and Sarah A. Wetter, "Responding to COVID-19: How to Navigate a Public Health Emergency Legally and Ethically," *Hastings Center Report* 50, no. 2 (2020): 8–12.

12. Evan D. Anderson and James G. Hodge Jr., "Emergency Legal Preparedness among Select U.S. Local Governments," *Disaster Medicine and Public Health Preparedness* 3, Supp. 2 (2009): S176–84.

13. "The Model State Emergency Health Powers Act," Center for Law and the Public's Health, accessed June 22, 2020, https://www.jhsph.edu/research/centers-and-institutes/center-for-law-and-the-publics-health/model_laws/MSEHPA.pdf.

14. "Report & Model," Global Health Security Index, accessed June 22, 2020, https://www.ghsindex.org/report-model/.

15. "Constitution of the World Health Organization," World Health Organization, accessed June 22, 2020, https://apps.who.int/gb/bd/PDF/bd47/EN/constitution-en.pdf?ua=1.

16. "What We Do," World Health Organization, accessed June 22, https://www.who.int/about/what-we-do.

17. "Classification of Diseases (ICD)," World Health Organization, accessed June 22, 2020, https://www.who.int/classifications/icd/en/.

18. "The Smallpox Eradication Programme—SEP (1966–1980)," World Health Organization, accessed June 23, 2020, https://www.who.int/features/2010/smallpox/en/.

19. "The WHO Programme Budget Portal," World Health Organization, accessed June 23, 2020, http://open.who.int/2020-21/home.

20. "How WHO Is Funded," World Health Organization, accessed June 22, 2020, https://www.who.int/about/planning-finance-and-accountability/how-who-is-funded.

21. World Health Organization, "How WHO Is Funded."

22. World Health Organization, *International Health Regulations* (Geneva: WHO Press, 2005).

23. World Health Organization, *International Health Regulations*, 9.

24. World Health Organization, *International Health Regulations*, 14–15.

25. Carlos Castillo-Chavez, Roy Curtiss, Peter Daszak, Simon A. Levin, Oscar Patterson-Lomba, Charles Perrings, George Poste, and Sherry Towers, "Beyond Ebola: Lessons to Mitigate Future Pandemics," *Lancet Global Health* 3, no. 7 (2015): E354–55.

26. John W. Kingdon, *Agendas, Alternatives, and Public Policies* (London: Pearson, 2010).

27. Frank R. Baumgartner, Christian Breunig, Christoffer Green-Pedersen, Bryan D. Jones, Peter B. Mortensen, Michiel Nuytemans, and Stefaan Walgrave, "Punctuated Equilibrium in Comparative Perspective," *American Journal of Political Science* 53, no. 3 (2009): 603–20.

28. Kingdon, *Agendas, Alternatives, and Public Policies*.

29. Coronavirus Aid, Relief, and Economic Security Act, H.R. 748, 116th Congress (2020).

30. "At Least 80 Million Children under One at Risk of Diseases Such as Diphtheria, Measles, and Polio as COVID-19 Disrupts Routine Vaccination Efforts, Warn Gavi, WHO, and UNICEF," World Health Organization, accessed June 23, 2020, https://www.who.int /news-room/detail/22-05-2020-at-least-80-million-children-under-one-at-risk-of-diseases -such-as-diphtheria-measles-and-polio-as-covid-19-disrupts-routine-vaccination-efforts -warn-gavi-who-and-unicef.

31. "COVID-19 Dashboard," Johns Hopkins Coronavirus Resource Center, accessed June 23, 2020, https://coronavirus.jhu.edu/map.html.

32. Xianding Deng et al., "Genomic Surveillance Reveals Multiple Introductions of SARS-CoV-2 into Northern California," *Science* (2020), doi:10.1126/science.abb9263.

33. "About Us: PEPFAR," US Department of State, accessed June 23, 2020, https:// www.state.gov/about-us-pepfar/.

34. "The Administration's Response to Ebola," White House of President Barack Obama (archival website), https://obamawhitehouse.archives.gov/ebola-response.

35. Greg Myre, "With Trump's Coronavirus Response, U.S. Forfeits Global Leadership Role," National Public Radio, last modified April 30, 2020, https://www.npr.org/2020/04 /30/848179346/pandemic-fuels-debate-trumps-america-first-or-u-s-global-leadership.

36. Gwendolyn L. Gilbert, "SARS, MERS, and COVID-19—New Threats; Old Lessons," *International Journal of Epidemiology* (2020), doi.org/10.1093/ije/dyaa061.

37. "The COVID-19 Crisis: Policy Lessons from East Asia," COVID-19 Policy Research Task Force, Reischauer Center for East Asian Studies, Johns Hopkins University School of Advanced International Studies, last modified April 2020, https://www.reischauercenter .org/reischauercenter/wp-content/uploads/The-COVID-19-Crisis-Policy-Lessons-from -East-Asia-FINAL.pdf.

38. David P. Fidler, *SARS, Governance and the Globalization of Disease* (New York: Palgrave Macmillan, 2004).

39. Institute of Medicine, *Learning from SARS: Preparing for the Next Disease Outbreak: Workshop Summary* (Washington, DC: National Academies Press, 2004).

40. Chelsea Clinton and Devi Sridhar, *Governing Global Health* (New York: Oxford University Press, 2017).

41. "WHO Timeline—COVID-19", World Health Organization, last modified April 2020, https://www.who.int/news-room/detail/27-04-2020-who-timeline—covid-19.

42. World Health Organization, "#China has reported to WHO a cluster of #pneumonia cases—with no deaths—in Wuhan, Hubei Province," Twitter, January 4, 2020, https://twitter.com/WHO/status/1213523866703814656?s=20.

43. "Pneumonia of Unknown Cause—China," World Health Organization, January 5, 2020, https://www.who.int/csr/don/05-january-2020-pneumonia-of-unkown-cause-china/en/.

44. "Statement on the Second Meeting of the International Health Regulations (2005) Emergency Committee regarding the Outbreak of Novel Coronavirus (2019-nCoV)," World Health Organization, last modified January 30, 2020, https://www.who.int/news-room/detail/30-01-2020-statement-on-the-second-meeting-of-the-international-health-regulations-(2005)-emergency-committee-regarding-the-outbreak-of-novel-coronavirus-(2019-ncov).

45. World Health Organization, "WHO Timeline."

46. Chris Buckley, "Chinese Doctor, Silenced after Warning of Outbreak, Dies from Coronavirus," *New York Times*, February 6, 2020, https://www.nytimes.com/2020/02/06/world/asia/chinese-doctor-Li-Wenliang-coronavirus.html.

47. World Health Organization, "WHO Timeline."

48. World Health Organization, *International Health Regulations*, 1.

49. World Health Organization, "How WHO Is Funded."

50. Laura Kelly, "China to Donate Additional $30M to WHO following U.S. Halt in Funding," *The Hill*, April 23, 2020, https://thehill.com/policy/international/494310-china-to-donate-additional-30m-to-who-following-us-halt-in-funding.

51. Michael D. Shear, "Trump Attacks W.H.O. over Criticisms of U.S. Approach to Coronavirus," *New York Times*, April 7, 2020, https://www.nytimes.com/2020/04/07/us/politics/coronavirus-trump-who.html.

52. "International Health Regulations Enter into Force," World Health Organization, last modified June 14, 2007, https://www.who.int/mediacentre/news/releases/2007/pr31/en/.

Chapter Six

Bioethics in a Post-COVID World

Time for Future-Facing Global Health Ethics

Jeffrey P. Kahn, Anna C. Mastroianni,
and Sridhar Venkatapuram

The global COVID-19 pandemic posed a multitude of ethics challenges as the realities of the public health emergency became apparent. Issues confronted ranged from the allocation of scarce medical resources to questions about the proper balance of civil liberties and public health–related restrictions to concerns over the harms and benefits of social distancing weighed against those of reopening certain parts of societies. Many faculty in academic bioethics programs across the United States and around the world were asked to help address these and other issues, creating an unprecedented demand for ethics input and analysis. Some issues were familiar to American bioethics scholars. Others were beyond the range of issues and contexts that they typically consider, leading to requests for help from colleagues and participation in collaborative efforts that reflected multidisciplinary perspectives necessary to tackle the problems' complexities. These efforts helped respond to the issues faced by institutions and states, and to

Jeffrey P. Kahn, PhD, MPH, is the Andreas C. Dracopoulos Director of the Johns Hopkins Berman Institute of Bioethics, the Levi Professor of Bioethics and Public Policy, and a professor in the Department of Health Policy and Management in the Johns Hopkins Bloomberg School of Public Health. Anna C. Mastroianni, JD, MPH, is a professor of law at the University of Washington School of Law and associate director of the University of Washington Institute for Public Health Genetics. Sridhar Venkatapuram, PhD, FFPH, is an associate professor of global health and philosophy at King's College London and director of global health education and training at King's Global Health Institute.

a limited extent the federal government, but left unaddressed issues at the international and global levels.

COVID-19 raises global challenges, however, and in this chapter we reflect on the need for the field to address the real and pressing challenges in the global arena. The pandemic has highlighted our interconnectedness and interdependency; it has compelled thinking about ethics and its relationship to health within and across countries, which requires greater coordination and cooperation in a world that seems geopolitically fractured. It has also exposed the limitations of the historically dominant approaches to bioethics, pointing to a need for approaches that take seriously and engage deeply the concerns of social justice and health equity—concerns that, during the COVID-19 response, have relevance for everything from decisions about the triage of lifesaving resources to global health policy. Bioethics needs to do better, and we argue in this chapter that this means a renewed focus on a global health ethics that recognizes and takes account of the realities highlighted by the pandemic: focusing on health, not just health care; health equity, not just allocation of scarce resources; and social justice, not just distributive justice.

Bioethics Challenges during the COVID-19 Pandemic

The pandemic has brought many issues to the surface that the majority of bioethics scholars were not mindful of or thought were not core to their work. The work of bioethics evolved for good reasons to focus on biomedical ethics and research ethics, mostly distinctive from the ethics of public health and health policy. As a function of the evolution of the field, the professionals working in it were primarily appointed in academic medical centers. In these environments the work of bioethics has been primarily, if not exclusively, focused on clinical ethics and on researching questions amenable to empirical research projects, and it has had little to do with scholars working on questions of health policy and public health practice, who are often appointed in completely different parts of universities. The field's functional divisions have created a false but understandable dichotomy between clinical or bedside ethics issues and issues of policy, thereby reifying unhelpful silos.

The effects of years of disconnection and narrow focus were made obvious when the pandemic and its consequences uncovered numerous urgent ethical issues that needed to be addressed, and bioethics scholars were asked to lend their expertise and, in some cases, to help guide the response. Some issues appeared on their surface to be familiar for bioethics, such as the allocation of resources made scarce by insufficient supply (such as personal protective equipment) or by unprecedented demand (such as ventilators and beds in intensive care units). Those are matters that parallel long-standing work on how to equitably distribute the limited number of solid organs available among the many patients whose lives could be saved by transplants. But while allocation of kidneys is amenable to a national waiting list, and access to livers relies on a system of increasing priority that allows patients to wait their turn until they become sickest and therefore first in line, COVID-19 required a plan for triage rather than allocation.

Physicians, nurses, hospital administrators, and clinical ethicists are steeped in prioritizing the best interests of individual patients and in promoting autonomous decision making by patients. But they were suddenly faced with the prospect of a surge in COVID-19 patients so large that it would swamp supplies of lifesaving resources and force triage decisions on a scale incompatible with patient-centered decision making. The questions that hospitals and health systems faced were more like population-level questions familiar to public health policy experts than like the decisions typically made in tertiary care medical centers. Discussions focused on how to balance the interests of individuals against societal goals such as saving the most lives possible. Those questions are much more tractable when applying utilitarian, communitarian, and other distributive and relational justice approaches to ethics than when applying mainstream bioethics principles such as respect for persons and beneficence. To take on these unprecedented challenges, teams with relevant expertise were rapidly convened. Clinicians, hospital leadership, attorneys, clinical ethicists, and scholars in ethics and public health policy worked together for the first time in their careers to take up questions of how to allocate scarce resources, whose input to seek, what frameworks to apply, how to implement the application of consensus approaches, how to do so consistently and across hospitals and systems, and how to resolve who should bear ultimate responsibility for what were likely to be life and death decisions.

The bioethics community has learned several important lessons as a function of the time spent working on these issues. First, connections between work on clinical ethics and hospital system or government health policy questions, which had seemed forced or manufactured at best, now seem critically entwined and integral to answering the ethical demands of the pandemic. Second, the dominant approaches to bioethics cannot adequately address questions that combine taking account of the individual needs of patients and the interests of others in society, including the gross inequities caused by health and income disparities. Doing so requires much deeper consideration and inclusion of community- and population-level perspectives and approaches for incorporating them. Those two lessons amount to a sort of reckoning for bioethics, demanding a reconsideration of how bioethics work is conceptualized, its proper areas of focus, and the approaches needed to address them.

A Pivot for Bioethics

We propose that the answer is health ethics, to encompass clinical ethics, research ethics, public health ethics, population health ethics, and global health ethics. Health, in this context, is not limited to health care but instead comprises a broader concept about populations and individuals being able to protect themselves from harm and be free from illness or injury. Such abilities are much more influenced by pervasive social determinants than by access to medical care.[1] That pivot requires applying a broader lens of a social contract and its implications for distributing the benefits and burdens of living together in a society; it encompasses more than individual rights and, in particular, more than the focus on negative rights (liberties) that is a feature of American social policy and public discourse. It means a renewed focus on health equity, on the social sources of health disparities and their disproportionate impacts, and on the issues of social justice that they invoke. The decades-long attention to global health security is germane in that it acknowledges the relevance and importance of securing the health of populations. But it is animated by interests of national security and a watchfulness for new and resurgent threats rather than by social justice for the populations experiencing endemic health deprivations and likely to be most affected by new health threats.

To make this pivot, however, requires increased social recognition of the importance of protecting and improving the health of individuals and populations on par with other social goals such as growing the economy, ensuring national security, and protecting civil liberties. The health of the American population lags behind that of most wealthy countries and is not commensurate with the outcomes expected from such lavish annual spending on health care. At over $3 trillion per year, the United States spends far and away more money on health care than any country in the world. Yet the average level of health and health inequalities is worse than in other countries, including some low- and middle-income countries (LMICs). Part of the reason is that not every citizen in the United States has access to health care, which is also where the US stands apart from all other industrialized countries. At the same time, good health is not the same as having access to health care. The persistence of health inequalities in other countries with universal access to health care evidences that lesson. It would be easy to say that the United States does not value health as much as it does other social goals such as economic growth or domestic and national security, but then why spend so much on health care? One possible explanation is that, in the United States, health has become a personal consumption good. That is, health is seen as something that is an attribute of the individual, and good or bad health is largely a function of the natural lottery combined with personal behavior. Health care is therefore a personal good to be consumed and is accessed by the ability to pay for it, either individually or through government provision. This account of the "American health disadvantage" gives little attention to the profound and pervasive social determinants of health.[2] This may in part explain why social support programs and public health infrastructure are relatively neglected. Research in the United States about the health impacts of social conditions and relationships has largely been a niche subject of public health academics, health foundations, and government reports.[3]

Mounting evidence of the health and social effects of the pandemic in the United States and around the world makes clear the need for new priorities that take into account how health disparities, food and housing security, employment, schools, and basic nutrition have an outsize impact on health separately and almost always in combination. From a traditional bioethics perspective, there are limited intellectual resources to analyze or support a focus on health ethics as we describe it, even with a focus just on the United States, let alone a transnational or global focus. Even with a more expansive intellectual scope, the traditional domain of American bioethics is health care and biomedical research done in institutions with policies discussed locally and nationally but rarely globally. What can bioethicists say about the relations within a country during an infectious outbreak or about how different countries and international organizations should relate to each other during a pandemic? To answer such questions we must first understand how bioethics came to focus on the range of issues it does.

The Limits of American Bioethics

Bioethics is a relatively young interdisciplinary field, with most accounts pointing to its emergence in the United States in the late 1960s.[4] It was a time of social, cultural, and political change in the aftermath of World War II, marked by many features including a new emphasis on individual rights—civil rights, consumer rights, patient rights—and their protection. The same postwar period also saw an explosion in government-funded biomedical research and an ensuing recognition of the need for ethics guidelines for its conduct.

An important aspect of the early history of American bioethics is how its emergence and evolution were greatly influenced by biomedical research scandals. Most notable is the 1972 exposé of a forty-year US government study of untreated syphilis in African Americans in the rural South, often referred to as the Tuskegee Syphilis Study.[5] The revelations that impoverished African American men were deceived into participating in a research project with no benefit to them and that the men involved were deprived of available treatment in the pursuit of biomedical knowledge about syphilis prompted the US Congress to pass the National Research Act of 1974 to address ethical oversight in human subjects research. This law included the establishment of the influential National Commission for the Protection of Human Subjects of Biomedical and Behavioral Research (1974–78), which was asked "to identify the basic ethical principles that should underlie the conduct of biomedical and behavioral research involving human subjects and to develop guidelines which should be followed to assure that such research is conducted in accordance with those principles."[6] The commission also produced a seminal document, commonly referred to as the *Belmont Report*, which articulated ethical principles that would not only inform the outcome of the commission's task but also would have an outsize influence on the evolution of the field.

In at least one telling, as the members of the commission trained in philosophy and theology worked to identify relevant basic ethical principles, they realized that their training and individual commitments to particular theoretical approaches to ethics made it unlikely that they could all agree on one conceptual approach that would then help in deriving basic principles.[7] Eschewing the selection of one ethical theory, they instead achieved consensus on midlevel principles that would be consistent with a range of theoretical approaches. These principles included respect for persons, beneficence (providing benefit and minimizing harm), and justice. This principle-based approach worked well in answering the particular research ethics questions posed to the commission, and an expanded and more deeply developed version was then used to address other applied ethics questions across biomedicine.[8]

As new rules were promulgated for research, new ethics requirements were also established for the accreditation of hospitals, and new educational requirements were established to include ethics in medical school curricula, often with the principle-based approach at their core (autonomy, beneficence, nonmaleficence, and justice). Bioethics as a field became professionally embedded in academic medicine, emphasizing issues arising in clinical ethics and research ethics. As professors of bioethics advanced in their careers as medical school faculty, success often required research funding from the US National Institutes of Health, which meant focusing on research priorities as articulated in calls for research, dominated by ethics and genomics and ethics and biomedical research. Bioethics faculty joined a growing group of professionals who could help apply policies, lead ethics committees, teach ethics to health professionals, and successfully compete for government grants, all while using the approach that had become dominant if not standard.

American bioethics, and to the extent it was adopted outside the United States, is in part a product of all these factors—its US origins in biomedical research and reactive policy making, the dominance of the principle-based approach, its emergence during a time of growth of individual rights, its professionalization, and its embeddedness in the academic biomedical enterprise. The demands and incentives created by those factors would affect the framing and choices in bioethics as a field in the coming decades—a framing that would, for the most part, ignore a conceptualization of bioethics approaches that could accommodate a more expansive view of health as a global and social justice issue. For example, issues of power, vulnerability, privilege, and systemic disadvantage have not been framed as central to the work of mainstream American bioethics. Many in bioethics have wrongly and comfortably assumed that the empowerment of individuals through informed consent processes and through applications of the ethical principle of respect for autonomy would adequately address power imbalances.[9] This presumably included systemic power differentials related to gender, race, disability, and other social categories of disadvantage. Feminist bioethics scholars, among others, have challenged the principle-based approach as it fails to adequately account for relationships of power and authority.[10] But even those challenges tended to be framed by issues of ethics and medicine, not health and society.

Appeals to broaden bioethicists' attention to a broader conceptualization of health and social justice have also come from individuals concerned about the racism and health inequities experienced by African Americans. Such pleas, for the most part, have been acknowledged but not been considered core issues to be addressed by mainstream bioethics. Annette Dula, for example, argued in 1991 for paying attention to issues of social equity, contending that the demographic makeup of bioethicists, dominated by "white, male, middle-class professionals and academics," narrowed the priorities and foci of the field to the exclusion of issues and perspectives relevant to racial and ethnic groups, poor people, and women.[11] And, prior to the pandemic, Marion Danis and colleagues used incidents of police violence against Blacks to draw attention to the urgent need for bioethicists to address structural injustice.[12]

Infectious diseases, with their potential for local impacts and global scope, were also overlooked in the formative period of bioethics, leaving bioethicists without the tools for their conceptual consideration.[13] HIV/AIDS offered opportunities to expand the remit of bioethics. But, surprisingly, few bioethicists engaged with HIV/AIDS or with its numerous social dimensions. With a few exceptions, the ethics of infectious diseases such as HIV/AIDS were initially shaped as domestic discussions and focused on confidentiality and professional obligations in a clinical context or on the ethics of HIV research in the developing world.[14] Later on, discussions about HIV/AIDS addressed research exploitation and the exportation of risk in LMICs.[15] Instead, the real ethical work around HIV/AIDS took place among activists and on the global stage. HIV/AIDS activists transformed the methodology of drug trials so that the drugs would reach patients faster, protested against governments that were unresponsive, and sought to ensure access to drugs by patients in LMICs. A global turning point was in 2001 when the United Nations General Assembly held a special session on HIV/AIDS, the first time for a health issue. It is here that HIV/AIDS became narrowly and politically framed as a global security threat, and so even at this level and opportunity, the first modern pandemic was not perceived as a bioethics issue.[16]

With some exceptions,[17] bioethics discussions about health as global and social justice issues were situated in public health schools and predominantly within the small field of public health ethics.[18] The focus of that work tended to be on domestic public health policy rather than global health. The few notable voices calling for global health ethics to be a focus of bioethics were received as identifying issues outside the mainstream and went largely unheeded.[19]

The field of bioethics was in large part disconnected from ongoing discussions, both domestically and on the world stage, of health policy issues such as rights to health care and certainly about rights to *health*. Those parallel discussions were happening, however, in political philosophy, human rights, law, and global development.[20] Reorienting bioethics—to attend more to health, not health care; to health equity, not allocation of scarce resources; to social justice, not distributive justice; to the effects of the pandemic, its emergence at a time of increasing nationalism, and its disparate racial impacts in the context of the Black Lives Matter movement—is required for a bioethics that is ready to address the challenges of a post-COVID world.

Global Health Ethics—a Bioethics for the Post-COVID World

It became clear by mid-March 2020 that the COVID-19 pandemic was going to be of a scale and nature very different from recent pandemics such as SARS, MERS, and H1N1. National responses to the pandemic in the form of shutting down most international trade and travel as well as many social activities through national "lockdowns" would be devastating to many countries in the short term and for years to come. As weeks progressed, it also began to be clear that diverse global and domestic dynamics could also have destabilizing impacts on the existing world order. That both Henry Kissinger and Mikhail Gorbachev, along with other senior statesmen and stateswomen around the world, published public statements about the need for giving attention to the global order signaled that responding to this phenomenon required more than science, money, and, even, pandemic ethics.[21] So, does the discipline of bioethics, and ethics more broadly, have something to contribute to analyzing and stabilizing the world order, or even to making it better? And, more specifically, can ethical resources and reasoning help address the role that health could or should have in stabilizing or reforming the world order?

Some international relations scholars may understand and integrate the pandemic as a new kind of global threat that requires mitigating and managing. That is, the pandemic is background music to the dominant issues of US-China relations or waning American influence in the global arena. There is another view that has more room for ethics, particularly related to human health and well-being. Gorbachev, as well as others, has come to recognize that world order needs to be reformed and centered on human well-being. He writes, "The overriding goal must be human security: providing food, water and a clean environment and caring for people's health."[22] And Dani Rodrik argues that "hyper-globalization" was too focused on trade and investment to the neglect of public health, and it was coming to an end even before the pandemic. A new, well-crafted globalization is needed that is centered on human rights, climate change, and public health.[23]

This focus on human well-being as the foundation of world order, or at least as a prominent part of global cooperation, is not novel. Emphasizing human well-being as the right target of global institutions and cooperation has motivated various efforts such as the United Nations' human security agenda advocated by the Japanese government.[24] And recent efforts to identify and promote cooperation around global public goods have been led by international agencies such as the United Nations Development Program, World Bank, and International Monetary Fund.[25] There have also been efforts to motivate national governments to go beyond aggregate macroeconomic indicators and focus on human well-being. These have included high-profile international commissions and the creation of new measures to assess the state and progress of countries, such as the Better Life Index of the Organisation for Economic Co-operation and Development.[26] While these efforts have aimed to put human well-being at the center of the work of international organizations, global cooperation agendas, and even national programs, they have not taken root. Growth in gross domestic product, international trade and investment, financial globalization, and, of course, national security have been hard to dislodge as primary concerns in the relations among countries.

Perhaps it is the depth of the near-universal shock to all governments and societies as well as to most international organizations that has created an opening to consider fundamental questions about the world order post-COVID. The lack of a robust, coordinated effort among nation-states and other global actors, and the continued neglect of public health in some of the weakest countries in the world, would mean more waves of the pandemic or would mean that the virus keeps circulating in the world, indefinitely threatening all countries. Epidemics and pandemics are also unpredictable. Depending on how the pandemic continues to evolve in the world, and how various countries respond domestically and abroad, this pandemic or worse pandemics to come could further destabilize geographic regions and world order.

The fast progression of the COVID pandemic is bewildering to bioethicists and global justice philosophers as much as it is to academics studying the world order. What is, or should be, apparent to all is that the spread of deadly infections makes patently visible the current state of interconnectedness of all human beings on this planet. Despite long-standing debates about globalization, it was largely understood as a phenomenon of trade and finance or, perhaps, of the clash of cultures. A virus being passed from person to person across borders makes global interconnectedness tangible, and personal vulnerability from being interconnected is immediately palpable. At the same time, it is a significant observation in itself that global interconnectedness helps transmit direct harms alongside many of the good things such as faster travel, exchange of ideas, greater economic prosperity, and alleviation of poverty.

A second related but distinct aspect that has become more visible is the interdependency of societies. Many Anglo-American global ethics and justice philosophers have up to now viewed the world as a group of distinct, self-contained entities. This is perhaps an understandable extension of theorizing about social justice in terms of self-contained individuals. As such, global ethics and justice have focused largely on possible rights and obligations across national borders, particularly between rich and poor countries. To state it simplistically, many global ethics and justice philosophers have focused on the question, What do we owe to distant strangers, particularly the poorest?[27] This pandemic challenges such a framing of the main problem in global ethics in a few ways. The pandemic has explicitly shown that all persons on this planet are interconnected across borders. And through those interconnections, we are made vulnerable to grievous harms and death. Moreover, it is likely that we have also passed on harms to other people in other countries. For example, by hosting one or more major international airports, wealthy countries—which previously were the benevolent actors in global ethics—have likely enabled the spread of the virus to other countries, particularly low-income countries that will suffer enormously.

And beyond receiving and transmitting harms, it is fairly well evident from the basic epidemiology of the pandemic that no single country or group of countries can contain the pandemic by themselves. No country can control the pandemic within its own borders and remain protected without all other countries also controlling the spread in their own countries. Interconnectedness, and interdependency, makes coordinated global action necessary to contain the pandemic everywhere. And not just the cooperation of a few countries but of all countries is needed to protect every country for as long as necessary. Benevolence or even humanitarian ethics is not the appropriate ethical resource to draw on in this situation. The necessity for and benefits of cooperative action at a global level have previously been identified regarding many other global issues such as climate change, nuclear proliferation, and illicit drug trafficking. But the distinctiveness of this pandemic is that it makes more prominent the interconnectedness and interdependency of all human beings, while producing a sense of urgency that is due to the imminent threat to bodily health, possibly leading to the deaths of untold thousands. And importantly, social interactions within and across borders will, in fact, be more necessary for societies to recover from the economic and social devastation.

It is this perspective of joint living on this planet, and of having intertwined destinies, that compels us to ask, So how should we live together? This is the mainstay of the philosophy of social and global justice and of particular theories of social contract and distributive justice. In the social contract tradition, a theory aims to identify the rules of social cooperation that fairly distribute benefits and burdens across all involved parties. The most famous modern Anglo-American proponent of the social contract approach to social justice was, of course, John Rawls.[28] Rawls identified a set of "primary goods," certain socially produced goods that serve as all-purpose means for every person to pursue their diverse life plans. Rawls also identified some rules for how these valuable goods should be distributed across individuals. But there are two significant weaknesses to Rawls's seminal theory. He had trouble with a global social contract, and he had trouble with health, even at the domestic level.[29] He pursued a methodology in which he theorized about social justice in a world where there is only one society. After he presented a theory of one ideal society, he then theorized the rules that might govern a world of many societies, each with diverse domestic arrangements, values, and cultures. As a result, he produced a set of minimal rules, and they were far from a global social contract. And regarding health, despite health being so valued by human beings and instrumental on a daily basis to their life plans, Rawls did not place health on the list of valuable goods. This is because he believed that health was a "natural good," something that one is born with or that is affected by personal behavior and luck. The possibility that health or disease and death could be produced or destroyed by social interactions, through the very rules he was seeking to devise, was not part of his reasoning. Such an understanding of health is not a failing unique to Rawls, nor is this social dimension of health just related to infectious diseases.

While a potentially fatal virus being passed from person to person across borders and within borders shows our interconnectedness and interdependency, the same also holds true for the spread of noncommunicable diseases. At the global level, along with many kinds of viruses and biological organisms that are passed across borders daily (e.g., flu), other health harms are also created and distributed through social relations, practices, norms, and neglect. International trade regulations that constrain the ability of countries to restrict or regulate things such as tobacco, alcohol, high-caloric low-nutritious foods, and so forth contribute to the causal chain of poor health of people in particular places—as do various kinds of transnational systems and practices that enable illicit financial flows out of LMICs or the emigration of health care workers. This type of interconnectedness, or causal chains, directly affecting health has been recognized and experienced for decades, particularly in LMICs. But this notion of our health as being affected by events in distant countries and by the functioning of global systems, practices, and institutions is being newly recognized by many citizens of industrialized countries, where the long global chain of causes may have been obfuscated.

The role of ethics in health and world order, then, is to provide moral guidance for the political processes and structures that distribute benefits and burdens across societies. It cannot simply be about how to distribute health care or conduct research in other places. And, unlike human rights law, which has also sought to provide guidance but has historically focused on the relationship between governments and their citizens, the scope of ethics can encompass a whole range of diverse actors that now exist and operate at the transnational global level. Nevertheless, while ethics or global ethics may be the right register from which to address issues regarding world order and the place of health, this is also the time to re-imagine global health ethics and bioethics. What does a theory of global ethics or justice look like that starts from interconnectedness and interdependency across borders and that puts human health and well-being at the foundation of global relations?

The existing approaches addressing health in foreign nations as a matter of charity and humanitarianism, or for commercial interest, or for national security have been at least inadequate and, arguably, misguided. We would not be here, in the middle of a global health emergency, if these previous approaches were effective. And global justice philosophers have also been waylaid by the issue of national sovereignty. The debates seemed to be polarized, with one pole centered on justice as being applicable only with a domestic political border and shared social institutions. The other pole is centered on the equal treatment of all individuals irrespective of where we find them, with substantial obligations across national borders to support the well-being of all people. While few if any global justice philosophers see national borders and sovereignty as an all-or-nothing issue, there has been little progress in over a decade on where the balance is between associative duties to compatriots versus general duties to foreigners as well as on the ideal system of global governance.[30]

The renewed recognition of the interdependency of all countries means that to protect ourselves we must also raise the level of health of the worst-off people and countries in the world, not for the sake of benevolence or to fulfill our obligations to ensure their minimal well-being. The continuation of their vulnerabilities to this present pandemic and future outbreaks means that they have the potential to become everyone's health threats. The present pandemic did not originate in some poor region in a poor country. It originated in a large city of a major economic power. There have been disease outbreaks in the United States, and with growing anti-vaccination movements, the likelihood of more is increasing. And, with that, there is the potential of spreading disease to other countries. So our interdependency requires good global citizenship, or reciprocity across all countries. Charity, commercial enterprise, or security approaches do not address all the sources of pandemic threats in other countries or other kinds of potential health threats. Rather, a recognition of shared mutual destinies, and fairness in the global distribution of benefits and burdens, has more likelihood of containing this pandemic and creating global resilience against future pandemics and health emergencies. It is also the right way to live together.

A shortsighted approach to our current global emergency and consideration of the effects on world order would be to understand it as a waiting game until a vaccine is found. At present, there is a global race under way to develop an effective vaccine against the coronavirus. Billions of dollars have been pledged for the research and development of a vaccine. And there is much rhetoric that the eventual vaccine(s) will be made available to all countries, in some way or another. A vaccine is indeed an urgent goal that must be pursued for the sake of preventing as many deaths and as much suffering as possible. But this is only one type of many deadly viruses that could either emerge or reemerge in the world. And this coronavirus is not the deadliest that is possible.[31] Even after containing this particular pandemic, national and global vulnerabilities to epidemics and pandemics will continue and perhaps increase even more. The economic and social devastation caused by the responses to this pandemic are erasing many hard-earned health gains in many LMICs, and many other infectious disease epidemics are ongoing. Low health and health resilience in any country, particularly as a result of this first wave of the pandemic, makes all countries vulnerable. And beyond vulnerability to another pandemic, it is now common knowledge around the world that the global relations among nation-states, the limited capacities of global institutions, and the lack of good global citizenship enable health harms to spread around the world. The current global order, in essence, is not good for the health of people. Indeed, as it stands, it is bad for certain countries and certain groups within countries.

It is because the pandemic has made evident both the structural inequities and inadequacies within countries and at the global level that we must reimagine global ethics. To avoid the error that Rawls made by starting with one society and then moving on to a world of societies, we must start with the global. The interconnectedness and interdependency across countries shape the health contexts within countries. That is, not only can health harms travel across countries; the world order, as it stands, creates and distributes harms within societies. Macroeconomists studying globalization and "economic contagion" have understood how economic harms travel from the global to the local for a while. And some epidemiologists, particularly social epidemiologists who study the global determinants of disease and death, also understand this. But global ethics and justice philosophers and bioethicists have been late to this realization. And even macroeconomists now recognize that they did not appreciate the public health dimension, assuming that investments in health meant health care. There is a profound role here for global political philosophy and ethics as a field to help build a better world order through reasoning about what the society of nations should be and how people in them should act toward each other, in light of their interconnectedness and shared destinies.

What can we do to fill the gaps and missing links and to enable people to do better global ethics and to put state-of-the-art knowledge about health at the center of the world order? There is an urgent need to build links at least among philosophical fields such as bioethics, public health ethics, and political philosophy. There also must be much stronger links between public health sciences and ethics. And importantly, there must be much better integration between public health schools and international relations departments, programs, and schools. As this pandemic has made clear, how disease spreads within countries is significantly affected by global institutions as well as by how various countries are willing or unwilling to cooperate across borders. Beyond the classroom, there need to be greater opportunities for internships and fellowships in professional settings across disciplines. For example, a bioethicist considers the research lab or hospital as a field site of training. Similarly, a public health ethicist or global ethics philosopher should have opportunities to spend time in settings where global policies are being shaped and implemented. This could be the US State Department or, indeed, the Global Fund or World Health Organization. And international relations practitioners should be able to spend time among bioethics and global health ethics scholars.

Conclusion

We have provided a brief description of the work that bioethics has been asked to take on in responding to the COVID-19 pandemic and the shortcomings in approaches to bioethics and political philosophy that the pandemic has exposed. The history and evolution of the field offer an explanation of the challenges that bioethics has faced in coming to grips with the global ethics issues that surfaced in the pandemic, and this explanation helps point the way toward an expanded scope for bioethics that includes global health ethics.

When the pandemic is under control, societies will be left with the knowledge that social structural inequities produce inequities in health, along with the understanding that global pandemic responses and resilience require governments and societies to be more just. Unfair global and social orders are not just bad for health. Health inequalities, and social responses necessary to sufficiently address pandemic threats, can devastate countries for years, affecting generations, and they threaten the global order. Health equity and human well-being must, therefore, be more of a central concern of global transformations under way and likely will need to be so for the foreseeable future.

NOTES

1. Donald M. Berwick, "The Moral Determinants of Health," *JAMA*, June 12, 2020, https://doi.org/10.1001/jama.2020.11129.

2. "Social Determinants of Health," World Health Organization, accessed July 7, 2020, http://www.who.int/social_determinants/en/.

3. Karen B. DeSalvo, Y. Claire Wang, Andrea Harris, John Auerbach, Denise Koo, and Patrick O'Carroll, "Public Health 3.0: A Call to Action for Public Health to Meet the Challenges of the 21st Century," *Preventing Chronic Disease* 14, no. 78 (2017), https://doi.org/10.5888/pcd14.170017; Secretary's Advisory Committee on National Health Promotion and Disease Prevention Objectives for 2020, "Healthy People 2020: An Opportunity to Address Societal Determinants of Health in the United States," US Department of Health and Human Services, last modified October 26, 2010; Paula Braveman and Laura Gottlieb, "The Social Determinants of Health: It's Time to Consider the Causes of the Causes," *Public Health Reports* 129, no. Suppl. 2 (2014): 19–31, https://www.ncbi.nlm.nih.gov/pmc/articles/PMC3863696/; "Social Determinants of Health," Robert Wood Johnson Foundation, accessed July 7, 2020, https://www.rwjf.org/en/our-focus-areas/topics/social-determinants-of-health.html; "Culture of Health Program," National Academy of Medicine, accessed July 7, 2020, https://nam.edu/programs/culture-of-health/.

4. See, e.g., Albert R. Jonsen, *The Birth of Bioethics* (New York: Oxford University Press, 2003).

5. James H. Jones, *Bad Blood* (New York: Simon and Schuster, 1993); Jonsen, *Birth of Bioethics.*

6. US Department of Health and Human Services, *Belmont Report*, last modified March 15, 2016, https://www.hhs.gov/ohrp/regulations-and-policy/belmont-report/index.html.

7. Tom L. Beauchamp, "The Origins and Evolution of the *Belmont Report*," in *Belmont Revisited: Ethical Principles for Research with Human Subjects*, eds. James F. Childress, Eric M. Meslin, and Harold T. Shapiro (Washington, DC: Georgetown University Press, 2005), 12–25; Tom L. Beauchamp, *Standing on Principles: Collected Essays* (New York: Oxford University Press, 2010).

8. Tom L. Beauchamp and James F. Childress, *Principles of Biomedical Ethics*, 7th ed. (New York: Oxford University Press. 2013).

9. Howard Brody, *The Future of Bioethics* (New York: Oxford University Press, 2009).

10. See, e.g., Susan Sherwin, *No Longer Patient: Feminist Ethics and Health Care* (Philadelphia: Temple University Press, 1992).

11. Annette Dula, "Toward an African-American Perspective on Bioethics," *Journal of Health Care for the Poor and Underserved* 2, no. 2 (Fall 1991): 259–69, https://doi.org/10.1353/hpu.2010.0399. See also Annette Dula and Sara Goering, eds., *"It Just Ain't Fair": The Ethics of Health Care for African Americans* (Westport, CT: Praeger, 1994).

12. Marion Danis, Yolonda Wilson, and Amina White, "Bioethicists Can and Should Contribute to Addressing Racism," *American Journal of Bioethics* 16, no. 4 (March 2016): 3–12, https://doi.org/10.1080/15265161.2016.1145283; Kayhan Parsi, "The Unbearable Whiteness of Bioethics: Exhorting Bioethicists to Address Racism," *American Journal of Bioethics* 16, no. 4 (March 2016): 1–2, https://doi.org/10.1080/15265161.2016.1159076.

13. Leslie P. Francis, Margaret P. Battin, Jay A. Jacobson, Charles B. Smith, and Jeffrey Botkin, "How Infectious Diseases Got Left Out—and What This Omission Might Have Meant for Bioethics," *Bioethics* 19, no. 4 (August 2005): 307–22, https://doi.org/10.1111/j.1467-8519.2005.00445.x; Margaret P. Battin, Leslie P. Francis, Jay A. Jacobson, and Charles B. Smith, *The Patient as Victim and Vector: Ethics and Infectious Disease* (New York: Oxford University Press, 2009); Michael J. Selgelid "Ethics and Infectious Disease," *Bioethics* 19, no. 3 (2005): 272–89, https://doi.org/10.1111/j.1467-8519.2005.00441.x.

14. R. Faden and N. Kass, "HIV Research, Ethics, and the Developing World," *American Journal of Public Health* 88, no. 4 (April 1998): 548–50, https://doi.org/10.2105/ajph.88.4.548; Francis, "How Infectious Diseases Got Left Out."

15. See, e.g., Ruth Macklin, *Double Standards in Medical Research in Developing Countries* (Cambridge: Cambridge University Press, 2004).

16. Stefan Elbe, *Strategic Implications of HIV/AIDS* (New York: Oxford University Press, 2003); John W. Dietrich, "The Politics of PEPFAR: The President's Emergency Plan for AIDS Relief," *Ethics & International Affairs* 21, no. 3 (2007): 277–92, https://doi.org/10.1111/j.1747-7093.2007.00100.x.

17. See, e.g., Dula, "Toward an African-American Perspective on Bioethics;" Dula and Goering, *"It Just Ain't Fair."*

18. See, e.g., D. E. Beauchamp, "Public Health as Social Justice," *Inquiry* 13, no. 1 (March 1976): 3–14; D. E. Beauchamp, "Community: The Neglected Tradition of Public Health," *Hastings Center Report* 15, no. 6 (December 1985): 28–36; Daniel I. Wikler, "Persuasion and Coercion for Health: Ethical Issues in Government Efforts to Change Life-Styles," *Milbank Quarterly* 56, no. 3 (1978): 303–38; Norman Daniels, *Just Health Care* (Cambridge: Cambridge University Press, 1985); J. D. Moreno and R. Bayer, "The Limits of the Ledger in Public Health Promotion," *Hastings Center Report* 15, no. 6 (December 1985): 37–41; R. Bayer and J. D. Moreno, "Health Promotion: Ethical and Social Dilemmas of Government Policy," *Health Affairs* 5, no. 2 (Summer 1986): 72–85, https://doi.org/10.1377/hlthaff.5.2.72; Ronald Bayer, *Private Acts, Social Consequences: AIDS and the Politics of Public Health* (New Brunswick, NJ: Rutgers University Press, 1989); S. R. Benatar, "Just Healthcare beyond Individualism: Challenges for North American Bioethics," *Cambridge Quarterly of Healthcare Ethics* 6, no. 4 (1997): 397–415, https://doi.org/10.1017/s0963180100008148; James F. Chil-

dress et al., "Public Health Ethics: Mapping the Terrain," *Journal of Law, Medicine & Ethics* 30, no. 2 (2002): 170–78, https://doi.org/10.1111/j.1748-720X.2002.tb00384.x; Ronald Bayer and Amy L. Fairchild, "The Genesis of Public Health Ethics," *Bioethics* 18, no. 6 (November 2004): 473–92, https://doi.org/10.1111/j.1467-8519.2004.00412.x; and Nancy E. Kass, "Public Health Ethics: From Foundations and Frameworks to Justice and Global Public Health," *Journal of Law, Medicine & Ethics* 32, no. 2 (2004): 232–42, https://doi.org/10.1111/j .1748-720x.2004.tb00470.x; Madison Power and Ruth Faden, *Social Justice: The Moral Foundations of Public Health and Health Policy* (New York: Oxford University Press, 2006).

19. See, e.g., Benatar, "Just Healthcare beyond Individualism"; S. Marchand, D. Wikler, and B. Landesman, "Class, Health and Justice," *Milbank Quarterly* 76, no. 3 (1998): 449–67, https://doi.org/10.1111/1468-0009.00098; Norman Daniels, Bruce P. Kennedy, and Ichiro Kawachi, "Why Justice Is Good for Our Health: The Social Determinants of Health Inequalities," *Daedalus* 128, no. 4 (1999): 215–51; Norman Daniels, "Equity and Population Health: Toward a Broader Bioethics Agenda," *Hastings Center Report* 36, no. 4 (2006): 22–35, https://doi.org/10.1353/hcr.2006.0058; Dan W Brock. "Broadening the Bioethics Agenda," *Kennedy Institute of Ethics Journal* 10, no. 1 (March 2000): 21–38; Solomon R. Benatar, Abdallah S. Daar, and Peter A. Singer, "Global Health Challenges: The Need for an Expanded Discourse on Bioethics," *PLOS Medicine* 2, no. 7 (July 2005): e143, https://doi .org/10.1371/journal.pmed.0020143; Joseph Millum and Ezekiel J. Emanuel, *Global Justice and Bioethics* (New York: Oxford University Press, 2012).

20. Amartya Sen, *Collective Choice and Social Welfare* (San Francisco: Holden Day, 1970); J. M. Mann, "Medicine and Public Health, Ethics and Human Rights," *Hastings Center Report* 27, no. 3 (1997): 6–13; Larry O. Gostin and Zita Lazzarini, *Human Rights and Public Health in the AIDS Pandemic* (New York: Oxford University Press, 1997); G. J. Annas, "Human Rights and Health—the Universal Declaration of Human Rights at 50," *New England Journal of Medicine* 339, no. 24 (December 10, 1998): 1778–81; Paul Farmer, *Pathologies of Power: Health, Human Rights, and the New War on the Poor* (Berkeley: University of California Press, 2003); Lawrence O. Gostin, *Public Health Law: Power, Duty, Restraint* (Berkeley: University of California Press, 2000); Henk ten Have, "The Activities of UNESCO in the Area of Ethics," *Kennedy Institute of Ethics Journal* 16, no. 4 (December 2006): 333–51, https://doi.org/10.1353/ken.2006.0024; Martha Nussbaum, *Frontiers of Justice: Disability, Nationality, Species Membership* (Cambridge, MA: Belknap Press of Harvard University Press, 2006); Sridhar Venkatapuram, *Health Justice: An Argument from the Capabilities Approach* (Cambridge: Polity Press, 2011).

21. Mikhail Gorbachev, "Mikhail Gorbachev: When the Pandemic Is Over, the World Must Come Together," *Time*, April 15, 2020, https://time.com/5820669/mikhail-gorbachev -coronavirus-human-security/; Henry A. Kissinger, "The Coronavirus Pandemic Will Forever Alter the World Order," *Wall Street Journal*, April 3, 2020, https://www.wsj.com /articles/the-coronavirus-pandemic-will-forever-alter-the-world-order-11585953005.

22. Gorbachev, "Mikhail Gorbachev: When the Pandemic Is Over."

23. Dani Rodrik, "Globalisation after Covid-19: My Plan for a Rewired Planet," *Prospect*, May 4, 2020, https://www.prospectmagazine.co.uk/magazine/dani-rodrik-glo balisation-trade-coronavirus-who-imf-world-bank.

24. Commission on Human Security, *Human Security Now* (New York: Commission on Human Security, 2003).

25. Richard G. Feachem, Jeffrey Sachs, and World Health Organization Commission on Macroeconomics and Health, *Global Public Goods for Health: The Report of Working Group 2 of the Commission on Macroeconomics and Health* (Geneva: World Health Organization, 2002); Inge Kaul, *Providing Global Public Goods: Managing Globalization* (New York: United Nations Development Project and Oxford University Press, 2003); Richard Smith, *Global Public Goods for Health: Health, Economic, and Public Health Perspectives* (Oxford: Oxford University Press, 2003).

26. Commission on the Measurement of Economic Performance and Social Progress, *Report of the Commission on the Measurement of Economic Performance and Social Progress*, last modified September 14, 2009, http://files.harmonywithnatureun.org/uploads/upload112.pdf; "OECD Better Life Index," Organisation for Economic Co-operation and Development, accessed 24 June, 2020, http://www.oecdbetterlifeindex.org/.

27. Deen K. Chatterjee, *The Ethics of Assistance: Morality and the Distant Needy* (Cambridge: Cambridge University Press, 2004).

28. John Rawls, *A Theory of Justice* (Cambridge, MA: Belknap Press of Harvard University Press, 1971); and John Rawls, *The Law of Peoples; with, The Idea of Public Reason Revisited* (Cambridge, MA.: Harvard University Press, 1999).

29. Norman Daniels, *Just Health Care* (New York: Cambridge University Press, 1985); Thomas Pogge, *Realizing Rawls* (Ithaca, NY: Cornell University Press, 1989).

30. Simon Caney, "International Distributive Justice," *Political Studies* 49, no. 5 (December 2001): 974–97, https://doi.org/10.1111/1467-9248.00351; David Miller, "The Ethical Significance of Nationality," *Ethics* 98, no. 4 (1988): 647–62, https://doi.org/10.1086/292997; Simon Caney, "Cosmopolitanism, Democracy and Distributive Justice," *Canadian Journal of Philosophy* 35, no. Suppl. (January 2005): 29–63, https://doi.org/10.1080/00455091.2005.10716849.

31. "Prioritizing Diseases for Research and Development in Emergency Contexts," World Health Organization, accessed July 7, 2020, https://www.who.int/activities/improving-treatment-for-snakebite-patients.

PART III / Transnational Issues: Technology, Climate, and Food

Chapter Seven

Global Climate and Energy Policy after the COVID-19 Pandemic

The Tug-of-War between Markets and Politics

Johannes Urpelainen

Before the COVID-19 pandemic of 2020, international climate diplomacy had settled into a regular yet disturbing routine. Every year, governments gathered to negotiate their climate commitments. Progress was haphazard and frustratingly slow, while economic growth and rising living standards contributed to the relentless growth of greenhouse gas emissions.

The pandemic changed everything. For the first time since the end of the Cold War, global greenhouse gas emissions decreased rapidly. In April 2020, they had fallen by 17% from their 2019 levels, with almost half of the reduction from transportation. Researchers estimate that this reduction would translate into a 4%–7% decrease for the entire year, depending on how quickly the world economy rebounds.[1]

Yet even this decrease, brought about by a massive economic shock, was barely in line with the emissions reductions needed to meet the goal of limiting global warming to 2 degrees Celsius by 2100. Climate scientists have shown that to achieve a 66% chance of limiting global warming to 2 degrees Celsius, net greenhouse gas emissions—subtracting carbon sequestered in oceans, forests, and so on—must reach zero by around 2070. To realize this goal, the emissions reductions driven by the COVID-19 pandemic would have to be repeated consistently over five decades.

Johannes Urpelainen is the Prince Sultan bin Abdulaziz Professor of Energy, Resources and Environment at the Johns Hopkins School of Advanced International Studies.

It is unlikely that such reductions would be driven by lockdowns and travel bans. A deeper change in the way people and firms create value will be necessary.

The stakes are high. If the international community fails to limit global warming during this century, serious climate disruption may follow. Massive wildfires, widespread flooding, and scorching heatwaves are among the dangerous climate impacts that we are already seeing. If climate change continues, these impacts will become more extreme over time. Islands and coastal areas, from Tuvalu to Bangladesh to Miami, will succumb to rising seas. Extreme weather events, such as droughts and floods, will ruin livelihoods. The resulting scarcity of food and water will trigger migration on a massive scale. These problems could be exacerbated by domestic unrest and international conflict.

After the pandemic, the outlook for dealing with climate disruption will be as unpredictable as ever. On the one hand, technological progress has contributed to decarbonization in the global power sector, and the rise of electric vehicles holds promise in transportation. If everything goes well in these sectors, the world could undergo a transition to an energy system that increasingly relies on electricity produced from low-carbon sources, such as wind and solar power. Low-cost batteries would store the energy generated when the wind blows and the sun shines, and electricity would replace gasoline, diesel, and natural gas for a wide range of purposes.

On the other hand, the deep undercurrents of international politics are distinctly unfavorable to effective, coordinated climate action. The rise of global right-wing populism and authoritarianism has brought to power leaders who have little interest in mitigating climate change and who disdain multilateral cooperation and globalization. COVID-19 has given rise to new geopolitical conflicts, as China and the United States compete for global influence and blame each other for the pandemic. In spite of the good news about clean technology, rapid climate action will be costly for the economy, at least in the short run. These costs are but a fraction of the global benefits of protecting our atmosphere, but major emitters must come to an agreement about burden sharing and then take costly action.

Ending the tug-of-war between politics and markets is essential for meaningful progress in the global effort to stop climate change before it is too late to avoid irreversible damage. Without a 180-degree change in the direction of international relations, today's great techno-economic opportunity will not save us from extreme climate disruption. Yet, there is still hope. When faced with a major crisis, governments and societies have time and again risen to the challenge.[2] From the world wars that roiled the twentieth century to the 1973 oil crisis that shook global energy markets, governments have shown remarkable resilience and boldness in doing things differently when the status quo was simply no longer an option.

Global Energy Markets: A Turbulent Future

Fossil fuels are both the lifeblood of the world economy and the primary driver of the climate crisis. Before the COVID-19 pandemic, approximately 80% of the world's final energy across all sectors came from fossil fuels (oil, gas, and coal). Oil continued to dominate the transportation sector, and coal continued to play an important role in the electricity sector, while the use of natural gas expanded in heating, industry, and electricity generation. Despite sharp decreases in the cost of renewable electricity generation, the share of fossil fuels in global energy consumption had not actually decreased at all. Fossil fuels accounted for slightly more than 80% of global energy consumption in 1971 and slightly less than 80% in 1989.

COVID-19 had an enormous impact on the global market for fossil fuels. Because the pandemic brought the world economy to a standstill, demand for energy decreased rapidly. Flights were cancelled, and people stopped going to the office. Bars and restaurants closed, and major events were called off. The economic shock also reduced manufacturing activity: global energy demand fell by 3.8% during the first three months of 2020. Based on this, the International Energy Agency (IEA), which closely monitors global energy markets, forecasts a 6% decrease in energy demand in 2020.[3]

Furthermore, according to the IEA, "the Covid-19 pandemic has set in motion the largest drop in global energy investment in history, with spending expected to plunge in every major sector this year—from fossil fuels to renewables and efficiency."[4] Global energy investment in 2020 is projected at slightly more than $1,500 billion. This total is $400 billion below that of 2019, with oil and gas accounting for 60% of the decline.

Oil markets have been particularly badly hit. While a barrel of oil in the European Brent oil market cost $56 in February 2020, the price fell to $32 in March, and in April it collapsed to $18. Given that the transportation sector was hit very hard by lockdowns and reduced travel, this is no surprise. Global oil supply had reached high levels before the COVID-19 crisis, and the sudden collapse in demand resulted in a glut. According to the IEA, oil demand in April 2020 was 29 million barrels per day (29%) lower than in April 2019.[5] For the year 2020, the year-on-year decrease would be 9.3 million barrels per day (9%).

The effect of the pandemic on natural gas and coal markets was less pronounced yet substantial. Natural gas demand is forecast to decrease by 5% in 2020, after ten years of uninterrupted, rapid growth.[6] Because natural gas is mostly used in power generation, industry, and heating, this reduction reflects a slowdown in economic activity. In the coming years, demand for natural gas is expected to grow especially outside the member countries of the Organisation for Economic Cooperation and Development (OECD) and for use outside the power sector.

The pandemic accelerated coal's difficulties. Demand for the most polluting of the fossil fuels is anticipated to decrease by 8% in 2020.[7] This is a much more significant decrease than for natural gas. Because power generation is the most important end use for coal, the slowdown in economic activity has been a major setback for the ailing industry. As demand for electricity dropped, coal suffered more than natural gas or renewables. While conventional economic analysis shows that low energy prices encourage consumption of fossil fuels, this temporary effect is less important than the destructive impacts of the COVID-19 pandemic on the fossil fuel industry. It is entirely possible that global oil consumption has peaked. The coal industry, which was struggling already before the pandemic, continues to lose money as cleaner fuels, notably renewables and natural gas, replace coal in the global power sector.

All these changes bode well for climate mitigation. Although the temporary energy demand reduction from the COVID-19 pandemic is not itself significant for mitigating climate change, the financial difficulties of the fossil fuel industry are significant. Even before the pandemic, fossil fuel producers faced a highly uncertain future. Oil producers worried about electric vehicles. Natural gas faced growing competition from renewable energy in the power sector. Coal could no longer compete with renewable energy and natural gas, and governments were slowly recognizing the need to impose stringent environmental regulations on coal-fired power generation. The pandemic hurt the fossil fuel industry, accelerating the global energy transition toward low-carbon alternatives.

This acceleration is essential because of the inertia in the energy system. Beginning with the invention of the steam engine, industrialized and, subsequently, emerging countries have spent centuries investing in infrastructure for fossil fuels. These investments have created a "carbon lock-in," a socio-technical system that favors the fossil fuels and leaves little room for alternatives.[8] Power plants, transmission lines, pipelines, tankers, coal mines, and oil fields are all elements of this system. If COVID-19 can weaken the once mighty fossil fuel industry and create opportunities for alternatives, then our chances of limiting global warming are significantly improved.

At the same time, the pandemic also revealed the impossibility of halting climate change without dramatic improvements in clean technology. As noted above, the global economic turmoil brought about by COVID-19 reduced global greenhouse gas emissions by 17% in early 2020. Even though the world economy came close to collapsing, the reduction in emissions was roughly in line with what we need to achieve *annually* to limit global warming to well below 2 degrees Celsius by 2100. Simply reducing energy demand is not sufficient. Climate mitigation requires deep structural changes in the production and consumption of energy.

No one can tell with any degree of certainty whether, and how quickly, the demand for fossil fuels will rebound. If the world economy continues to struggle, the demand for fossil fuels will likely remain subdued. But even if the world economy recovers, it is possible that behavioral and organizational changes will suppress the growth in demand for fossil fuels. Oil, in particular, is facing heavy pressure. The pandemic forced organizations to allow their employees to work from home, and a major shift toward flexible working arrangements could reduce oil consumption in transportation. Similarly, lingering fears about infection might reduce air travel for both business and leisure.

On the other hand, a recovery is also possible. COVID-19 has suppressed demand for travel and many other economic commodities. If the structural changes seen in commuting, business travel, and tourism prove to be temporary, emissions could quickly rebound. One might imagine, for example, the travel industry advertising the attractiveness of long-range tourism after people spent months upon months in their homes. Similarly, widespread awareness about contagious diseases could drive people away from public transit and toward increased car ownership and use.

In the long run, a combination of renewable energy and electric vehicles could reduce emissions, regardless of how the pandemic plays out. Even if people around the world decide to purchase cars on a large scale and drive them over long distances, emissions need not increase. Electric vehicles, powered by affordable solar and wind power, would allow enhanced mobility. Because electric vehicles have batteries, they offer a natural end use for intermittent solar and wind power. Repeating this success in trucking and aviation will be more difficult.

All told, the post-pandemic era offers an enormous opportunity for rebuilding a resilient and sustainable world economy, but doing so will require decisive action. The bad news is that the outlook for such decisive action is bleak.

International Climate Policy: Will We Always Have Paris?

The primary engine and achievement of pre-pandemic climate policy was the Paris Agreement. In December 2015, the international community negotiated this flagship treaty in Paris at a United Nations summit. Unlike its predecessor, the widely criticized Kyoto Protocol of 1997, the Paris Agreement was built on countries designing and submitting their National Determined Contributions (NDCs). The Paris Agreement did not impose negotiated emission targets but instead let each country formally announce their climate action plans. These plans would then be collectively reviewed over time, with the goal of encouraging governments to ratchet up their climate action plans under peer review and public scrutiny.

Success in ratcheting up is necessary for the Paris Agreement to mitigate climate change. Today's NDCs are not ambitious enough to avoid rapid global warming. According to the Climate Action Tracker, a nonprofit that monitors the Paris pledges, the current NDCs would lead to a global warming of 2.3–3.5 degrees Celsius by 2100.[9] This is only slightly below where current policies would lead us, with a range of 2.3–4.1 degrees Celsius. Unless governments significantly increase their ambition levels, take rapid action, and meet their targets, the international effort to halt climate disruption can be considered a failure.

The Paris Agreement was the result of decades of negotiations. The 1997 Kyoto Protocol imposed emissions reductions exclusively on industrialized countries, with the presumption that the developing world was not yet ready to act on climate change, both because of resource constraints and because of low baseline emissions. While this idea was reasonable in 1997, a decade later it seemed anachronistic, as China's stupendous economic expansion began to dominate global emissions trends.

In 2007, governments convened in Bali, Indonesia, to develop an action plan for a globally binding treaty. They then tried to negotiate it in 2009 in Copenhagen, Denmark, but the talks failed and the outcome, the Copenhagen Accord, simply listed the voluntary efforts that different countries would agree to undertake. It took the international community another six years to regroup, so that the 2015 Paris Agreement would show a new direction for global climate cooperation.

The Paris Agreement was built on the notion that national sovereignty is an inviolable foundation of international law. Earlier, global cooperation on climate change had produced underwhelming results because major emitters simply refused to commit to deep emissions reductions. The Kyoto Protocol did not impose specific requirements on any developing countries, including China and India. The

United States decided not to ratify the agreement, and Canada left in 2011. Recognizing the impossibility of a legally binding global treaty, negotiators switched gears and lowered their expectations. The goal was no longer to have countries meet top-down targets to limit global warming but to enable countries to set their own targets and increase the stringency of these targets over time.

In practice, the Paris Agreement is a fair-weather agreement. It is easy for governments to announce ambitious NDCs when they are already reducing carbon emissions and their economies are prospering. But if emissions are growing rapidly or if the economy is in recession, commitments that could be costly or difficult to meet pose a significant reputational risk for the negotiators. In 2017, only two years after the Paris negotiations, a group of scholars noted that industrialized countries, which were supposed to lead climate mitigation efforts, were not on track with their commitments.[10] In the United States, President Donald J. Trump was not following the previous administration's plans to decarbonize the power sector with the Environmental Protection Agency's Clean Power Plan. In the European Union, the Emissions Trading Scheme reduced electricity usage and industrial emissions, but progress in the other 55% of European emissions has been lackluster.

President Trump's abrupt withdrawal from the Paris Agreement in June 2017 illustrates these challenges.[11] The 2015 Paris negotiations were significantly boosted by the November 2014 bilateral agreement on climate change cooperation between China and the United States. Combine that with a high level of enthusiasm among the EU countries and India's newfound passion for renewable energy, and the Paris talks started from a position of strength. But when Trump succeeded Barack Obama as president, the United States was out. Developing countries, for example, were furious when they realized that the $100 billion a year that the industrialized countries had promised by 2020 to finance climate mitigation and adaptation would not be available.

The pandemic has also demonstrated that fair-weather agreements struggle when the storm comes. The immediate effect of the COVID-19 pandemic was the postponement of the 2020 United Nations Climate Change Conference to 2021. But it also reduced attention to climate change, as people, businesses, and governments focused on the more urgent problems of a global public health crisis and an economic recession. If 2019 was the year of climate change, then 2020 was the year of the pandemic, with little attention devoted to climate change. Nonetheless, because the Paris Agreement is built on the primacy of domestic climate policy, it provides a suitable framework for amplifying the impact of national and even subnational climate initiatives. Under the Paris Agreement, major emitters can lead with domestic action and encourage others to match their ambition.

To salvage climate cooperation under the Paris Agreement, major powers must agree on a common green stimulus strategy. When the pandemic triggered a global recession, private sector investment in the energy sector decreased rapidly. Under these circumstances, public finance must play a critical role not only in economic recovery but also in moving the world toward a low-carbon economy. Moreover, historically low interest rates (negative interest rates in some cases) offer a unique opportunity for massive public investment in clean technology. If a critical mass of major emitters were to embrace a common green stimulus, other countries would have strong incentives to follow. A coordinated green stimulus backed by the world's largest economies would create new opportunities for clean technology. Governments would seek to exploit these opportunities both as a strategy for economic recovery and to bolster their reputations.

In a virtuous cycle, a massive green stimulus strategy will enable governments to extend the accidental emissions reductions caused by the pandemic recession. The COVID-19 emission reductions are not a good model for climate cooperation, but they do buy governments some time. A successful green stimulus strategy would first avoid a rapid rebound and then launch a wave of emissions reductions in key sectors, from energy to transportation. Furthermore, a successful green stimulus would also contribute to economic growth, as governments are rightly concerned about their debt burden even in a climate of generally low interest rates.

Over time, a green stimulus could trigger a complete restructuring of the world economy. We already have most of the technology required for a low-carbon economy. Renewable energy could provide most of our electricity. Energy for transportation, industry, and buildings could increasingly be produced with the help of wind and solar power. In these areas, green stimulus should focus on aggressive deployment of clean technology and building political coalitions that lobby and vote for continued investments in low-carbon industry.

In those areas where technology is not yet ready, such as steel production or aviation, green stimulus packages should promote innovation. Because energy technologies tend to crawl from the laboratory to market, generous support for innovation is essential. Major emitters could invest in everything from laboratory research to public-private partnerships and international demonstration projects.

The problem with this strategy lies in the difficulty of international cooperation. For the Paris Agreement to limit global warming to well below 2 degrees Celsius by 2100, major emitters from China and India to Russia and the United

States must devise and implement astonishingly ambitious climate policies over decades.

Discord in the Era of Climate Disruption

Cooperation on climate change has always been a near-impossible challenge. Each country's government is not only concerned about the costs of climate mitigation but also understands that other countries reap many of the gains.[12] While US emissions reductions are necessary to save Bangladesh from destructive sea-level rise, Americans will reap few direct gains from this achievement. Moreover, emissions reductions can be costly, and many of the costs will be incurred by vested interests such as fossil fuel producers and heavy industry.[13]

In recent years, the Paris Agreement's pragmatism and rapid technological progress gave new hope to climate advocates. Between 2014 and 2016, the trajectory of global emissions reached a plateau, largely thanks to China's increased investment in clean energy and the decline of coal use in the OECD countries.[14] This plateau augured a bright future, as the Paris Agreement drove countries toward ever more ambitious emissions reductions in the tailwinds of a clean technology revolution.

But this hope has not yet translated into deep emissions reductions. Before COVID-19, the total effect of the NDCs fell far short of what is needed to achieve the Paris Agreement's goal. In 2017–2019, global emissions again resumed a rising trajectory. In the absence of the pandemic, emissions might have continued to increase in 2020 despite the growing competitiveness of renewables and the growing use of electric vehicles. Simply put, adding renewable electricity generation capacity and electric vehicles is not enough without substantial progress in other sectors of the global energy system.

Worse, already before the pandemic, the megatrends of international affairs pointed in a disturbing direction. Donald Trump's surprise election as president of the United States revealed an important change in politics, as people grew frustrated with the liberal, multilateral elites and voted for outsiders who challenged conventional ideas with populism. Great Britain's exit from the European Union, China's turn toward authoritarian centralization, India's Hindu nationalism, and Brazil's return to right-wing authoritarianism suggest that this change is global in nature and not limited to American politics.

This era of populist nationalism is not fertile ground for multilateral cooperation. Dealing with a "wicked" problem such as climate change is a complex social challenge that requires trust in science, effective bargaining over burden sharing, commitment to international rules over long periods of time, and rapid adaptation to change.[15] Today's populist leaders despise scientists, favor aggressive unilateralism over multilateral cooperation, break rules when it is convenient, and fail to adapt to new realities. President Trump's "America First" campaign and his failure to react to the COVID-19 pandemic in a timely manner illustrate these tendencies, and climate change is a far more complicated problem than the coronavirus pandemic.

COVID-19 made everything worse in global politics. The novel coronavirus began to spread in the Chinese city of Wuhan, and President Trump did not miss a beat in seizing the opportunity to blame the public health crisis on China. Instead of a global effort to contain the coronavirus, led by the World Health Organization, governments played the blame game and focused on protecting their own interests. This behavior contributed to a more general decrease in international cooperation, as governments increasingly distrusted each other and saw international affairs as a zero-sum game.

This deterioration of cooperation can already be seen in climate change. After COVID-19, China's role in international climate cooperation has become increasingly complicated. China's relationship with the United States has continued to deteriorate as President Trump blames China for the pandemic. At the same time, the precipitous decline in international trade has yet again led China to seek energy security in coal, the most polluting of all fossil fuels. The growth of nationalism and calls for national self-reliance have also made governments around the world worry about their dependence on China, which could reduce imports of Chinese clean technology.

The global community therefore faces a vexing dilemma. On the one hand, time is running out. The destructive effects of climate change are increasingly clear, with wildfires raging in California and rural populations in India leaving areas that are no longer suitable for agriculture. Every year that goes by without decisive action by the majority of significant emitters makes achieving any meaningful and timely emissions reductions increasingly unlikely. While there is no specific deadline for climate action, the global community cannot lose much more time, or climate change will cause massive and irreversible destruction.

On the other hand, cooperation is more challenging than at any time since the end of the Cold War. Cooperation on climate change was difficult enough in the 1990s and early 2000s; it will be much more difficult in the competitive, zero-sum world order that is currently emerging. Major emitters will be reluctant to trust each other in the spirit of reciprocity when they are competing for global influence and trying to undercut other nations in the realms of national security and economic diplomacy.

Conclusion

International climate policy is at a crossroads. Both paths eventually lead to a low-carbon world economy, but only one of them will avoid dangerous climate disruption.

In the continued tug-of-war between markets and politics, the global energy system will eventually reduce its dependence on carbon fuels. However, the transition will be far too slow to avoid serious climate disruption. While governments scramble to respond to the COVID-19 pandemic and talk about green stimulus, their responses are too fragmented and unambitious to bend the emissions curve. Markets continue to deliver less expensive clean technology, but without government support, progress will be slow. At the time of this writing, this outcome appears likely. When major emitters finally realize that they must act, their historical emissions will have already committed us to a far less hospitable global climate. If global cooperation on climate change were to accelerate a decade after the COVID-19 pandemic, climate disruption would be all but unavoidable. Governments would have to invest in more exotic and uncertain solutions, such as geo-engineering, which aspires to offset global warming through innovative techniques like ocean fertilization or reflecting sunlight back into space, or negative emissions, which remove carbon dioxide from the atmosphere. These techniques might or might not provide some relief. Adaptation to climate change—sea walls, resilient infrastructure, drought-resistant crops, and so on—will be necessary in any case, but without an effective mitigation effort, adaptive measures will be both expensive and difficult.

But if the tug-of-war ends now, rapid progress is possible. If the COVID-19 pandemic were to bring major emitters together to rebuild a sustainable and resilient world economy, government action could significantly accelerate progress in the development and deployment of clean technology. Substantial, coordinated investments in clean technology would usher in an era of low-carbon development, with fossil fuels rapidly losing ground. Public finance would catalyze private investment. This would produce a much better global outcome, but moving in that direction is not possible without a 180-degree change in the way major emitters approach global cooperation. As long as these countries continue to be ruled by authoritarian or proto-authoritarian leaders who hold international law in contempt, this outcome is unlikely.

In the long run, the COVID-19 pandemic will affect both markets and politics. The impact on markets will be through behavioral change, such as people working from home or rejecting public transit, and favors the survival of the fittest in an economic recession. These behavioral changes could accelerate or halt progress in clean technology innovation and deployment, but they will not fundamentally break our dependence on fossil fuels. Wealthy people will continue to use large amounts of fossil fuels to support their lifestyles, and their less affluent counterparts will aspire to increase their energy consumption.

The impact on politics is more complex and more profound. Governments respond to crises, but the nature of the response is difficult to predict. It could be destructive, with governments opting for nationalism and isolation. It could be constructive, as governments recognize the impossibility of progress without a much higher level of international cooperation. The past centuries have shown that governments can and will do the right thing, but only after they have no other choice.

Of the two impacts, on markets and politics, the latter is more important. Behavioral changes will have at best marginal effects on greenhouse gas emissions. Political changes, however, could change the direction of international climate policy and give governments one last chance to avoid climate disruption, after four decades of inaction. The odds are not in civilization's favor, but failure is not yet a foregone conclusion.

NOTES

1. Corinne Le Quéré et al., "Temporary Reduction in Daily Global CO2 Emissions during the COVID-19 Forced Confinement," *Nature Climate Change* 10 (2020): 647–53, https://www.nature.com/articles/s41558-020-0797-x.

2. Michaël Aklin and Johannes Urpelainen, *Renewables: The Politics of a Global Energy Transition* (Cambridge, MA: MIT Press, 2018).

3. International Energy Agency, *World Energy Investment 2020* (Paris: International Energy Agency, 2020).

4. International Energy Agency, "The Covid-19 Crisis Is Causing the Biggest Fall in Global Energy Investment in History," May 27, 2020, https://www.iea.org/news/the-covid-19-crisis-is-causing-the-biggest-fall-in-global-energy-investment-in-history.

5. International Energy Agency, *Oil Market Report April 2020* (Paris: International Energy Agency, 2020).

6. International Energy Agency, *World Energy Investment 2020*.

7. International Energy Agency, *World Energy Investment 2020*.

8. Gregory C. Unruh, "Understanding Carbon Lock-In," *Energy Policy* 28, no. 4 (2000): 817–30.

9. Climate Action Tracker, https://climateactiontracker.org/ (accessed June 17, 2020).

10. David G. Victor, Keigo Akimoto, Yoichi Kaya, Mitsutsune Yamaguchi, Danny Cullenward, and Cameron Hepburn, "Prove Paris Was More Than Paper Promises," *Nature* 548, no. 7665 (2017): 25.

11. Johannes Urpelainen and Thijs Van de Graaf, "United States Non-Cooperation and the Paris Agreement," *Climate Policy* 18, no. 7 (2018): 839–51.

12. Scott Barrett, "Self-Enforcing International Environmental Agreements," *Oxford Economic Papers* 46, Supplement (October 1994): 878–94.

13. Llewelyn Hughes and Johannes Urpelainen, "Interests, Institutions, and Climate Policy: Explaining the Choice of Policy Instruments for the Energy Sector," *Environmental Science and Policy* 54 (December 2015): 52–63.

14. Thomas Spencer, Michel Colombier, Oliver Sartor, Amit Garg, Vineet Tiwari, Jesse Burton, Tara Caetano, Fergus Green, Fei Teng, and John Wiseman, "The 1.5 C Target and Coal Sector Transition: At the Limits of Societal Feasibility," *Climate Policy* 18, no. 3 (2018): 335–51.

15. Kelly Levin, Benjamin Cashore, Steven Bernstein, and Graeme Auld, "Overcoming the Tragedy of Super Wicked Problems: Constraining Our Future Selves to Ameliorate Global Climate Change," *Policy Sciences* 45, no. 2 (May 2012): 123–52.

Chapter Eight

No Food Security, No World Order

Jessica Fanzo

While food insecurity and malnutrition remain significant challenges, over the last two decades, the global hunger rate decreased 25%.[1] Much of that decline is attributed to decreases in poverty. In the last 30 years, populations living in extreme poverty (defined as those living on less than $1.90 per day) decreased from 2 billion in 1990 to 700 million in 2015. These gains have in large part been attributed to stronger social protection programs, increased basic service coverage, and income and private sector growth.

However, in the last four years, the number of people who go to bed hungry has risen from 796 million to 821 million.[2] Immediate or acute hunger increased by 70% over the same period, from 80 million to 135 million, with the majority of those populations living in Africa or conflict-affected countries.[3] Why has hunger increased, undermining years of progress? Most of the rise is due to climate change and conflict.[4] Sixty percent of people facing hunger live in war-torn countries such as Afghanistan, the Democratic Republic of Congo (DRC), Nigeria, Syria, Venezuala, and Yemen.[5] Climate change, too, has played a significant role; climate-related natural disasters have significantly tested the efficiency and functioning of global food systems.[6]

The failure to address near-term food insecurity and hunger will block progress in mitigating the COVID-19 pandemic—not only in the present moment but as the

Jessica Fanzo is a Bloomberg Distinguished Professor of Global Food Policy and Ethics at Johns Hopkins University.

pandemic spreads around the world over the next one to three years. The United Nations World Food Programme (WFP) estimates that the number of people facing acute food insecurity will rise to 265 million by the end of 2020, up by 130 million from 135 million in 2019, as a result of the economic impact of COVID-19.[7] The United Nations University World Institute for Development Economics Research estimates that 85 million people will fall into the "extreme poverty" category because of the pandemic, putting more people at risk for food insecurity and malnutrition. The World Bank estimates that 40 million to 60 million people will fall into extreme poverty in 2020, due to potential economic shocks resulting from the pandemic.[8]

There is deep concern about sub-Saharan Africa in particular. While some countries have made significant progress in alleviating poverty, civil wars and armed conflict continue to destabilize the region, disrupting agriculture and food production, destroying food supply chains and trade, and leading to internal displacement and migration. Almost 80 million people have been forced to move.[9] Floods and droughts plague the continent, and now East Africa is dealing with severe locust swarms that are decimating food crops.[10]

This essay focuses on how the COVID-19 pandemic is affecting global food security and the repercussions for future world order if we do not address food insecurity in the short and long term. There will be no world order at all without food security.

Consequences of Hunger and Food Insecurity

In the short term, hunger and food insecurity destabilize individuals, households, communities, and nations; over the long term, they give rise to social unrest, disenfranchisement, and political instability. While food insecurity can contribute to or exacerbate nutrition deficits, it is also linked to chronic diseases and conditions for people of all ages.[11] Food insecurity is especially detrimental to the health, development, and well-being of children.[12]

Food-insecure populations are especially vulnerable to poor nutrition and obesity due to additional risk factors associated with inadequate household resources.[13] Many of the same people who struggle with hunger also struggle with obesity. This may sound like an paradox, but both are often rooted in poverty. Food-insecure adults in the United States are 32% more likely than others to be obese—especially if they are women, black, non-Hispanic or Hispanic.[14] Children living in food-insecure households also have a greater-than-average chance of being overweight or obese, and they have poor diets and eating habits.[15] Food-insecure children also tend to display behavioral problems, disrupted social interactions, poor cognitive development, and marginal school performance. These challenges, in turn, increase children's risk of becoming obese adults.[16] There is also a significant body of epidemiological and mechanistic evidence which suggests that hunger *in utero* and in early life can put individuals at higher risk for being overweight in adult life.[17]

Obesity and other noncommunicable diseases (NCDs) are worsening around the world and are considered significant risk factors for COVID-19 hospitalizations and complications in both young and older patients.[18] Diets are one of the significant risk factors for obesity and NCDs, and the ability to access food and healthy diets is being directly targeted by the COVID-19 pandemic because of an inefficient global food system.[19] Much of that has to do with the design and reorientation of agriculture following the Second World War.

The first international commitment to ending hunger was made in 1943 at the UN Conference on Food and Agriculture at Hot Springs, Virginia. That conference set the goal of "freedom from want of food, suitable and adequate for the health and strength of all peoples" that should be achieved "in all lands within the shortest possible time."[20] After the war, the immediate focus was on reviving agriculture in Europe and East Asia. This rebirth of agriculture focused on positioning the food supply to produce basic food staples, consisting of energy-dense cereals, in order to feed a growing population. With an escalating Cold War and Malthusian fears that food shortages would stoke Communism, the UN Food and Agriculture Organization (FAO), the Rockefeller Foundation, and the United States War against Hunger called the 1960s the "fighting hunger decade."[21] Throughout the 1970s and the 1980s, this "green revolution" spread to Asia and enabled cereal production to stay ahead of population growth.[22]

Although the green revolution made major contributions to reducing undernutrition, other forms of malnutrition, such as obesity, began to rise.[23] Policies favoring the production of major cereals during the green revolution persisted during the decades following, undermining incentives to supply more diversified diets that contribute to better nutrition and health.[24] What we are left with in 2020 is a "syndemic" in which 1 billion people still suffer from hunger, 2 billion have some form of micronutrient deficiency due to low diet diversity, and 2.1 billion are overweight or obese.[25]

Food Security and International Security

Food security is highly correlated with international security. Lasting food insecurity has been shown to lead to social unrest, food riots, radicalization, instability, and conflict.[26] Most countries currently experiencing conflict are classified by the FAO as "low-income food deficit," and they have high burdens of under-nourishment. Nearly 75% of children under five who experience chronic under-nutrition live in countries affected by conflict that can last for generations after war is over.[27] It is therefore crucial for all countries to ensure that food security is a central priority in ensuring their own national security as well as international security and cooperation.

Many conflicts that lead to food insecurity and famine are human-made, stemming from natural resource competition, poverty, or health system shocks, such as epidemics like HIV/AIDS, malaria, or Ebola. Conflict generates food insecurity by affecting food availability, access, and use. Food systems that are repeatedly put under stress by conflict tend to move from predictable food-value chains to instability and volatility.[28] Violent armed conflict can lead to the destruction of crops, livestock, land, and water systems, as well as disruptions in infrastructure such as roads and other transportation modalities, markets, and the human capacity required for food production, processing, distribution, and safe consumption.[29] Sometimes hunger is not only an indirect result of conflict but is itself used as a weapon of war.[30] Many geopolitical conflicts cross the borders of different food systems. Fragile and failed nation-states influence, and are in turn influenced by, global market forces, and food security is often one of the first factors to be affected.

While most conflicts result from human action, the trigger for conflict or crisis may be natural, such as a prolonged drought, or economic, such as the change in the price of a country's major staple or cash crop. Price volatility can spark disorder and social unrest among urban communities unable to afford basic staples.[31] On the other hand, hunger may also be viewed as a cause of conflicts, a perspective that has been far less studied.[32]

COVID-19 Began as a Food System Risk

Like H1N1 influenza, SARS-CoV-2 (the virus that causes the COVID-19 disease) infected people through a zoonotic spillover event, probably from a bat, although another animal may have been involved. At first, case trace-back from the December outbreak of pneumonia in Wuhan, China, implicated a "wet food market" in which wildlife and other live animals are bought and sold for consumption. These food markets are risky places from a pandemic preparedness perspective since stressed wild animals from many different areas are brought together—circumstances that encourage a pathogen to jump species. As China reopened in early June 2020, COVID-19 cases surged again in Beijing. The government tracked seventy-nine new infections and again traced cases back to a bustling food market in the south of the city where live animals are sold.

Regardless of SARS-CoV-2's precise trajectory, experts agree that COVID-19 is a zoonosis, a disease that jumped from animals to humans. Sixty percent of emerging infectious diseases are zoonotic, and of that 60%, 72% originate in wildlife.[33] Humanity has experienced a long history of zoonotic diseases including rabies, Lyme, anthrax, SARS, Ebola, West Nile, Zika, Rift Valley fever, AIDS, and the bubonic plague that killed a third of the world's population in the 1300s.

The question remains as to why viruses jump from animals to humans and become insidious diseases. Food plays a large part in the transmission. Zoonotic disease spread and spillover events usually occur when animals are put in close proximity to humans, either because their natural habitat has shrunk or been destroyed or because they are removed from their habitats.[34] As a result of the reconfiguration of the planet's landscape—through urbanization, deforestation, intensive agriculture, and mining—many wild animals are forced to venture into the built environments of human populations. The excessive hunting and trade of wildlife for consumption, fiber and fur, or medicinal uses significantly increase the likelihood of cross-species mingling and infection. Modern transportation, by trains, planes, and automobiles, can accelerate the spread of pathogens around the world. According to a *New York Times* article, "other animals' diseases have not so much leapt onto us as flowed into us through channels we supplied."[35]

Human activity is the biggest instigator of change, much of it related to agriculture. No other species has so profoundly changed the planet and the ecosystems that support species diversity in such a short span of time.[36] Given that nearly all of earth's systems show signs of human impact, many scientists suggest that we have entered a new geological era, the Anthropocene, which is characterized by the influence of humans on the planet.[37] A preponderance of global evidence shows that atmospheric, geologic, hydrologic, biospheric, and other planetary system processes are now altered by humans.[38] Of the human behaviors driving the Anthropocene, agriculture and food production contribute significantly to climate change and other environmental stressors.

Just two centuries ago, only about 5% of the world's arable land was devoted to agriculture. That changed dramatically due to the reconstruction of agricultural systems in the wake of the Second World War. To feed the 8 billion people currently living on the planet, of whom 55% to 85% reside in urban areas, we now use 40% of the earth's landmass for agriculture.[39] This growth is driven by population pressure and the demand for animal-source foods.[40] In turn, much of the increase in the animal and livestock sector to feed that demand promotes the spread of viruses between humans, livestock, and wildlife.[41] This growth has resulted in a very efficient global agriculture system that is producing enough food to feed the world in aggregate, but it has also resulted in extreme human, environmental, and social equity costs.[42]

Along with deforestation, the biodiversity loss of animal and plant species is accelerating at 100 to 1,000 times the pre-human extinction rate.[43] This lost biodiversity has been replaced with a homogenous food system dominated by a handful of food crops, including maize, rice, wheat, soy, chickens, and cattle.[44] This profound loss of diversity exposes the planet to a multiplicity of risks, including climate, nutrition, and zoonotic risks.

COVID-19: A Food System Shock

Food systems encompass the activities of producing, processing, distributing, preparing, and consuming food as well as the people who influence those activities.[45] Food systems are highly interconnected—any policy intervention that addresses one part of the system will affect other parts. These interconnections have implications for health, politics, society, the economy, and the environment. While food systems come in all shapes and sizes, the COVID-19 pandemic has shown how extraordinarily interconnected they are. The pandemic has also shown that food supply chains have become far more resilient and adaptive than they would have been fifty or even twenty years ago due to globalization, trade, and technology.[46] Early data suggest that global markets of staple grains remain steady and robust for now, due mainly to abundant harvests in 2019.[47] This means that stocks of most staple food products are stable.

While stocks are adequate, the downstream effects along the food supply chain are showing vulnerabilities and disruptions; some are calling to move away from long globalized food supply chains to short local supply chains.[48] When a shock, such as a pandemic, affects food systems, the consequences are immediate, with potential long-term implications.[49] The pandemic implicates actors in all parts of the food system. The deep global economic shocks caused by COVID-19 will continue to affect the movement of cash and small and medium-size agribusinesses' access to financial institutions. There is early evidence that COVID-19 is also decreasing production capacity, slowing or limiting market access, limiting remittances as safety nets, lowering employment opportunities, and triggering unexpected medical costs.

Farming is a particularly vulnerable livelihood given the older age profile of farmers and their risk of higher morbidity and mortality with COVID-19 incidence. It is also a livelihood that is heavily reliant on mobile workforces. Border restrictions and lockdowns are slowing harvests in some parts of the world, leaving seasonal workers unable to get to farms to support their livelihoods. These restrictions also affect the ability of farmers to obtain the tools and technology they need, including pesticides, seeds, and equipment to plant and harvest crops.

Physical distancing, curfews, and lockdowns affect the costs of moving food around, within countries and across borders, leading to food loss and empty markets. Some boats full of food sit at ports waiting for clearance, leaving food vulnerable to rot.[50] Where farmers can grow crops, lockdown restrictions are regularly preventing them from transporting produce and livestock to markets. These supply chain disruptions have resulted in farmers burying perishable produce or dumping milk.[51] Meat processing plants and food markets are being forced to close in many locations due to COVID-19 outbreaks among workers; in the United States, meat processing plants are seeing incidences of COVID-19 cases at twice the national average.[52] As a result, many people struggle to obtain fresh fruits and vegetables, dairy, meat, and fish. Even staple grains can be hard to come by; rice imports to sub-Saharan Africa that were intended to compensate for the shortfall have been disrupted or stopped, driving up prices of this staple.[53]

Government-imposed shelter-in-place orders further restrict individuals' ability to earn wages; as a result, the purchasing power of many families that were already struggling with poverty has been compromised. One study projected that up to 20 million jobs could be lost in sub-Saharan Africa due to the COVID-19 crisis.[54] A Michigan State University survey of five South Asian countries—Bangladesh, India, Nepal, Pakistan, and Sri Lanka—found that about 37% of households reported that at least one person in the household had either lost a job or experienced a significant reduction in work hours during the past month.[55] As a rough approximation, data suggest that 75% of unemployment in March and April 2020 can be linked directly or indirectly to the COVID-19 pandemic.

High levels of unemployment, loss of income, and rising food costs are also making access to food difficult for many. The prices of basic foods have begun to rise in some countries at a time when people have less money in their pockets.[56] Food price volatility also generates uncertainty. More food staples and unhealthier, highly processed foods that are cheaper and have longer shelf lives will be consumed as a result of price hikes and shortages. More nutritious foods are expensive, hard to come by, and perishable.[57] The trend toward suboptimal dietary patterns affects the quality of diets and their contributing risk to longer-term chronic disease, with significant health, economic, and societal costs.[58]

In the long term, the COVID-19 health crisis may exploit the food system to worsen the global impact of the disease. Disruptions to health care and the ability to deliver essential services will significantly affect maternal and child health. Estimates suggest that in 118 low-income and middle-income countries, even a small reduction in the coverage of maternal and child health services could lead to 42,240 additional child deaths and 2,030 additional maternal deaths per month, with worst-case scenario disruptions resulting in 1,157,000 child deaths and 56,700 maternal deaths over six months.[59] The editors of the *Lancet Global Health* observed that "these indirect effects will reach far beyond the disease itself, with long-term social and economic consequences for individuals and society."[60]

Also in the long term, unresolved agendas will have consequences. Climate change is one such consequence. The syndemic that preceded COVID-19—continued conflicts, climate change, more violent and less predictable natural disasters, and the massive burden of malnutrition—has been undermining food security in many contexts.[61] Agriculture and associated changes in land use account for nearly one-quarter of greenhouse gas emissions, making the sector the second-largest industrial emitter of greenhouse gases after the energy sector.[62] If we stay on a business-as-usual course, extreme weather, food and water shortages, and increased prevalence of disease and other climate-related maladies are projected to cause an additional 529,000 deaths per year.[63]

The bi-directional relationship between agriculture and climate change has implications for healthy diets and adequate food supplies. Agriculture is a driver of climate change, but it is also significantly affected by the changing climate. Although the precise impacts of climate change on agriculture are uncertain, projections suggest that the current practices and intensity of food production will be unsustainable under climate change.[64] The environmental challenges posed by climate change may require the production of even more food. Climate-induced stressors on the agricultural system will likely contribute to a reduction in crop yields and nutritional quality, especially in equatorial regions. These projections vary substantially, however, between regions and crops.[65] Climate change is adding a double layer of challenges for food access and distribution, affordability, and safety.[66]

Early Lessons of COVID-19 for Food Systems

Some early food system lessons have begun to emerge from the COVID-19 pandemic. These lessons have limited evidence and data, but they are attended with much speculation and sensationalism. There is great uncertainty about how food systems will continue to react and function depending on how long the pandemic lasts and whether, in the absence of a vaccine or herd immunity, countries retreat into lockdowns in the near future.

Food systems do not operate independently; they are linked to complex societal systems. The functionality of health systems can greatly impact food systems and vice versa. COVID-19 and other infectious diseases, such as Ebola, have demonstrated that a shock to the health system can have severe ramifications on the functioning of food systems, sometimes completely dismantling them.[67] These shocks can have effects within a system, but they also cut across other systems. For example, the health system has taken a heavy toll as it deals with COVID-19. While attention has been diverted, other diseases have been left unaddressed, and a rise in cases of measles and dengue has been documented.[68] The question is how to make systems more reactive, adaptive, and resilient in order to address multiple large challenges at once.

Second, surprisingly, governments can be nimble and act quickly. For years, the international development community has been pushing agendas such as poverty reduction, ending hunger, and mitigating climate change. While some of these agendas have led to global commitments, such as the Sustainable Development Goals and the Paris Agreement, governments are inconsistent as to how much political will and financial resources they are willing devote to these global targets; they are often slow to react and often fall short of what is needed. COVID-19 has shown that governments can act quickly to shut down borders and mandate curfews and lockdowns. While the slowdown in globalization has mitigated the spread of the disease in some places, allowing health systems to catch up, the quick reaction and dramatic alteration of the way the world normally works has had profound consequences for other sectors. The lesson is that when countries and states are faced with a significant threat, such as that of a highly infectious disease with potentially large-scale mortality, governments can take notice, act with speed, and act in their own interest.

Third, food supply workers have always been an undervalued segment of the workforce, but they have been thrust into the spotlight with COVID-19. A policy brief on COVID-19 and food released by the UN secretary-general shows that the highest proportion and greatest number of jobs lost during the pandemic are in the "middle" of the food supply chain (Table 1).[69] These workers—grocery store clerks, packagers, processors, distributors, and those who deliver food to markets and households—are at the frontlines, and they are at high risk of exposure to

Table 1   Impacts of COVID-19 on Food System Livelihoods (in millions)

	Food Systems		COVID-19			
	Jobs	Livelihoods	At-risk jobs	% of food systems jobs	At-risk livelihoods	% of food systems livelihoods
Primary production	716.77	2,023.80	152.35	21	404.76	20
Food processing	200.73	484.54	120.44	60	290.72	60
Food services	168.97	339.44	101.38	60	203.66	60
Distribution services	96.34	241.48	57.81	60	144.89	60
Transportation services	41.61	101.05	16.64	40	40.42	40
Machinery	6.51	13.18	1.72	26	3.48	26
Inputs	4.89	11.06	1.29	26	2.92	26
R&D	0.13	0.29	0.02	15	0.03	10
Total	1,280.93	3,214.84	451.64	35	1,090.89	34

Source: United Nations Policy Brief: The Impact of COVID-19 on Food Security and Nutrition (New York: United Nations, June 2020), 11, incorporating unpublished Food and Agricultural Organization / IFPRI estimates, based on International Labor Organization 2020—ILO extrapolation scenario. Not annualized. Jobs represent formal employment; livelihoods cover a broad array of self-employed, informal, migrant, and seasonal labor.

the coronavirus. The pandemic has also shed light on the reliance of agriculture on immigrant populations. In the United States alone, 50% of the agricultural workforce is composed of undocumented immigrants, whose livelihoods have been disrupted by the pandemic and who have no social support system or safety net in place.[70]

Finally, safety nets, in the form of cash or food, are critical for the most vulnerable, the poorest, and the smallholder farmers and food workers in all sectors during the pandemic.[71] Studies show that social protection programs improve both the quantity and the quality of food consumed by beneficiaries. The average social protection program increases the value of food consumed relative to expenditure by 13% and caloric acquisition by 8%.[72] Social protection programs should be more closely linked to promoting the consumption and production of nutritious food, not just preventing food insecurity.[73]

Achieving Resilient Food Systems for World Order

What would it take to achieve resilient food systems? Seven technical and coordination actions are presented below to address both the short- and the long-term effects of the COVID-19 pandemic on food systems and to recommend measures to avoid catastrophic future zoonotic pandemics.

First, the short-term priority is to stabilize food systems and keep trade open and flowing. To do this, it is important to recognize that all workers across food supply chains are critical in keeping the food system moving. There is a need to support these workers, producers, and entrepreneurs and to ensure they are healthy so that they can keep the world fed. They need personal protective equipment including proper face masks, fair living wages, and decent work. While at work, measures need to be put into place to ensure that coronavirus testing is made available, spaces are designed for social distancing, and hand sanitizers and proper infrastructure for washing hands and maintaining hygiene are in place. Low-touch, low-contact equipment must be a priority investment by business. Workers should also be trained on how infectious disease spreads and how they can protect themselves and their customers. Unlike other shocks to food systems, such as climate change, this is a fast-spreading infectious disease that requires a complete new understanding of how pathogens spread through a highly interconnected food system involving many workers.

Second, there is a case to make for ensuring that our global food supply is safe, nutritious, and equitable. Diabetes and other noncommunicable diseases are risk factors for COVID-19 mortality, and additional attention should be devoted to preventing the former because of the latter.[74] The major driver of poor metabolic health, which increases the risk of hospitalization and death from COVID-19, is a diet that relies heavily on starchy staples, sugar, salt, and unhealthy fats largely in the form of highly processed foods and that is low in unprocessed food, vegetables, fruits, whole grains, beans, seafood, nuts, and seeds.[75] Poor metabolic health also explains some of the risks of hospitalization and death disproportionately impacting low-income and minority populations. African Americans account for 70% of COVID-19 deaths in the United States.[76] Multisectoral policies for better diets and nutrition should be a top priority for governments and businesses; these include strengthening health systems, improving school and workplace food environments (particularly in impoverished neighborhoods), implementing transparent and informative food labeling and dietary guidelines, and devising economic incentives for the private sector and consumers to produce and consume healthy foods.[77]

Third, wildlife habitats are threatened and affected by land-use changes and deforestation, often due to agriculture expansion. Trade in wildlife is common, and it is available for purchase in wet markets in many parts of the world. This is shifting viral reservoirs and contact-rates between virus-carrying animals and humans. Local authorities must formulate and enforce regulations governing the illegal sale of wildlife in global food trade and food markets while balancing respect for cultural food practices with public health prevention measures. Social behavior change strategies that focus on mitigating the risks of secondary infections and the handling of animals should be prioritized and scaled up. Campaigns in Sierra Leone with Lassa fever and in the DRC with Ebola increased awareness of how the disease is transmitted in the handling and exposure of animals as food or through food contamination by animals.

Fourth, social protection programs should be linked to promoting the consumption and production of nutritious food and addressing food insecurity. Supporting developing countries with increased availability and rapid deployment of funds to support their food security policy programs is essential. The secretary-general of the United Nations has called for a debt standstill and debt restructuring for low-income countries. David Beasley, the World Food Programme's executive director, recommends that international lending institutions work with low-income countries to strengthen health, education, and other social safety nets during and after this crisis. The World Food Programme and its partners need support to continue to provide food assistance and other services in what is now a global economic and food crisis.

Fifth, researchers and development practitioners must recognize that the health of people, animals, and our shared environment are tightly interconnected. There is a need for a greater understanding of how our food system relates to climate change and the environment and how changes in ecosystems where animals live are driving the circulation of viral spread in real time.[78] Public health issues are environmental issues, and taking a "One Health" approach to science is critical to avoid future zoonotic spillovers. Governments should not fall silent and turn inward on their global commitments. Instead, they should double down on fostering opportunities to re-engage and collaborate on issues that will require global cooperation such as climate change, sustainable development, ending hunger, and developing resilient ecosystems and oceans.

Sixth, there is no systematic global effort to monitor pathogens emerging from animals that put human populations at risk. The WHO should lead this effort, but it needs support from its member states. With the United States turning its back on the WHO during what may be one of the most crucial global health issues of the century, multilateral cooperation is imperiled. There is a need for even more surveillance through traceability technologies in the food system to track potential zoonotic and food-borne illnesses that threaten food systems and the health of our global population. One Health approaches—those at the intersection of human health, animal health, and environmental health—are critical as we respond to COVID-19, recover and learn from its impacts, and prepare for the next zoonotic pandemic.

Finally, financial backing is crucial if we are to ensure that hunger does not become the prevailing pandemic. The United Nations established a COVID-19 Global Humanitarian Response Plan that is estimated to cost $2 billion. These funds would enable agencies such as the WHO, the United Nations International Children's Fund (UNICEF), and the World Food Programme to provide basic services to the most vulnerable populations including food, water and sanitation, vaccinations, and COVID-19 testing materials and medical equipment. Only 46% of the required amount has been received.[79] Fending off a potential hunger pandemic will require not just public investment in these essential services and social protection but also a greater long-term private sector investment in sectors such as agriculture.[80]

The Necessity of World Order for Food Security

None of these technical recommendations to fix food systems is sustainable in the current fractured and sclerotic global politically enabling environment. For food systems to function effectively, equitably, and sufficiently during the pandemic and long after, the political environment must embrace global cooperation and inclusion, support private sector engagement, and minimize political polarization and geopolitical competition.

Climate change, for example, is a wide-reaching, large-scale transnational challenge in which every country is threatened and every country must act with others, in a coordinated fashion, on a short time-scale to mitigate the threat. The same is true for the COVID-19 pandemic. It requires a coordinated effort because of its inherent infectious nature and because of the interconnected globalized world in which the virus can spread. The adage "we are all in this together" requires strong public institutions at national and supranational levels. However, what we currently see is a world splintering geopolitically and ideologically. This trend does not bode well for an internationally coordinated response to the global COVID-19 crisis and the health, food, and economic systems that the pandemic has battered.

To ensure that food systems keep functioning, leadership, cooperation, and capacity are critical. Francis Fukuyama observed that "countries with dysfunctional states, polarized societies, or poor leadership have done badly, leaving their citizens and economies exposed and vulnerable."[81] It is not surprising that states led by populist, inward-facing leaders such as the United States, Brazil, and Mexico are not sufficiently addressing the pandemic. This has led to dire consequences for the citizens living in these countries, many of whom struggle with food insecurity and high COVID-related morbidity and mortality.

The COVID-19 response has also displayed the weaknesses of the multilateral system and existing institutions.[82] Within this, the global food architecture is often slow and outdated. For example, there is no overarching international governance structure that deals with food shocks. UN agencies involved in food systems decision making, such as the WHO, the FAO, UNICEF, and the World Food Programme, now more than ever need to coordinate and not worry so much about mission creep. The FAO (formed in 1945) and the WHO (formed in 1948) were created during a time when alliances were indispensable, but these organizations are perhaps now out of date and in need of an overhaul. The CGIAR (formerly the Consultative Group on International Agricultural Research), a potentially influential global partnership that unites international organizations engaged in research about food security, is in the middle of yet another reform process. This process must quickly come to closure, with a renewed effort to lead agriculture into the 21st century. The World Bank and the International Fund for Agricultural Development (IFAD), along with the bilateral organizations, need to step up their financial commitments. Currently, nutrition and agriculture receive less than 5% of official development assistance, which is largely inadequate.[83]

However, cooperation can happen in times of crisis. In 2008, the world food price crisis exposed millions of people to food insecurity and poverty and sparked food-related riots. The international community was ill prepared to respond, due to lethargic coordination of food policy and governance efforts. Yet, rising from the ashes, the G20 governments launched the Global Agriculture and Food Security Program (GAFSP), a multilateral fund to support low-income countries and increase investment in agriculture. Since its inception in 2010, GAFSP has invested $1.6 billion supporting more than 13 million smallholder farmers. Perhaps more efforts to scale GAFSP up and out should be considered to address food insecurity with the current pandemic.

Some are calling for a well-funded public health–oriented treaty organization that organizes a coordinated response during pandemics.[84] This too is needed within the food governance architecture. The UN Food Summit in 2021 might be a moment to create a global strategy for food governance that is nimble, modern, and inclusive, backed by a body modeled on the Intergovernmental Panel on Climate Change that provides evidence and science to support actions.

Conclusion

Governments, communities, and businesses around the world are learning to cope with the COVID-19 pandemic. The short-term priority is to stabilize food systems to ensure that hunger, poor diets, and failing health do not cause a complete economic collapse. But it is in times of great crisis that fundamental reforms are born. The United Nations, the World Bank, the International Monetary Fund, and the welfare state were developed following the Second World War as governments came together to move toward a path of global cooperation, stability, and peace. The FAO and the WHO were formed as specialized agencies within the United Nations to address issues with international implications such as global hunger, poverty, and infectious diseases like smallpox and polio, under the assumption that global cooperation was imperative.

The world, however, has changed over the last fifty-plus years, and we face new challenges. The COVID-19 pandemic has become a food, economic, and social crisis, and it has exacerbated disease burdens. There is a need to reshape our food systems for tomorrow—to deal with the COVID-19 crisis as well as with the much larger diet-related health crisis, which has been with us for decades. This is the time to foster greater collaboration between governments, civil society, the multilateral system, and the private sector to reshape a post-crisis narrative about how the global food architecture and governments can better work together to improve access for all to safe, nutritious foods.

NOTES

1. UN Food and Agriculture Organization, International Fund for Agricultural Development, and World Food Programme, *The State of Food Insecurity in the World, 2015* (Rome: FAO, 2015), http://www.fao.org/3/a-i4646e.pdf.

2. UN Food and Agriculture Organization, International Fund for Agricultural Development, and World Food Programme, *The State of Food Insecurity in the World, 2019* (Rome: FAO, 2019), http://www.fao.org/3/ca5162en/ca5162en.pdf.

3. World Food Programme, *2020: Global Report on Food Crises*, April 20, 2020. https://www.wfp.org/publications/2020-global-report-food-crises.

4. FAO, *The State of Food Insecurity in the World, 2019.*

5. World Food Programme, *2020: Global Report on Food Crises.*

6. FAO, *The State of Food Insecurity in the World, 2019*; Walter Willett et al., "Food in the Anthropocene: The EAT-Lancet Commission on Healthy Diets from Sustainable Food Systems," *Lancet* 393, no. 10170 (2019): 447–92.

7. World Food Programme, "COVID-19 Will Double Number of People Facing Food Crisis Unless Swift Action is Taken," WFP news release, April 20, 2020, https://www.wfp.org/news/covid-19-will-double-number-people-facing-food crises-unless-swift-action-taken.

8. World Bank, "Poverty," accessed June 25, 2020, https://www.worldbank.org/en/topic/poverty/overview.

9. UNHCR, "Figures at a Glance," June 18, 2020, https://www.unhcr.org/en-us/figures-at-a-glance.html.

10. Lancet Global Health Editors, "Food Insecurity Will Be the Sting in the Tail of COVID-19," *Lancet Global Health* 8, no. 6 (2020): e737, https://doi.org/10.1016/S2214-109X(20)30228-X.

11. Craig Gundersen and James P. Zilliak, "Food Insecurity and Health Outcomes," *Health Affairs* 34, no. 11 (2015): 1830–39, https://doi.org/10.1377/hlthaff.2015.0645.

12. Jung Sun Lee, Craig Gundersen, John Cook, Barbara Laraia, and Mary Ann Johnson, "Food Insecurity and Health across the Lifespan," *Advances in Nutrition* 3, no. 5 (September 2012): 744–45, http://10.3945/an.112.002543; Priya Shankar, Rainjade Chung, and Deborah A. Frank, "Association of Food Insecurity with Children's Behavioral, Emotional, and Academic Outcomes: A Systematic Review," *Journal of Developmental & Behavioral Pediatrics* 38, no. 2 (2017): 135–50, https://doi.org/10.1097/dbp.0000000000000383.

13. Christian A. Gregory and Alisha Coleman-Jensen, "Food Insecurity, Chronic Disease, and Health among Working-Age Adults," United States Department of Agriculture, Economic Research Service, Economic Research Report no. 235 (July 2017), https://www.ers.usda.gov/webdocs/publications/84467/err-235.pdf?v=3858.

14. Liping Pan, Bettylou Sherry, Rashid Njai, and Heidi M. Blanck, "Food Insecurity Is Associated with Obesity among US Adults in 12 States," *Journal of the Academy of Nutrition and Dietetics* 112, no. 9 (2012): 1403–9, https://doi.org/10.1016/j.jand.2012.06.011.

15. Lauren E. Au, Sonya M. Zhu, Lilly A. Nhan, Kaela R. Plank, Edward A. Frongillo, Barbara A. Laraia, Klara Gurzo, and Lorrene D. Ritchie, "Household Food Insecurity Is Associated with Higher Adiposity among US Schoolchildren Ages 10–15 Years: The Healthy Communities Study," *Journal of Nutrition* 149, no. 9 (2019): 1642–50, https://10.1016/j.jand.2012.06.011.

16. Edward A. Frongillo and Jennifer Bernal, "Understanding the Coexistence of Food Insecurity and Obesity," *Current Pediatrics Reports* 2, no. 4 (2014): 284–90, https://link.springer.com/content/pdf/10.1007/s40124-014-0056-6.pdf.

17. Laura C. Schulz, "The Dutch Hunger Winter and the Developmental Origins of Health and Disease," *Proceedings of the National Academy of Sciences* 107, no. 39 (2010): 16757–58, https://doi.org/10.1073/pnas.1012911107.

18. Global Nutrition Report, 2020, https://globalnutritionreport.org; Hans Henri P. Kluge, Kremlin Wickramasinghe, Holly L. Rippin, Romeu Mendes, David H. Peters, Anna Kontsevaya, and Joao Breda, "Prevention and Control of Non-communicable Diseases in the COVID-19 Response," *Lancet* 395, no. 10238 (2020): 1678–80, https://10.1016/S0140-6736(20)31067-9; David A. Kass, Priya Duggal, and Oscar Cingolani, "Obesity Could Shift

Severe COVID-19 Disease to Younger Ages," *Lancet* 395, no. 10236 (2020): 1544–45, http://10.1016/S0140-6736(20)31024-2; Jennifer Lighter, Michael Phillips, Sarah Hochman, Stephanie Sterling, Diane Johnson, Fritz Francois, and Anna Stachel, "Obesity in Patients Younger Than 60 Years Is a Risk Factor for COVID-19 Hospital Admission," *Clinical Infectious Diseases*, ciaa415 (April 2020), https://doi.org/10.1093/cid/ciaa415.

19. Ashkan Afshin, Patrick John Sur, Kairsten A. Fay, Leslie Cornaby, Giannina Ferrara, Joseph S. Salama, Erin C. Mullany et al., "Health Effects of Dietary Risks in 195 Countries, 1990–2017: Systematic Analysis for the Global Burden of Disease Study 2017," *Lancet* 393, no. 10184 (April 2019): 1958–72, https://doi.org/10.1016/S0140-6736(19)30041-8.

20. US Department of State, *United Nations Conference on Food and Agriculture: Final Act and Section Reports* (Washington DC: Government Printing Office, 1943), http://resource.nlm.nih.gov/2511080R.

21. Derek Byerlee and Jessica Fanzo, "The SDG of Zero Hunger 75 Years On: Turning Full Circle on Agriculture and Nutrition," *Global Food Security* 21 (2019): 52–59, https://10.1016/j.gfs.2019.06.002.

22. Robert E. Evenson and Douglas Gollin, "Assessing the Impact of the Green Revolution, 1960 to 2000," *Science* 300, no. 5620 (2003): 758–62, https://10.1126/science.1078710; Prabhu L Pingali, "Green Revolution: Impacts, Limits, and the Path Ahead," *Proceedings of the National Academy of Sciences* 109, no. 31 (2012): 12302–8, https://doi.org/10.1073/pnas.0912953109.

23. Prabhu L. Pingali, "The Green Revolution and Crop Biodiversity," in *The Routledge Handbook of Agricultural Biodiversity*, ed. Danny Hunter, Luigi Guarino, Charles Spillane, and Peter C. McKeown (Abington: Routledge, 2017): 213–23, https://doi.org/10.4324/9781317753285.

24. Pingali, "The Green Revolution"; Colin K. Khoury, Anne D. Bjorkman, Hannes Dempewolf, Julian Ramirez-Villegas, Luigi Guarino, Andy Jarvis, Loren H. Rieseberg, and Paul C. Struik, "Increasing Homogeneity in Global Food Supplies and the Implications for Food Security," *Proceedings of the National Academy of Sciences* 111, no. 11 (2014): 4001–6, https://10.1073/pnas.1313490111.

25. Boyd A. Swinburn, Vivica I. Kraak, Steven Allender, Vincent J. Atkins, Phillip I. Baker, Jessica R. Bogard, Hannah Brinsden et al., "The Global Syndemic of Obesity, Undernutrition, and Climate Change: the Lancet Commission Report," *Lancet* 393, no. 10173 (2019): 791–846, https://www.thelancet.com/commissions/global-syndemic.

26. Marc F. Bellemare, "Rising Food Prices, Food Price Volatility, and Social Unrest," *American Journal of Agricultural Economics* 97, no. 1 (2015): 1–21, https://doi.org/10.1093/ajae/aau038; Adesoji Adelaja, Justin George, Takashi Miyahara, and Eva Penar, "Food Insecurity and Terrorism," *Applied Economic Perspectives and Policy* 41, no. 3 (2019): 475–97; Cullen S. Hendrix and Stephan Haggard, "Global Food Prices, Regime Type, and Urban Unrest in the Developing World," *Journal of Peace Research* 52, no. 2 (2015): 143–57, https://doi.org/10.1177/0022343314561599; Ore Koren and Benjamin E. Bagozzi, "From Global to Local, Food Insecurity Is Associated with Contemporary Armed Conflicts," *Food Security* 8, no. 5 (2016): 999–1010, https:// 10.1007/s12571-016-0610-x/.

27. UN Food and Agriculture Organization, International Fund for Agricultural Development, and World Food Programme, *The State of Food Insecurity in the World, 2017* (Rome: FAO, 2017), http://www.fao.org/3/a-I7695e.pdf.

28. High-Level Expert Forum, UN Food and Agriculture Organization, *Food Insecurity in Protracted Crises—An Overview* (Rome: FAO, 2012), http://www.fao.org/fileadmin /templates/cfs_high_level_forum/documents/Brief1.pdf.

29. Alex De Waal, *Mass Starvation: The History and Future of Famine*, 1st ed. (Cambridge, MA: John Wiley & Sons, 2017).

30. Ellen Messer, Marc J. Cohen, and Thomas Marchione, "Conflict: A Cause and Effect of Hunger," *Enviromental Change and Security Program*, no. 7 (2001): 1–16, https://www .wilsoncenter.org/sites/default/files/media/documents/publication/ECSP7-feature articles-1.pdf.

31. Marc F. Bellemare, "Rising Food Prices, Food Price Volatility, and Social Unrest," *American Journal of Agricultural Economics* 97, no. 1 (2015): 1–21.

32. De Waal, *Mass Starvation*.

33. Kate E. Jones, Nikkita G. Patel, Marc A. Levy, Adam Storeygard, Deborah Balk, John L. Gittleman, and Peter Daszak, "Global Trends in Emerging Infectious Diseases," *Nature* 451, no. 7181 (February 2008): 990–93, https://https://doi.org/10.1038/nature06536.

34. World Wildlife Foundation Global Science, "Beyond Boundaries: Insights into Emerging Zoonotic Diseases, Nature, and Human Well-Being: Internal Science Brief" (unpublished paper).

35. Ferris Jabr, "How Humanity Unleashed a Flood of New Diseases," *New York Times*, June 25, 2020, https://www.nytimes.com/2020/06/17/magazine/animal-disease-covid .html.

36. World Wildlife Foundation Global Science, "Beyond Boundaries."

37. Simon L. Lewis and Mark A. Maslin, "Defining the Anthropocene," *Nature* 519, no. 7542 (2015): 171–80, https://doi.org/10.1038/nature14258.

38. Andrew P. Schurer, Gabriele C. Hegerl, Michael E. Mann, Simon F. B. Tett, and Steven J. Phipps, "Separating Forced from Chaotic Climate Variability over the Past Millennium," *Journal of Climate* 26, no. 18 (2013): 6954–73, https://doi.org/10.1175/JCLI-D -12-00826.1.

39. Willett et al., "Food in the Anthropocene."

40. Tim Searchinger, Richard Waite, Craig Hanson, Janet Ranganathan, Patrice Dumas, and Emily Matthews, "Creating a Sustainable Food Future: A Menu of Solutions to Feed Nearly 10 Billion People by 2050," *World Resources Report*, December 2018, https:// files.wri.org/s3fs-public/creating-sustainable-food-future_2.pdf.

41. James M. Hassell, Michael Begon, Melissa J. Ward, and Eric M. Fèvre, "Urbanization and Disease Emergence: Dynamics at the Wildlife-Livestock-Human Interface," *Trends in Ecology and Evolution* 32, no. 1 (2017): 55–67, https://10.1016/j.tree.2016.09.012.

42. FAO, *The State of Food Insecurity in the World, 2019*.

43. Samuel T. Turvey and Jennifer J. Crees, "Extinction in the Anthropocene," *Current Biology* 29, no. 19 (2019): R982–R986, http://10.1016/j.cub.2019.07.040; Gerardo Ceballos, Paul R. Ehrlich, and Peter H. Raven, "Vertebrates on the Brink as Indicators of Biological Annihilation and the Sixth Mass Extinction," *Proceedings of the National Academy of Sciences* 117, no. 24 (2020): 13596–602, https://doi.org/10.1073/pnas.1922686117.

44. Colin K. Khoury et al., "Increasing Homogeneity in Global Food Supplies and the Implications for Food Security," *Proceedings of the National Academy of Sciences* 111, no. 11 (2015): 4001–6.

45. UN Food and Agricultual Organization, *Nutrition and Food Systems,* September 2017, http://www.fao.org/3/a-i7846e.pdf; Kelly Parsons, Corinna Hawkes, and Rebecca Wells, "What Is the Food System? A Food Policy Perspective," in *Rethinking Food Policy: A Fresh Approach to Policy and Practice* (London: Centre for Food Policy, 2019).

46. Jill E. Hobbs, "Food Supply Chains during the COVID-19 Pandemic," *Canadian Journal of Agricultural Economics,* special issue (April 2020): 1–6, https://doi.org/10.1111/cjag.12237; Jessica Fanzo, Namukolo Covic, Achim Dobermann, Spencer Henson, Mario Herrero, Prabhu Pingali, and Steve Staal, "A Research Vision for Food Systems in the 2020s: Defying the Status Quo," *Global Food Security* (in press, 2020); Máximo Torero, "Without Food, There Can Be No Exit from the Pandemic," *Nature* 580, no. 7805 (2020): 588–89, https://10.1038/d41586-020-01181-3.

47. Torero, "Without Food, There Can Be No Exit from the Pandemic."

48. Michael Pollan, "The Sickness in Our Food Supply," *New York Review of Books* 67, no. 10 (June 2020): 1–6, https://www-nybooks-com.proxy1.library.jhu.edu/articles/2020/06/11/covid-19-sickness-food-supply/; Alessio Cappelli and Enrico Cini, "Will the COVID-19 Pandemic Make Us Reconsider the Relevance of Short Food Supply Chains and Local Productions?" *Trends in Food Science & Technology* 99 (May 2020): 566–67, https://doi.org/10.1016/j.tifs.2020.03.041.

49. Christopher B. Barrett, "Actions Now Can Curb Food Systems Fallout from COVID-19," *Nature Food* 1 (2020): 319–20, https://doi.org/10.1038/s43016-020-0085-y.

50. Torero, "Without Food, There Can Be No Exit from the Pandemic."

51. Pollan, "The Sickness in Our Food Supply."

52. Sarah Graddy, Soren Rundquist, and Bill Walker, "Investigation: Counties with Meatpacking Plants Report Twice the National Average Rate of COVID-19 Infections," *Infections: Environmental Working Group,* https://www.ewg.org/news-and-analysis/2020/05/ewg-map-counties-meatpacking-plants-report-twice-national-average-rate.

53. Lancet Global Health Editors, "Food Insecurity Will Be the Sting in the Tail of COVID-19."

54. "Impact of the Coronavirus (COVID-19) on the African Economy," *Africa Union,* https://au.int/sites/default/files/documents/38326-doc-covid-19_impact_on_african_economy.pdf

55. Mywish Maredia, "Key Findings of the 2020 South Asia Survey on the Effects of COVID-19," World Technology Access Program, Michigan State University, June 23, 2020, https://www.canr.msu.edu/news/key-findings-of-the-2020-south-asia-survey-on-the-effects-of-covid-19.

56. Stella Nordhagen, "Covid-19 and Food Prices: What Do We Know So Far?" *Gain Health,* May 4, 2020, https://www.gainhealth.org/media/news/covid-19-and-food-prices-what-do-we-know-so-far.

57. Kalle Hirvonen, Yan Bai, Derek Headey, and William A. Masters, "Cost and Affordability of the EAT-Lancet Diet in 159 Countries," *Lancet Global Health* 8, no. 1 (January 2020): E59–E66, http://dx.doi.org/10.2139/ssrn.3405576; Manika Sharma, Avinash Kishore, Devesh Roy, and Kuhu Joshi, "A Comparison of the Indian Diet with the EAT-Lancet Reference Diet," *BMC Public Health* 20, no. 812 (2020): 1–13, https://doi.org/10.1186/s12889-020-08951-8.

58. Matthias B. Schulze, Miguel A. Martínez-González, Teresa T. Fung, Alice H. Lichtenstein, and Nita G. Forouhi, "Food-Based Dietary Patterns and Chronic Disease Prevention," *BMJ* 361 (2018): 1–6, https://doi.org/10.1136/bmj.k2396; Renata Micha, Jose L. Peñalvo, Frederick Cudhea, Fumiaki Imamura, Colin D. Rehm, and Dariush Mozaffarian, "Association between Dietary Factors and Mortality from Heart Disease, Stroke, and Type 2 Diabetes in the United States," *JAMA* 317, no. 9 (2017): 912–24, https://10.1001/jama .2017.0947; Dariush Mozaffarian, Sonia Y. Angell, Tim Lang, Juan A. Rivera, "Role of Government Policy in Nutrition—Barriers to and Opportunities for Healthier Eating," *BMJ* 361 (2018): 1–11, https://doi.org/10.1136/bmj.k2426.

59. Timothy Roberton, Emily D. Carter, Victoria B. Chou, Angela R. Stegmuller, Bianca D. Jackson, Yvonne Tam, Talata Sawadogo-Lewis, and Neff Walker, "Early Estimates of the Indirect Effects of the COVID-19 Pandemic on Maternal and Child Mortality in Low-Income and Middle-Income Countries: A Modelling Study," *Lancet Global Health* 8, no. 7 (May 2020): e901–908, https://doi.org/10.1016/S2214-109X(20)30229-1.

60. Lancet Global Health Editors, "Food Insecurity Will Be the Sting in the Tail of COVID-19."

61. Khoury et al., "Increasing Homogeneity in Global Food Supplies."

62. Searchinger et al., "Creating a Sustainable Food Future."

63. Marco Springmann, Daniel Mason-D'Croz, Sherman Robinson, Tara Garnett, H. Charles J. Godfray, Douglas Gollin, Mike Rayner, Paola Ballon, and Peter Scarborough, "Global and Regional Health Effects of Future Food Production under Climate Change: A Modelling Study," *Lancet* 387, no. 10031 (2016): 1937–46, https://10.1016/S0140-6736 (15)01156-3.

64. Searchinger et al., "Creating a Sustainable Food Future."

65. Willett et al., "Food in the Anthropocene."

66. Jessica Fanzo, Claire Davis, Rebecca McLaren, and Jowel Choufani, "The Effect of Climate Change across Food Systems: Implications for Nutrition Outcomes," *Global Food Security* 18 (2018): 12–19, https://doi.org/10.1016/j.gfs.2018.06.001.

67. Barrett, "Actions Now Can Curb Food Systems Fallout from COVID-19."

68. Kirk Semple, "In Some Nations, Coronavirus Is Only One of Many Outreaks, *New York Times,* May 30, 2020, https://www.nytimes.com/2020/05/30/world/americas /virus-central-america-dengue.html?action=click&module=RelatedLinks&pgtype=Ar ticle; Jan Hoffman and Ruth Maclean, "Slowing the Coronavirus Is Speeding the Spread of Other Diseases," *New York Times,* July 1, 2020, https://www.nytimes.com/2020/06/14 /health/coronavirus-vaccines-measles.html?action=click&module=RelatedLinks&pgtyp e=Article.

69. United Nations Policy Brief, *The Impact of COVID-19 on Food Security and Nutrition* (June 2020), https://www.un.org/sites/un2.un.org/files/sg_policy_brief_on_covid_impact _on_food_security.pdf.

70. United States Department of Agriculture, Economic Research Service, "Farm Labor," accessed June 30, 2020, https://www.ers.usda.gov/topics/farm-economy/farm-labor/.

71. Rafael Pérez-Escamilla, Kenda Cunningham, and Victoria Hall Moran, "COVID-19 and Maternal and Child Food and Nutrition Insecurity: A Complex Syndemic," *Maternal & Child Nutrition* 16, no. 3 (2020): e13036, https://doi.org/10.1111/mcn.13036.

72. Melissa Hidrobo, John Hoddinott, Neha Kumar, and Meghan Olivier, "Social Protection, Food Security, and Asset Formation," *World Development* 101 (2018): 88–103, https://doi.org/10.1016/j.worlddev.2017.08.014.

73. Stephen Devereux and Jonas Nzabamwita, "Social Protection, Food Security and Nutrition in Six African Countries," IDS Working Paper 518 (2018), https://opendocs.ids.ac.uk/opendocs/handle/20.500.12413/14091.

74. Philip B. Maffetone and Paul B. Laursen, "The Perfect Storm: Coronavirus (Covid-19) Pandemic Meets Overfat Pandemic," *Frontiers in Public Health* 8 (2020): 135, https://doi.org/10.3389/fpubh.2020.00135.

75. Mozaffarian, "Association between Dietary Factors and Mortality."

76. Clyde W. Yancy, "COVID-19 and African Americans," *JAMA* 323, no. 19 (2020): 1891–92, https:// doi:10.1001/jama.2020.6548.

77. Dariush Mozaffarian, "Dietary and Policy Priorities to Reduce the Global Crises of Obesity and Diabetes," *Nature Food* 1, no. 1 (2020): 38–50, https://doi.org/10.1038/s43016-019-0013-1.

78. Willett et al., "Food in the Anthropocene"; Intergovernmental Panel on Climate Change, *Climate Change and Land,* January 2020, https://www.ipcc.ch/site/assets/uploads/sites/4/2020/02/SPM_Updated-Jan20.pdf.

79. Lancet Global Health Editors, "Food Insecurity Will Be the Sting in the Tail of COVID-19."

80. David Beasely, "The Looming Hunger Pandemic," *Foreign Affairs* 99, no. 4 (July/August 2020), https://www.foreignaffairs.com/articles/world/2020-06-16/looming-hunger-pandemic.

81. Francis Fukuyama, "The Pandemic and Political Order: It Takes a State," *Foreign Affairs* 99, no. 4 (July/August 2020): 26–32, https://www.foreignaffairs.com/articles/world/2020-06-09/pandemic-and-political-order.

82. Fukuyama, "The Pandemic and Political Order."

83. Derek Byerlee and Jessica Fanzo, "The SDG of Zero Hunger 75 Years On," *Global Food Security.*

84. Michael Osterholm and Mark Olshaker, "Chronicle of a Pandemic Foretold: Learning from the COVID-19 Failure—Before the Next Outbreak Arrives," *Foreign Affairs* 99, no. 4 (July/August 2020): 10–24, https://www.foreignaffairs.com/articles/united-states/2020-05-21/coronavirus-chronicle-pandemic-foretold.

Flat No Longer

Technology in the Post-COVID World

Christine Fox and Thayer Scott

E ven before the world faced a pandemic crisis, the bloom was already coming off the rose of globalization. Nowhere is this more true than in the high-technology arena—an arena that had been at the forefront of breaking down barriers and transcending the traditional antagonisms between nations. Technology, commerce, and connectivity would move on apace regardless of what governments did or said. Fields such as telecommunications, computing, artificial intelligence (AI), and biotechnology have all benefited from the relatively open exchange of people and products since the Cold War ended.

By the time the COVID-19 pandemic struck, the globalist system of technology commerce and research was already starting to fray. The United States was in the midst of using its semiconductor advantages to slow the spread of Chinese telecommunications infrastructure—efforts that would intensify after the outbreak. The COVID-19 crisis revealed the United States' deep and disturbing dependence on China for key pharmaceuticals and medical equipment, sparking calls for more self-sufficiency and less reliance on foreign suppliers. The kind of globalism extolled by Thomas Friedman and others after the Cold War now looks much less inevitable—and attractive—in the wake of COVID-19.[1]

Christine Fox is assistant director for policy and analysis at the Johns Hopkins University Applied Physics Laboratory. Thayer Scott is a public policy writer and consultant.

The authors are grateful for the contributions of Melissa Terlaje and Jessica Dymond to this essay.

China has moved quickly and opportunistically to further upend a liberal world order that had been conducive to technology innovation—and to American interests. For example, the Chinese government is leveraging its existing Belt and Road Initiative (BRI) relationships and transport hubs to provide medical equipment, supplies, and treatment to many of the same countries as part of a new "Health Silk Road." China is also aggressively deploying its own 5G telecommunications systems and enabling electronic surveillance in ways that are appealing to authoritarian governments within the BRI and elsewhere. Where the United States has withdrawn—through a combination of hostility and indifference—from global institutions, most notably the World Health Organization (WHO), China has jumped in to fill the gap. This dynamic extends to international bodies that set standards for the next generation of technology. Recently, China's president, Xi Jinping, presented China as an exemplar nation, promoting a "community of common destiny for mankind."[2] The United States appears to be entering a period of retrenchment, on course to unravel supply chains for medical equipment, computing, telecommunications, and more.

Retrenchment and disentanglement pose significant risks, as the United States could end up with less access to international technology talent, innovation, and markets. Before the pandemic, the Chinese government had set ambitious plans and made significant investments in critical technologies—efforts redoubled in the wake of COVID-19.[3] China is poised to expand its influence by more widely deploying its telecommunications infrastructure, encouraging the de facto splintering of what had been a World Wide Web, and reaping the fruits of massive investments in domestic research and development and manufacturing. China's aggressive engagement with international standards setting could further advance and validate its authoritarian model in much of the world.

Many important technology products and discoveries trace their origins to when the US government, in the context of the Cold War, played a much larger role in funding and research. In recent decades, the commercial sector has been the driving force behind technology innovation. American technology leaders often cite the relatively light, or absent, hand of national governments as a key to success. But the past couple of years have also shown the limits of laissez-faire—for telecom and pharmaceuticals especially. To mitigate some of these dependencies in a way that minimizes negative economic and scientific impacts, the US government will need to play a more active and more competent role in ensuring reliable sourcing on everything from 5G to antibiotics. Attempting to do so unilaterally will almost certainly fail and leave us worse off. Without trying to replicate an inefficient and centralized Chinese model, the governments of advanced democracies must collaborate more—with each other and between each country's public and private sectors.

These partnerships are needed to hinder Chinese attempts to achieve technology market dominance and, with it, the ability to intimidate and coerce other nations. The approach must be nuanced enough to allow for, and even encourage, research collaborations in fields that benefit the world such as AI and biotech. This strategy will be difficult to design and carry out—it must build up domestic capacity while pursuing global engagement in ways that shape international norms and values. But continuing on this present course will lead to a post-COVID-19 world order that will look considerably different—and much less hospitable—to American needs and aspirations.

This essay explores these challenges—along with recommended government responses—with respect to the potential disintegration of the global internet, the unraveling of global supply chains for semiconductors and telecommunications, and the risks and opportunities posed by biotechnology.

The Coming Splinternet

The internet is a network of independently managed networks—a network of networks—that enables the global sharing of information, communications, and our digital economy. The internet is also at the core of modern disputes over freedom of expression, privacy, transnational crime, internal security, intellectual property, trade, and economic regulation.[4] It has been blamed for the rise of terrorism, the destruction of individual privacy, increased intellectual property theft, and the spread of misinformation. It is also seen as having the potential to sway elections and even topple governments, as evidenced by the Arab Spring.[5] The issues associated with internet governance—technical standards, censorship, privacy, intellectual property—reflect a wider global balkanization. Contravening the internet's origins and ideals, many nations are seeking to impose controls on what populations can see and do online within their borders, in effect fragmenting the internet into different camps with different rules. Eric Schmidt coined the term "splinternet" several years ago, and it stuck.[6] Were this to happen, the World Wide Web that we have grown so accustomed to would be gone, or at least significantly less "world wide." Without a universal internet, national governments would be able to decide what their citizens can access online from inside or outside the country—products, services, information, or ideas. This is not a world that is easy for us to envision today, yet it is a world that we may be heading for.

In some cases, concerns over privacy, health, and safety are creating localized rules and regulations. France, for example, has required Google to remove thousands of search results under a "right to be forgotten" law. France is also leading the European Union (EU) in pushing for new copyright protections that could result in websites banning users from uploading files.[7] But the world's most stringent set of data protection rules comes from the EU's General Data Protection Regulation (GDPR),[8] which went into effect in 2018. These rules place limits on what organizations can do with personal data. And these rules have teeth: the GDPR enables regulators to impose huge fines on businesses for noncompliance.[9] The GDPR is often heralded as a model for personal privacy protections, but it also contributes to segmentation of the internet. It creates a new set of regulatory hurdles and costs for internet transactions. If other countries follow suit, we could end up with an overlapping regulatory environment that puts a damper on international business flow. Smaller businesses in particular would struggle to navigate a complex web of compliance laws.[10]

For other groups of nations, the prime motivation is information control. Russia's "sovereign internet" law of May 2019 mandates that all internet traffic flow through government-controlled choke points, allowing authorities to censor the information before it reaches the Russian people. Russia's internet is not designed technically for this type of choke-point control, however. Hundreds of networks come together in Russia, and many of them are supplied by international network providers.[11] Experts suggest that attempts to employ choke points and block content in this complex network will result in instabilities that will make Russia's internet slower and less reliable.[12] Nonetheless, for the Russian leadership, controlling the internet's content is more important than the quality of internet service received by its people.

China, on the other hand, built its internet from the start on a series of state-run network operators, leading to what is commonly called the Great Firewall of China.[13] It allows the Chinese central government to censor the information available to its citizens more easily than Russian leadership can. China's president, Xi Jinping, does not consider his blatant efforts to control the internet to be a source of embarrassment or something to hide. Rather, he openly discusses this system with pride and sees his vision as a model for other countries,[14] one that advances commerce and innovation without fostering dissent that leads to political change.

Because the existing internet does not align with national borders, governments desiring this kind of internal control must, in effect, build their own internets with their own rules. China is working on a new root name server—a mechanism for translating domain names into numeric internet protocol (IP) addresses—and a corresponding operating organization. Currently there are at least a dozen virtual root name servers based in the United States, Europe, and Japan—but none in China.[15] Control of root name servers translates into control of the distribution of IP addresses and domain names.[16] In a December 2019 statement announcing this effort by the China Academy of Information and Communications Technology (CAICT), the Chinese government said, "While ensuring the stable operation of the server and providing quality service to users, the CAICT should also protect users' information security and safeguard national interests."[17] This new root name server could further splinter the internet and provide other governments an alternative to the current system.

A splintered internet will lead inevitably to an even more splintered big-tech enterprise. US companies are still the overall global leaders in internet services and search engines—except in China. While Google holds more than 90% of the worldwide search engine market, it holds less than 5% of the market in China.[18] Baidu, China's top seach engine provider, is focused primarily on the domestic market and as a result has little market penetration elsewhere. Those metrics should give no comfort to American companies—or US leaders. Consider that in the first quarter of 2020, China had more than 900 million internet users, and that number was growing at a rate of 5% annually. In fact, China has more internet users than the United States and the European Union combined.[19]

If China is successful at creating a separate splinter of the internet, Baidu, along with Alibaba and Tencent, collectively known as "BAT," will be ready with the corresponding search engines and internet services. Over time, this Chinese version of the internet and aligned technology companies could become favored by Digital Silk Road countries and authoritarian governments elsewhere. If successful, they could eat into the international market currently dominated by the United States and its corresponding technology giants, including Facebook, Apple, Amazon, Netflix, and Google. No longer "citizens of the world," major US technology companies would need to operate more like "national champions." Under this scenario, Americans would continue to access quality technology goods and services from US providers and partners, but with less choice and at a higher price.

The inherent strengths of the West and its democratic allies worldwide nonetheless provide a foundation for continued success. The concern is less commercial than ideological. The Chinese governing model—state direction and subsidy of a technology industry subsequently used to control its population—may gain more purchase elsewhere. A "digital curtain" could divide up much of the world into competing (and increasingly incompatible) camps for information and communications. China could be poised to take a larger share of emerging economies with growing populations in the BRI nations of Central Asia, Latin America, Africa, the Middle East, and possibly even southeastern Europe. This scenario does not bode well for US ideals or interests over the long term.

Mitigating the downside of a fragmented technology world will require cooperating in ways that run counter to current trends, with nations turning inward in the name of self-reliance and security. It will also require a commitment by the United States to international standard-setting organizations that, mostly out of the public eye, can make decisions with long-term consequences. As noted by Lindsay Gorman of the Cyberspace Solarium Commission, China has set an explicit goal of becoming "a standards-issuing country." Gorman adds, "China coordinates national standards-work across government, industry and academia as part of its push to increase international influence."[20] A March 2020 letter signed by seventeen US senators spanning the political and ideological spectrum voiced concern over China's use of international bodies to enshrine its preferred norms and rules for advanced surveillance technology. "China is currently working to use standards setting bodies to gain the imprimatur of international legitimacy and support across a range of emerging technologies . . . in service of [its] antidemocratic vision for technology."[21]

Over time China's well-coordinated and aggressive advocacy for international standards that reflect its interests and values will bear fruit at America's expense—and those of our European and Asian allies as well. Solarium's Gorman notes that, by contrast, the US approach to standardization has been bottom-up, stakeholder driven, and generally resistant to central planning. "For years, U.S. technological dominance in internet technologies meant that a lack of a coordinated approach did not seriously stifle U.S. competitiveness. . . . This hands-off approach may no longer be sufficient."[22]

The Showdown in Semiconductors and the Future of Telecom

Although other nations in Europe and Asia—including China—have developed successful semiconductor industries, the United States remains the dominant provider and player in the design and production of the most technically advanced chips used for many technologies, most notably telecommunications (5G) and AI. America's electronic design automation (EDA) vendors have held a lead in this market for three decades.[23] The United States also continues to dominate the production of semiconductor capital equipment. American companies generate more than half the global revenue for chip manufacturing equipment compared with Japan's 27% and Europe's 17%.[24]

Recently the United States has not been shy about exploiting some of these advantages, particularly in the area of telecommunications. In May 2019, President Donald J. Trump signed an executive order prohibiting US companies from using foreign telecommunications equipment deemed to be a national security risk.[25] Six months later, the Federal Communications Commission (FCC) barred American rural customers from tapping into an $8.5 billion government fund to buy from Huawei or other Chinese providers. The executive order was extended in May 2020 with what seemed a nuclear option for the telecommunications global supply chain: in addition to severing direct access to US suppliers, the order cut off Huawei's access to equipment manufactured overseas using American technology and software.[26] This meant that Huawei could no longer obtain semiconductors from its largest and most important supplier in Taiwan. The Commerce Department has since "clarified" the order to allow cooperation with Huawei on standards setting.[27] Huawei had reportedly been stockpiling chips for months in anticipation of the US action, but it faces a wrenching supply challenge in the future.

The Chinese government has been keenly aware of these hardware dependencies and is working to develop alternatives to American capital equipment and EDA tools. The barrier to entry is steep—the cost of creating manufacturing plants for the most advanced chips can run into the multiple billions. Huawei's ability to mitigate the effects of US restrictions will largely depend on its ability to develop international alternatives. Given the attractiveness of Huawei's market, this might be possible in just a few years.[28]

Irrespective of where the battle over semiconductors leads, the telecommunications sector is on an inexorable path toward fragmentation, and the COVID-19 crisis is accelerating it. The industry is heading back to the days of separate and competing global standards and a lack of interoperable equipment. We may see the effective dismantling of a truly global supply chain, replaced by more government-sanctioned sourcing arrangements between groups of like-minded countries, potentially leading to a new telecommunications cold war. Nations would be forced to choose either China's 5G capabilities, which entails buying into China's authoritarian-friendly standards framework, or a more expensive and potentially less capable alternative.

Again, this is starting to happen. Last year, the United States launched a campaign—mostly fruitless—to convince NATO members to exclude Huawei from new 5G networks. The economic benefits of transitioning to Huawei 5G, however, outweighed the security concerns raised by the United States. But the scale of China's deception at the onset of the pandemic caused a number of European allies to rethink prior decisions to allow Huawei to compete for all, or even part, of their future telecom infrastructure. According to news reports, the British government is proposing a 5G alliance of ten democracies to explore alternatives to Huawei. The alliance comprises the countries in the Group of Seven (G7)—Canada, France, Germany, Italy, Japan, the United Kingdom, and the United States—as well as Australia, South Korea, and India.[29] The alternate Chinese-led bloc will presumably consist of BRI and Digital Silk Road countries, among other authoritarian-leaning states. The challenge for the next decade will be to counter China's 5G technology advantages, not with punitive (and often counterproductive) sanctions, but with sustainable and effective alternatives.

In China there is no expectation of separation among the private, public, and nonprofit sectors—academia, business, and the military. This is not a model the United States can or should seek to emulate. Nonetheless, the post-COVID-19 technology order will require the return of a robust role for government—direction, regulation, funding, and linkage to policy goals—that would have been anathema to Silicon Valley as late as a decade ago. But to produce more than just headlines and disruption, the US government will need to overhaul its "whack-a-mole" approach to dealing with foreign companies, people, and research in sensitive technology areas. Today, expertise and authorities are scattered throughout the federal government within the major cabinet departments and in subordinate or independent agencies such as the FCC, the National Telecommunications and Information Administration, the Food and Drug Administration (FDA), and more.

The United States will need to rethink—reimagine even—the governing structure for supervising its technology industry, monitoring the activities of foreign companies, and representing its interests and values to allies in an international setting. In early June, the Senate Permanent Subcommittee on Investigations published a bipartisan report criticizing the executive branch's oversight of foreign telecommunications companies.[30] Within the Trump administration, that responsibility had fallen to an ad hoc "Team Telecom" created by an April 2020 executive order. It was heavily weighted toward national security equities: the secretary of defense, the attorney general, and the secretary of homeland security were formal members of the committee. Other "advisory" members, without executive authority, included the State Department, the Department of Commerce, and the Department of Treasury as well as the Council of Economic Advisers.[31] Despite this security orientation, the subcommittee report found that Team Telecom provided "minimal oversight" of Chinese state-owned telecommunications companies operating in the United States. Significantly, the report recommends that Congress turn Team Telecom into a statutorily authorized committee. Its existence and authority would be formalized into US law and thus overseen by Congress. Among other powers, this statutory body would have the authority to recommend that the FCC revoke existing licenses. The Lawfare blog considered it an "important signal that Congress may get more involved in empowering and monitoring the executive branch's supply-chain security process for foreign telecoms."[32]

We should empower and consolidate an elite cadre of professionals—drawing on the best talent from industry, government, and academia—to oversee America's international technology collaborations from a holistic perspective: from research centers to supply chains to connectivity standards. They can also more ably represent US interests in venues such as the International Telecommunication Union, which, like the WHO, has come under significant Chinese influence. The Arms Control and Disarmament Agency, separated from the State Department in 1961, provided a base of institutional knowledge on the arcane details of nuclear weapons and treaty negotiations; it was disbanded in 1999 after the end of the Cold War. The answer to sorting through these thorny technology questions—in a way that avoids crude and counterproductive restrictions providing little security benefit—may lie in a similar independent agency or an empowered organization nested within an existing department. Foreign governments—not just China, but those in Europe—are set up much more effectively to advance national equities and share international decision making in the technology realm. The US government, as many have observed, is still largely organized around a 1947 model designed during the smokestack era.

Biotech Maneuvering and Mastery

Even before the COVID-19 pandemic galvanized the world, China had set a clear goal to dominate the biotechnology market—everything from pharmaceuticals to medical equipment to genetic engineering. During a Senate hearing in November 2019, Tara J. O'Toole, senior fellow and executive vice president at In-Q-Tel, said that "China has said repeatedly and forcefully . . . that they intend to own the bio-revolution. And they are building the infrastructure, the talent pipeline, the regulatory system, and the financial system they need to do that."[33]

Until a few years ago, the Chinese pharmaceutical industry was producing generic drugs of varying quality under a difficult regulatory system riddled with corruption and cronyism.[34] The Chinese government responded with multibillion-dollar investments and by revamping its drug approval and quality control process to more closely resemble that of the United States

China now possesses the second-largest pharmaceutical market in the world.[35] It also controls the global supply of the ingredients for thousands of essential generic medicines. The trauma of the COVID-19 crises exposed Americans and Europeans to their overdependence on one country. According to Rosemary Gibson, author of *China Rx: Exposing the Risks of America's Dependence on China for Medicine*, fully 90% of the chemical ingredients for generic drugs in the United States to care for people with serious coronavirus infections requiring hospitalization are sourced from China.[36]

In a 2019 speech predating the pandemic, Chinese economist Li Daokiu said, "We are at the mercy of others when it comes to computer chips, but we are the world's largest exporter of raw materials for vitamins and antibiotics. Should we reduce the exports, the medical systems of some western countries will not run well."[37] In a March editorial widely quoted and criticized in the United States, China's official news agency reportedly asserted, "If China announces that its drugs are for domestic use and bans exports, the United States will fall in the hell of a new coronavirus epidemic."[38]

As a result of this vulnerability, many are calling for the United States to "reshore" its capacity to manufacture vital pharmaceuticals and even, in some cases, to outlaw importation from China altogether.[39] But we are not reliant solely on China. India is the world's second-largest exporter of active pharmaceutical ingredients.[40] As the intensity of the pandemic grew in March, the Indian government, looking to the needs of its people, ordered its pharmaceutical manufacturers to stop exporting twenty-six drugs, most of them antibiotics.

At this point, it is not clear whether rebuilding a robust domestic pharmaceutical production capacity is even possible. The issue is not technical capability but rather the cost and time necessary to build the infrastructure. Undeterred, President Trump recently used executive order authority to award a $354 million, four-year contract to a new company called Phlow to manufacture pharmaceutical ingredients and generic medicines used in treating patients hospitalized for COVID-19.[41] When asked about the challenges ahead, White House trade adviser Peter Navarro said, "If we have strong Buy American procurement, that will establish a robust base level of demand that provides the appropriate incentives for our pharmaceutical manufacturers to invest and locate domestically."[42] Despite these efforts, it is likely that the United States will remain dependent on China and other nations for key pharmaceuticals for a long time. Thomas Cosgrove, a former senior FDA official, said it will take "decades and billions" to bring the pharmaceutical supply chain back to the United States.[43]

In addition to pharmaceutical production, the US medical equipment industry went all in on globalization in pursuit of cost savings and shareholder value. Those decisions, allowed if not encouraged by US government policy, were reasonable at the time from a business perspective, but they proved nearly fatal, literally, when the United States faced the same major bio-threat and pharmaceutical requirements at the same time as the rest of the world.

By 2018 China provided nearly half of all US imports of personal protective equipment (PPE).[44] When coronavirus cases were initially surging in spring 2020, many other afflicted nations stopped exporting masks and protective gear, including South Korea, Germany, India, and Taiwan.[45] Instead of dropping exports of PPE, China rapidly stepped up production to twelve times its supply before the outbreak of the pandemic.[46] This effort was marred later by reports of quality problems with some of the Chinese products,[47] but the speed and scale of China's response still resonated, especially in contrast with the efforts of the United States and other Western countries. In early May, Andrew Cuomo, governor of the state hit hardest by the virus at the time, announced that New York hospitals must build a ninety-day supply of PPE to prepare for another outbreak. Cuomo said, "You can't be dependent on China to have the basic equipment to save lives in the United States."[48]

To regain and sustain a major domestic sourcing capacity for PPE, US industry needs more clarity regarding the magnitude and time frame of the expected need. Companies want to avoid a repeat of what occurred during the 2009 swine flu outbreak, when a number of providers doubled staff and purchased new equipment only to find the crisis over. One in particular, Prestige Ameritech, came to the brink of bankruptcy as a result.[49] On top of relying on global sources for key protective equipment, successive administrations and congresses neglected the national PPE stockpile after the 2009 H1N1 outbreak.[50] Without purchase guarantees from the government, companies will be reluctant to invest in production capabilities of medical supplies like PPE in the face of so many uncertainties.

Despite struggling with the effects of COVID-19, China has spent the last several months cementing and expanding its existing global relationships using its Belt and Road Initiative and Health Silk Road. By taking full advantage of the world's struggles with COVID-19, China is promoting yet more widespread reliance on its products while, as with telecom and the internet, offering an alternative model to the West.

China introduced its Health Silk Road model in the WHO back in 2017.[51] The message was that 21st-century health challenges require a more high-tech approach and that China was the country to lead the world in delivering those technologies, including 5G telecommunications. When the COVID-19 pandemic struck, global media were flooded with images of 5G-enabled technologies helping combat the virus, including health consultants employing telemedicine, robots taking temperatures, and drones delivering face masks.[52]

China is also using COVID-19 to strengthen its humanitarian reputation. China's Jack Ma and Alibaba Foundations have delivered supplies to dozens of countries, including the United States.[53] As the United States pulled inward to deal with the impact of the pandemic and its economic repercussions, China stepped into the void. When the United States froze its funding to the WHO in April 2020, China significantly increased its contributions. Recently, China announced that it would donate $2 billion over two years to help nations respond to the pandemic.[54]

Of course, the Belt and Road Initiative, and now the Health Silk Road, are a means for China to deploy its telecommunications and surveillance infrastructure globally. Without alternatives, struggling nations will accept these offers of "benevolent" assistance. China's technology companies and telecommunications and surveillance infrastructure will become ingrained in every aspect of these nations' workings, opening doors to greater data collection, increased leverage, and ultimately strong influence over the recipient nations' policies. The very nature of authoritarian governments allows them to control their populations, track movements, and trace contacts, whether to prevent the spread of disease or, very often, the spread of unwelcome ideas and viewpoints. In the pandemic response, authoritarian governments and democracies alike cannot avoid the necessity of using technology for public health and public safety. But how these powerful tools are used and viewed varies greatly. For a good number of countries—in Africa, Latin America, Central Asia, the Middle East, and even eastern and southern Europe—the COVID-19 experience validates a more aggressive approach to technology and governance. China already had a foothold in some of these countries, providing automated tools for internal security—facial recognition, drones, AI, and more. These tools can spread further in the name of public health.

When faced with today's coronavirus pandemic or an unknown pandemic of the future, it is vital to have cooperative research on a global scale that enables preparedness, treatment, and ultimately eradication. According to an Ohio State University study, collaborations between US and Chinese scientists have actually intensified despite the geopolitical tensions between the two countries. China has significantly increased its funding for COVID-19 research and is participating in research teams with US and UK scientists.[55] This is happening despite Donald Trump's recent presidential proclamation aimed at limiting the entry of Chinese graduate students to the United States.[56]

Political concerns are nonetheless creeping into the process, and we can expect a further decline in cooperation—and thus advancement—in the scientific realm. China has introduced new policies that require scientists to obtain approval to publish their results. Some suggest that this measure is designed to prevent what happened early in the pandemic, when some poor-quality Chinese COVID-19 studies were posted online. Others are concerned that this is primarily an effort by the Chinese government to control and limit information that may not reflect well on its response to the outbreak.[57]

On the US side, officials are warning American companies to be extremely careful to protect their research against potential Chinese attempts to steal it. The race for a COVID-19 vaccine—along with other treatments neglected during the crisis—could suffer if national pride and perceived self-interest thwart collaboration. In this respect biotechnology may more closely resemble the recent course of AI—a previously open field now being targeted for controls and restrictions justified on national security grounds. The basic foundations of AI algorithms—forms of mathematics available from open sources—are virtually uncontrollable across borders. Biotechnology is more vulnerable to restriction and, accordingly, to the potential loss of needed advances in medicine and public health.

The global response to COVID-19 has shown a great need for international cooperation and, at the same time, revealed the challenges of achieving that cooperation when all nations are struggling with the same problem. There are many reasons why China's reputation should be marred by the world's coronavirus experience: there is strong evidence that the government suppressed attempts to alert others to the threat of COVID-19, and there is evidence that the Chinese government continues to underreport cases. Yet, even taking undercounting and potential deception into account, China's death rate per capita is almost certainly lower than that of the United States.[58] In late June, the EU released a list of non-European countries whose citizens would be allowed onto the continent, which included Canada, Australia, and South Korea. China is on the list pending confirmation that EU travelers will be allowed to reciprocally enter mainland China. Citizens and residents of the United States, Brazil, and Russia were barred because of the continued spread of the virus in those countries.[59] China holds the cards in many of the needed medical capabilities and is using that advantage to extend its global reach by offering medical assistance *along with* 5G technology. When the world looks back on this pandemic, China's strategic, opportunistic response may emerge as the turning point for the new world order.

Conclusion

The experiences of a global pandemic have caused the American public and its leaders across the political spectrum to look more skeptically—and fearfully—at the highly globalized system of technology commerce and innovation. With widespread sickness, job loss, or worse looming, it seemed as if the United States had lost the ability to take care of its own people. Foreign dependencies impeded a rapid and effective national response, highlighting our limitations in knowledge, capacity, and essential materials and supplies. This pandemic came at a time when the United States and China were already growing estranged and on the path to decoupling in many areas of technology. In the wake of the COVID-19 outbreak, the United States has made it a priority to become more self-sufficient and less dependent on China for critical medical equipment and supplies. China is leveraging the needs of other nations to expand its telecommunications infrastructure and model of internet governance. The combination of attitudes—one self-focused and the other opportunistic—could lead to a new digital cold war, in which the technology path chosen by a country comes with a corresponding set of norms, standards, and practices conducive to either democratic values, supported by the United States and the West, or an authoritarian model, underwritten by China.

The United States needs a more comprehensively planned and funded government strategy on critical materials and technologies. This strategy will need to be nuanced—it must foster research collaborations while loosening China's grip on essential drugs and medical supplies and ensure that we are not again caught flat-footed and scrambling by another Chinese advance like 5G.

We must sustain America's leading position in technology innovation by participating in international research collaborations and sustaining the use of technology through global standards and norms. Even as we work in concert with like-minded partners and support an international research environment conducive to the well-being of all, the legitimate needs of individual nations for independence and national security must be respected. The United States must strengthen the voice of democratic values in a world where technology is increasingly used to suppress information, spread disinformation, and control populations.

It is tempting to use current American strengths in manufacturing sectors, such as semiconductors, to hold China back and, presumably, advantage our position over time. But these policies could backfire. They provide China with a platform from which to argue that it is the open, engaged, and forward-leading player on the world stage while the United States and the West cling to the past. Through a combination of necessity and national pride, China will be further incentivized to enhance its own capabilities to the point where the advantage, and thus leverage, we do have in certain technologies fades away. It is generally a better bet to build on our strengths than try to weaken others.

Those US strengths include human capital educated in the world's top research institutions; an environment that attracts the most talented people to learn, stay, and invest here; and a vibrant commercial technology enterprise that is helping revive high-value manufacturing in this country.[60] But government cannot simply get out of the way. It must invest in a more pragmatic strategy for technology that transcends the pandemic and sustains US leadership in the post-COVID-19 world.

NOTES

1. Thomas Friedman, *The World Is Flat* (New York: Farrar, Straus and Giroux, 2005).

2. Kirk Lancaster, Michael Rubin, and Mira Rapp-Hooper, "Mapping China's Health Silk Road," *Asia Unbound* (blog), Council on Foreign Relations, April 10, 2020, https://www.cfr.org/blog/mapping-chinas-health-silk-road.

3. Chad P. Bown, "COVID-19: China's Exports of Medical Supplies Provide a Ray of Hope," Peterson Institute for International Economics, March 26, 2020, https://www.piie.com/blogs/trade-and-investment-policy-watch/covid-19-chinas-exports-medical-supplies-provide-ray-hope.

4. Milton Mueller, "Internet Governance," in *Oxford Research Encyclopedias: International Studies* (International Studies Association and Oxford University Press, 2017), https://oxfordre.com/internationalstudies/internationalstudies/view/10.1093/acrefore/9780190846626.001.0001/acrefore-9780190846626-e-245.

5. Mueller, "Internet Governance."

6. Gordon M. Goldstein, "The End of the Internet?" *The Atlantic*, July/August 2014, https://www.theatlantic.com/magazine/archive/2014/07/the-end-of-the-internet/372301/.

7. Jeff John Roberts, "The Splinternet Is Growing," *Fortune*, May 29, 2019, https://fortune.com/2019/05/29/splinternet-online-censorship/.

8. Matt Burgess, "What Is GDPR? The Summary Guide to GDPR Compliance in the UK," *Wired*, March 24, 2020, https://www.wired.co.uk/article/what-is-gdpr-uk-eu-legislation-compliance-summary-fines-2018.

9. Burgess, "What Is GDPR?"

10. Mehdi Daoudi, "Beware the SplinterNet—Why Three Recent Events Should Have Businesses Worried," *Forbes*, July 12, 2018, https://www.forbes.com/sites/forbestechcoun cil/2018/07/12/beware-the-splinternet-why-three-recent-events-should-have-businesses -worried/#59ad890a2c00.

11. Merrit Kennedy, "New Russian Law Gives Government Sweeping Power over Internet," NPR, November 1, 2019, https://www.npr.org/2019/11/01/775366588/russian-law -takes-effect-that-gives-government-sweeping-power-over-internet.

12. Elizabeth Schulze, "Russia Just Brought in a Law to Try to Disconnect Its Internet from the Rest of the World," CNBC, November 1, 2019, https://www.cnbc.com/2019/11/01 /russia-controversial-sovereign-internet-law-goes-into-force.html.

13. Schulze, "Russia Just Brought in a Law."

14. Elizabeth C. Economy, "The Great Firewall of China: Xi Jinping's Internet Shutdown," *Guardian*, June 29, 2019, https://www.theguardian.com/news/2018/jun/29/the -great-firewall-of-china-xi-jinpings-internet-shutdown.

15. "FAQ," root-servers.org, accessed June 24, 2020, https://root-servers.org/faq.html.

16. Wei Sheng, "China's Imaginary Root Server to Fix Imaginary Threat," *TechNode*, December 24, 2019, https://technode.com/2019/12/24/chinas-imaginary-root-server-to-fix -imaginary-threat/.

17. Xinhua News Agency, "China Greenlights Establishment of Root Server," December 8, 2019, http://www.xinhuanet.com/english/2019-12/08/c_138613999.htm.

18. "Search Engine Market Share Worldwide," Statcounter GlobalStats, accessed June 24, 2020, https://gs.statcounter.com/search-engine-market-share.

19. "Number of Internet Users in China from December 2008 to March 2020," *Statista*, released April 2020, https://www.statista.com/statistics/265140/number-of-internet-users -in-china/#:~:text=As%20of%20the%20first%20quarter,app%20market%20in%20 the%20country.&text=In%202018%2C%20China%20accounted%20for,four%20bil lion%20internet%20users%20worldwide.

20. Lindsay Gorman, "The U.S. Needs to Get in the Standards Game with Like-Minded Countries," *Lawfare*, April 2, 2020, https://www.lawfareblog.com/us-needs-get-standards -game-minded-democracies.

21. Rob Portman et al., letter to US Secretary of State Michael R. Pompeo, March 11, 2020, https://www.portman.senate.gov/sites/default/files/2020-03/China%20Warren%20 AI%20Letter_0.pdf.

22. Gorman, "U.S. Needs to Get in the Standards Game."

23. Doug Fuller, *Cutting off Our Nose to Spite Our Face: US Policy towards China in Key Semiconductor Industry Inputs, Capital Equipment, and Electronic Design Automation Tools* (forthcoming July 2020).

24. Fuller, *Cutting off Our Nose.*

25. Eric Geller, "Trump Signs Order Setting Stage to Ban Huawei from U.S.," *Politico*, May 15, 2019, https://www.politico.com/story/2019/05/15/trump-ban-huawei-us-1042046.

26. Carrie Mihalcik, "FCC Bars Huawei, ZTE from Billions in Federal Subsidies," *CNET*, November 22, 2019, https://www.cnet.com/news/fcc-bars-huawei-zte-from-billi ons-in-federal-subsidies/.

27. Sean Keane, "Huawei Ban Timeline: US Companies Allowed to Work with Huawei on 5G Standards," *CNET*, June 17, 2020, https://www.cnet.com/news/huawei-ban-full-timeline-us-restrictions-china-trump-executive-order-security-threat-5g-commerce/.

28. Fuller, *Cutting off Our Nose.*

29. Justin Sherman, "The UK Is Forging a 5G Club of Democracies to Avoid Reliance on Huawei," Atlantic Council (blog), June 2, 2020, https://www.atlanticcouncil.org/blogs/new-atlanticist/the-uk-is-forging-a-5g-club-of-democracies-to-avoid-reliance-on-huawei/.

30. David McCabe, "Senate Faults Oversight of Chinese Telecom Companies in U.S.," *New York Times*, June 9, 2020, https://www.nytimes.com/2020/06/09/technology/senate-china-telecom-security.html.

31. Harris, Wiltshire and Grannis LLP, "President Trump Formalizes Team Telecom Process for Reviewing Foreign Investments in U.S. Telecommunications Market," HWG advisory, April 9, 2020, https://www.hwglaw.com/president-trump-formalizes-team-telecom-process-for-reviewing-foreign-investments-in-u-s-telecommunications-market/.

32. Justin Sherman, "Senate Report Finds Poor Executive Branch Oversight of Chinese State-Owned Telecoms," *Lawfare* (blog), June 17, 2020, https://www.lawfareblog.com/senate-report-finds-poor-executive-branch-oversight-chinese-state-owned-telecoms.

33. Claudia Adren, "Chinese Biotechnology Dominates the U.S. Senate Hearing on Biological Threats," *Hometown Preparedness News*, November 19, 2019, https://homelandprepnews.com/countermeasures/40093-chinese-biotechnology-dominates-u-s-senate-hearing-on-biological-threats/

34. "The Next Biotech Superpower," *Nature Biotechnology* 37, no. 11 (November 2019): 1243, https://www.nature.com/articles/s41587-019-0316-7.

35. "The Next Biotech Superpower."

36. "The Coronavirus and America's Small Business Supply Chain," testimony of Rosemary Gibson before the US Senate Committee on Small Business and Entrepreneurship, March 12, 2020, https://www.sbc.senate.gov/public/_cache/files/1/c/1c39a1bc-f22c-4178-951e-29b92dcb2182/3AD9C94FB267763A83913E2303A6A772.gibson-testimony.pdf.

37. Jeff Ferry, "It's Time to Rebuild Domestic Drug Production in the US, for Both Health and Economic Reasons," *IndustryWeek*, March 17, 2020, https://www.industryweek.com/the-economy/article/21126380/its-time-to-rebuild-domestic-drug-production-in-the-us-for-both-health-and-economic-reasons.

38. "Coronavirus and America's Small Business Supply Chain," testimony of Rosemary Gibson.

39. Ferry, "It's Time to Rebuild Domestic Drug Production."

40. World Health Organization, *China Policies to Promote Local Production of Pharmaceutical Products and Protect Public Health* (Geneva: World Health Organization, 2017), https://www.who.int/phi/publications/2081China020517.pdf?ua=1.

41. Michael Rea, "An 'America First' Pharma Supply Chain Sounds Good. But It Won't Work," *STAT*, June 17, 2020, https://www.statnews.com/2020/06/17/an-america-first-pharma-supply-chain-sounds-good-but-it-wont-work/; "HHS, Industry Partners Expand U.S.-based Pharmaceutical Manufacturing for COVID-19 Response," MedicalCountermeasures.gov, accessed June 24, 2020, https://www.medicalcountermeasures.gov/newsroom/2020/phlow-us-manufacturing/.

42. Ana Swanson, "Coronavirus Spurs U.S. Efforts to End China's Chokehold on Drugs," *New York Times*, March 11, 2020, https://www.nytimes.com/2020/03/11/business/economy/coronavirus-china-trump-drugs.html.

43. Rea, "'America First' Pharma Supply Chain."

44. Bown, "COVID-19."

45. Rea, "'America First' Pharma Supply Chain."

46. Bown, "COVID-19."

47. Alice Su, "Faulty Masks, Flawed Tests: China's Quality Control Problem in Leading Global COVID-19 Fight," *Los Angeles Times*, April 10, 2020, https://www.latimes.com/world-nation/story/2020-04-10/china-beijing-supply-world-coronavirus-fight-quality-control.

48. Emma Newburger, "Cuomo Calls PPE Shortages a National Security Issue: 'You Can't Be Dependent on China,'" CNBC, May 3, 2020, https://www.cnbc.com/2020/05/03/coronavirus-cuomo-warns-against-dependence-on-china-for-ppe.html.

49. Caleb Watney and Alec Stapp, "Masks for All: Using Purchase Guarantees and Targeted Deregulation to Boost Production of Essential Medical Equipment," policy brief, Mercatus Center, George Mason University, April 8, 2020, https://www.mercatus.org/publications/covid-19-crisis-response/masks-all-using-purchase-guarantees-and-targeted-deregulation.

50. Nick Miroff, "Protective Gear in National Stockpile Is Nearly Depleted, DHS Officials Say," *Washington Post*, April 1, 2020, https://www.washingtonpost.com/national/coronavirus-protective-gear-stockpile-depleted/2020/04/01/44d6592a-741f-11ea-ae50-7148009252e3_story.html.

51. Kristine Lee and Martijn Rasser, "China's Health Silk Road Is a Dead-End Street," *Foreign Policy*, June 16, 2020, https://foreignpolicy.com/2020/06/16/china-health-propaganda-covid/.

52. Lee and Rasser, "China's Health Silk Road."

53. Lancaster, Rubin, and Rapp-Hooper, "Mapping China's Health Silk Road."

54. Lee and Rasser, "China's Health Silk Road."

55. Jeff Grabmeier, "Chinese, American Scientists Leading Efforts on COVID-19," *Ohio State News*, May 26, 2020, https://news.osu.edu/chinese-american-scientists-leading-efforts-on-covid-19/.

56. Stuart Anderson, "Inside Trump's Immigration Order to Restrict Chinese Students," *Forbes*, June 1, 2020, https://www.forbes.com/sites/stuartanderson/2020/06/01/inside-trumps-immigration-order-to-restrict-chinese-students/#4d29bf4b3bec.

57. Andrew Silver and David Cyranoski, "China Is Tightening Its Grip on Coronavirus Research," *Nature*, April 15, 2020, https://www.nature.com/articles/d41586-020-01108-y.

58. Gavin Yamey and Dean T. Jamison, "U.S. Response to COVID-19 Is Worse than China's, 100 Times Worse," *Time*, June 10, 2020, https://time.com/5850680/u-s-response-covid-19-worse-than-chinas/.

59. Matina Stevis-Gridneff, "E.U. May Bar American Travelers as It Reopens Borders, Citing Failures on Virus," *New York Times*, June 23, 2020, https://www.nytimes.com/2020/06/23/world/europe/coronavirus-EU-American-travel-ban.html?smid=tw-nytimes&smtyp=cur.

60. Richard Danzig, John Allen, Phil DePoy, Lisa Disbrow, James Gosler, Avril Haines, Samuel Locklear III, James Miller, James Stavridis, Paul Stockton, and Robert Work, *A Preface to Strategy: The Foundations of American National Security* (Laurel, MD: Johns Hopkins University Applied Physics Laboratory, 2018), https://www.jhuapl.edu/Content/documents/PrefaceToStrategy.pdf.

PART IV / The Future of the
Global Economy

Chapter Ten

Models for a Post-COVID US Foreign Economic Policy

Benn Steil

T he COVID-19 pandemic has intensified centrifugal forces in the global economic order, forces which have been growing in strength over recent years. The crisis has animated governments to impose sweeping new restrictions on the movement of people and goods, and many of these are likely to remain well after it has passed.

More than 70% of the world's air, sea, and land ports of entry restrict access to foreigners. In the United States, politicians from both major parties are demanding new "Buy American" rules for government health spending. French President Emmanuel Macron is seeking "full independence" in critical medical supplies by year's-end. Almost ninety countries are now blocking the export of medical goods. Twenty-nine are doing so with food.

Japan is paying companies to move factories home from China; the Trump administration may soon follow suit. The European Union (EU) is imposing new restrictions on foreign investment and takeovers. Even notable free-trade champions, such as Pascal Lamy, former director-general of the World Trade Organization (WTO), are now emphasizing the need to shift international supply-chain management away from an efficiency focus and toward "resilience"—that is, duplication and renationalization—to minimize the consequences of disruption.

Benn Steil is director of international economics at the Council on Foreign Relations and the author, most recently, of *The Marshall Plan: Dawn of the Cold War.*

"National security" will become the umbrella logic for all manner of government intervention in this and other areas of commerce.

Not all countries are pulling back from globalization in all its aspects. New Zealand and Singapore, for example, are leading a coalition to *expand* trade in medical products through tariff reduction[1]—the idea being that the crisis shows the need for more commitment to cooperation, not a retreat into autarky. The School of Advanced International Studies project that gave rise to this volume used online communications technology, rather than planes, to bring experts together; this will likely become the global norm in knowledge-based industries. Still, that technology is itself becoming a leading battlefield of national conflict, as so-called fifth-generation (5G) wireless technology ruptures between Chinese and western-led versions.

If the crises of World War I and the Spanish flu of 1918 are anything to go by, the challenges and conflicts raised by COVID-19 are likely to be long-lived. It took a second world war a quarter-century later before de-globalization was stopped and a half-century before it returned to pre–World War I levels.

As the COVID crisis passes, the fraying current order is unlikely to revive itself unaided. Government action will be needed to rebuild or replace it. This essay looks at three models the United States might pursue in order to reshape its relationship to the future global economy.

Orders Old and New

History over the quarter-century following World War I provides useful guideposts for thinking about the types of economic order available to the United States. Broadly, they may be labeled Isolationism, One-Worldism, and Two-Worldism.

Isolationism was the dominant US model from the end of World War I until the Japanese attack on Pearl Harbor in 1941. Its central motif was that the United States must not allow itself to become entangled in the problems of other nations, as that must inevitably act to limit its scope for independent action and drag it into conflicts peripheral to its interests.

One-Worldism was the postwar vision of President Franklin D. Roosevelt, repudiating Isolationism. It presumed that there was sufficient commonality of interest among the United States, the United Kingdom, the Soviet Union, and China to construct mutually beneficial global structures for regulating commerce and political relations. Its cornerstone institutions, conceived in the early 1940s, were to be the United Nations (UN), the International Monetary Fund (IMF), the World Bank, and an international trade organization.

Two-Worldism was the corrective put in train by President Harry S. Truman, based on the belief that fundamental differences in interests and ideology existed between the United States and the Soviet Union which made a political and economic division of Europe unavoidable. Its founding structures were to be two off-shoots of the Marshall Plan—the European Coal and Steel Community (a precursor to the EU) and the North Atlantic Treaty Organization (NATO)—along with the General Agreement on Tariffs and Trade (a precursor to the WTO).

Following the end of the Cold War three decades ago, Two-Worldism, now stripped of its ideological basis, morphed into a One-Worldism based largely on the structures created by the United States in the late 1940s. Not surprisingly, a certain triumphalism pervaded Washington, a sense that we had arrived at "The End of History."[2]

Over the past decade, however, growing economic and political conflict between the United States and China, political conflict between the United States and Russia, and the election of a nationalist US president in 2016 have conspired to undermine the viability of this "One World" order. The COVID-19 pandemic, which has given rise to a surge in US-China tensions and global trade and migration barriers, is accelerating its destruction. The recent resignation of WTO director-general Roberto Azevêdo is emblematic of this fact. It is therefore essential for US policy makers now to examine critically whether they wish to arrest its demise or to replace it with a different model for US engagement.

Model 1: One World

A "One World" economic model for the future is premised on the belief that the United States and China can coexist on a mutually beneficial basis within a set of common rules, norms, and institutions governing economic exchange. This was the premise that underlay American thinking when China acceded to the WTO in 2001. That premise was itself based on the belief that China was evolving in a liberal direction, one in which the state would play a progressively lesser role in the economy.

Since the emergence of Xi Jinping as paramount leader in 2012, however, China has moved decidedly in the opposite direction. The Communist Party of China eliminated term limits to accommodate Xi's indefinite rule, and state-owned enterprises (SOEs) have come to play a far larger and more critical role in the economy—not the smaller one that had been anticipated a decade prior. This phenomenon has had a profound effect not just on China but on economics and politics in the United States.

To boost state-led investment, China pursues policies to restrict the income flowing to workers and retirees. Taxes are regressive, social safety nets minimal, and the rights of urban-dwelling rural migrants few. SOEs do not pay dividends, and bank deposit rates are capped. This latter policy enables banks to borrow cheaply and lend on to SOEs at a modest markup, secure in the knowledge that the government will not allow default—irrespective of how bad the investments prove to be. With returns on savings miserly and government support nominal, Chinese households have the lowest consumption rate (as a share of output) in the world, and the nation as a whole has the highest savings rate of any in history.

China's surplus savings and persistent state-generated overproduction spill over abroad, most notably into the world's most open national economy: the United States. The US absorbs it by fueling excess credit creation (through the proliferation of "CDOs-cubed" and the like), which seeds financial crisis, as well as by accelerating de-industrialization and manufacturing job loss.

These effects do not owe entirely to Chinese policy, and surely many segments of American society have benefited from cheaper credit and cheaper goods. But the political ramifications of the concomitant dislocations are distinctly hostile to the perpetuation of One World. The election of US President Donald J. Trump in 2016 on a platform of heavily taxing Chinese imports, however ineffective a response to the underlying problem, was a powerful sign that China's model is unsustainable under the current architecture of international economic relations.

In order for One World to survive, it will have to be reincarnated along different lines. At the broadest level, China will need to allow household income to rise at the expense of investment. Whereas such change may sound technocratic and innocuous, it would be highly consequential. It would curtail SOE expansion and the political power that local governments enjoy in directing it. If banks, for example, were merely obliged to compete for savers' deposits, the relentless funneling of underpriced savings to over-indebted enterprises would begin to dry up.

At present, gross domestic product (GDP) in China is not the output of a largely self-regulating economic system, as it is in the developed world, but a political *input* that determines how much borrowing, lending, and production there must be to satisfy government wants. When China declares a 6% GDP growth target and then meets it, it does so only by stoking the inexorable growth of bad loans that goes along with it. With China's true debt likely running at about 300% of national income, the country is nearing its debt capacity.[3] It needs to change course in its own economic interests as well as those of the wider world.

A rebalancing of the Chinese system in favor of households, sufficient to halt the flow of surplus goods and savings to the United States, would require the shrinking of overextended Chinese enterprises, massive loan write-offs, slower growth, and less government control over who makes what for what end. It would, in effect, mean nothing less than a reversal of Xi's vision for China's next stage of development. It is for this reason that it has not happened.

China's production and dumping of excess goods and savings in the United States is but an element in the growing economic frictions between the countries. Systematic Chinese commercial espionage, intellectual property theft, forced technology transfer, and open intervention on behalf of domestic firms have all contributed mightily to American disenchantment with the growing integration between the two countries. The enormous economic and political implications of the global shift toward 5G wireless technology only raise the stakes for a continuation down the current path.

The past decade has also witnessed growing tensions between the United States and China over One World economic institutions. Misguided foot-dragging by Congress over governance reform at the IMF and World Bank during the Obama administration—reforms that increased China's voice but left the United States with sole veto power—acted as a powerful impetus for China to promote new alternative institutions: the Asian Infrastructure Investment Bank (AIIB), the New Development Bank (or "BRICS" Bank), and the Belt and Road Initiative (BRI). The last of these, BRI, has seen China lend hundreds of billions of dollars for infrastructure development to mostly developing nations, affording it growing political influence. Extended without the sort of transparency and conditionality required by the World Bank, these loans were initially greeted warmly by recipient governments. Charges by the United States that the initiative amounted to "debt-trap diplomacy," however, may soon be borne out as BRI borrowers, having entered recession with the COVID crisis, approach default and plead for write-offs.

Also worrying for the One World model is the way in which the United States has brought WTO dispute settlement to a standstill by refusing to allow appointments to the appellate body. The resignation of Director-General Roberto Azevêdo in May 2020 clearly signaled his view that the organization, which has not concluded a round of multilateral trade liberalization since 1994, has been reduced to a state of impotence.

Saving One World is now a tall order. Even if 2021 sees a change in the US administration and outlook that keeps the WTO on life support and seeks to reengage

China constructively, China appears set on a path that makes a mockery of what the WTO was established to do: lower trade barriers among market economies. When China's economy was, at its accession, less than 10% the size of what it is today, this mattered much less—particularly since China seemed to be headed in the right direction. Now, however, it is undermining the stability of the global economy and creating dangerous political frictions.

Since the potential benefits of One World dwarf those of Isolationism, and exceed those of "Two Worlds" with a lower risk of military conflict, the United States should, in its own interest, make a sincere effort to save it. The way to do so is to restock the WTO appellate body with judges and to join with allies in Europe and Asia to challenge China's policies in four broad areas: intellectual property protection and enforcement, trade secrets protection, forced technology transfer, and state subsidies.

Such cases will be difficult to prosecute, and the outcome is highly uncertain. Yet if the United States and its allies win all or most of them, China, which has a respectable record on implementing WTO decisions[4] and cares deeply about world opinion, may decide—wholly in calculation of its own interest—to change course and comply. In fact, China losing at the WTO would give it a face-saving way to make shifts in policy that might otherwise prove impossible to engineer owing to the appearance of caving to unilateral US threats and demands.

If China loses and does not comply, the United States and its allies would win the legal right to "suspend concessions or other obligations"—that is, to retaliate with tariffs, quotas, and the like. This too may fail to motivate Chinese compliance. Given the legal complexities inherent in such cases, the US and its allies may also lose one or more of them. In the case of Chinese noncompliance or US losses, Washington may reasonably conclude that the WTO—and the One World model on which it was built—has outlived its usefulness. It might then look to set up alternative regimes together with like-minded nations, or to go it alone—a model to which I now turn.

Model 2: Isolationism

The term "Isolationism" does not mean ignoring the outside world. Rather, it is a "doctrine of isolating one's country from the affairs of other nations by declining to enter into alliances, foreign economic commitments, [or] international agreements."[5] If this is not the stated meta-policy of the Trump administration, it is clearly the destination toward which it has been headed since 2017.

The attractions of Isolationism are obvious. All else being equal, governments prefer the freedom to act, unencumbered, and to stand aloof, unentangled. And since the United States is the world's richest and most powerful nation, it can, at least in many circumstances, benefit from a strategy of divide-and-conquer—that is, dealing with weaker nations bilaterally and on a narrow transactional basis.

Yet all else is not equal, and there are obvious costs to this strategy. When the United States forswears commitments to others, others forswear commitments to the United States. Those countries may, of course, also choose to bind together with alternative suitors to pursue aims antithetical to US interests. In turning away from multilateralism, the United States liquidates moral capital accumulated over decades, capital built on the foundation of long-standing commitment to the values of political and economic liberalism—values which transcend its narrow national interests. This commitment is the basis of what Harvard's Joseph Nye has called America's "soft power"—its ability, without applying force or coercion, "to get others to do what they otherwise would not."[6] No other nation, certainly not China or Russia, combines economic and military power with a compelling vision for the organization of human society. There is clear value to the United States in being able to leverage moral authority in crafting agreements and not simply presenting itself as just another self-interested brute.

Curiously, the Trump administration has not argued that America's historic multilateral initiatives were misguided (even if Trump himself may believe so). Instead, it has argued that the conditions which made them successful no longer apply. The 2017 National Security Strategy, for example, while stating that "putting America first is the duty of [its] government and the foundation for U.S. leadership," actually pays homage to the country's postwar multilateralist diplomacy—in particular, the creation of the Marshall Plan in 1947 and NATO in 1949. It claims, however, that over recent decades others have "exploited the international institutions we helped to build."[7]

Whereas this claim has merit in the case of China's demands, under the umbrella of the WTO, for the right to access markets abroad freely while closing them at home, it is deeply misguided with respect to other countries and institutions. On the security front, alliances have lowered the cost of US political and military action abroad.[8] NATO's Article 5 collective defense provision has been invoked only once in the alliance's history—by America's allies, supporting it after the September 11, 2001, Al Qaeda terrorist attacks on New York and Washington. On the economic front, multilateral institutions have accorded Washington far greater influence than is justified by its role in the global economy. When the United States designed the IMF and World Bank back in 1944, for example, it accounted for half the world's output. Today it accounts for under a quarter. Could anyone imagine the United States today, under such vastly less favorable circumstances, creating powerful international institutions in which it could grant itself the sole right of veto? It is unthinkable. Yet the fact that it retains such outsize influence in the so-called Bretton Woods institutions is testimony both to its foresight at the time and to its responsible stewardship (with notable exceptions) of the liberal order since then.

Indeed, the Truman administration, working with a Republican Congress, pushed America out on the multilateralist path not just for short-term benefit but with the expectation that it would pay dividends for generations. "The recovery of Western Europe," wrote Republican senator Henry Cabot Lodge, Jr. in 1947, "is a twenty-five to fifty-year proposition, and the aid which we extend now and in the next three or four years will in the long future result in our having strong friends abroad." Forty-two years later, with the fall of the Berlin Wall, we saw just how right he was. Moscow's Warsaw Pact collapsed almost overnight, whereas those alliances Washington forged as offshoots of the Marshall Plan—NATO and the European Union—rose to new heights of popularity, with the freshly liberated countries of central and eastern Europe clamoring for entry.

The isolationist path along which the United States has been moving since 2017, in contrast, has generated bitterness and resentment abroad while achieving none of its goals at home. On the economic front, it was supposed to have revived domestic manufacturing and manufacturing employment. Yet after nearly four years of ever-widening and greater import tariffs—that is, taxes on Americans buying abroad—these efforts have shown no signs of success. Take steel and aluminum tariffs, which President Trump imposed on contrived "national security" grounds. Whereas imports of both metals declined after the tariffs took effect, the import of products *using* them soared in consequence—prompting the president to impose another round of tariffs to contain the damaging effect on American metal-using industries.

The net result of tariffs has been to make US firms relying on foreign parts less competitive globally, to raise costs for US consumers, and to harm US exporters—particularly farmers—whose products have been hit with foreign retaliation.[9] Meanwhile, the protected industries, which remain behind the global curve on automated production, continue to stagnate or decline. China, the main target of the president's tariff strategy, has, notwithstanding the so-called Phase One trade deal in 2019, neither materially increased US imports nor made any significant structural and market-access reforms. (In fact, the deal obliges China to apply *more* state direction.)[10] The Trump administration and its congressional supporters now speak of new "reshoring" initiatives, such as domestic-content requirements, partly in response to COVID-induced shortages. But these are certain only to further erode US competitiveness; there are more sensible and cost-effective ways to promote supply-chain resilience.[11]

Furthermore, in renouncing the (now-)11-nation Trans-Pacific Partnership (TPP) agreement, the Trump administration has abandoned the chance to shape the rules and norms of economic exchange in Asia. Putting aside the well-documented economic benefits of liberalizing trade multilaterally,[12] the United States has ceded the initiative on regional trade to China—an aspiring hegemon with interests increasingly at odds with those of the US. And once the nations of the region build up an alternative panoply of mutual commitments, even if motivated by fear rather than opportunity, it will become difficult, if not impossible, for the United States to reclaim influence. Washington's aim, in short, should therefore be not to isolate America further, through tariffs or "reshoring" requirements, but to revive or reconstitute multilateralism in a more effective form.

Model 3: Two Worlds

In April 1947, six weeks prior to Secretary of State George Marshall's Harvard speech setting out the background to what would become the Marshall Plan, a joint State, War, and Navy department staff committee report concluded that minimizing "the costs and duration of United States economic assistance" to revive western Europe would "require a substantial increase in trade with Soviet-dominated areas" in the east. For this and many other reasons, they thought it vital to press for an understanding with Moscow over the future political and economic architecture of Germany and Europe. But American trade with the east, the committee added, could *only* be "arranged on terms compatible with the economic and political independence of western-oriented areas."[13] And once Marshall concluded that Stalin would never allow this condition to be met, he laid down requirements for American aid—in particular, economic integration among the participant nations—that he knew the Soviet dictator would never abide. Thus was the shift from the FDR's "One World" vision to Truman's "Two World" policy initiated reluctantly but decisively.

We are at precisely such a crossroads with regard to America's relations with China. Though China does not oppose the One World model, it uses it to its advantage by exploiting, rather than embracing, the developed world's commitment to open markets. It seeks not to replace One World institutions but to increase its influence over them and, in areas, to counterbalance them with schemes of its own (like BRI). In President Xi's words, China seeks "a future where we will win the initiative and have the dominant position."[14]

This is not just rhetoric. In service of its "Made in China 2025" industrial policy, which pledges the government to pursue Chinese supremacy in areas of strategic economic and security importance, China has committed at least $1.4 trillion in public funds over the coming five years to investments in artificial intelligence, data centers, mobile communications, and other technology-related projects—all of which are to be based on domestic firms.[15] Governments that criticize Chinese policy—such as Germany over Huawei and 5G, Sweden over human rights, Norway over the Nobel Peace Prize, and Australia over COVID—have been met with import bans, or threats thereof, from Beijing.[16]

For the United States, continuation down a One World path while China persists in distorting the global economy and orchestrating its dominance of strategic technologies will only heighten economic dislocation, political polarization, and security risks. If China, like the Soviet Union in 1947, rejects the basic American vision of a liberal order, then the United States must be prepared to initiate a shift to a Two Worlds model.

To effect it will require persuading allies to join in a progressive *multilateral decoupling*—an escalating quarantining of Chinese firms and industries that persist in either illegal activities (such as espionage and theft) or unfair trade practices (like dumping to eliminate competition). Simultaneously, it should seek to construct a new multilateral trade regime, populated by nations that meet basic standards for respecting fair and open markets. A mass withdrawal from the WTO by such nations, followed by the erection of a parallel organization based on stronger open-market principles, would be the cleanest way to move forward. However, it may be legally and practically sufficient for those same nations simply to operate a new trade rubric side by side with a moribund WTO. This rubric might combine elements of TPP and the mothballed Transatlantic Trade and Investment Partnership (TTIP), covering tariffs on goods and services, intellectual property rights, e-commerce rules, inward investment, regulatory cooperation, labor and environmental standards, and dispute resolution. The United States should, further, initiate a "Manhattan Project" with allies in Europe and Asia to massively accelerate 5G and 6G wireless technology development. Such an initiative is necessary in order to leapfrog China in an arena of vital strategic importance, covering capabilities as diverse as threat detection, feature and facial recognition, and health care.[17]

This agenda would result in what has been called a "splinternet," and, as former Google CEO Eric Schmidt has rightly emphasized, it is far less desirable than finding a way to coexist peacefully and profitably with China under one set of standards and a genuinely global market for technology and communications. But much the same was said about the division of Europe in 1947. Two Worlds was, however, clearly a less-bad option than trying to appease Stalin. And if China is going to grow both more authoritarian and more ubiquitous in the global economy, it is bound to result in yet more political turmoil, both within the United States and internationally. In this case, Two Worlds, for all its manifest limitations, is the better way to go.

Whereas a Two World agenda may have sounded extreme a year ago, it has already taken embryonic shape. The European Union, for example, has embarked on an effort to assert "strategic autonomy" from China, which includes plans to bar foreign companies that have received large grants, loans, tax credits, or other state aid from buying EU companies or competing with them for EU contracts. The agenda has been accelerated by the COVID pandemic, which has triggered fears of China and others exploiting the crisis at the expense of European firms. Paradoxically, the biggest barrier to cooperation on the initiative with Washington has been the Trump administration's tariff and other aggressive trade threats against the EU.[18] It is high time for Washington to get its priorities straight and to coordinate a determined multilateral response to Beijing's challenge.

Of course, the United States must always be prepared to act alone to protect its core interests, but that should become the *last* resort—no longer the first. The new strategy must be based on nurturing and acquiring allies, not on disparaging and punishing them. Creating allies is precisely the strategy the United States employed so successfully in the aftermath of World War II.

Final Thoughts on the Role of COVID

Whereas the COVID pandemic is hardly the genesis of spiraling economic conflict between the United States and China, it has clearly exacerbated that conflict. Beijing's lack of candor and transparency, if not outright dishonesty, as the virus spread through Wuhan in late 2019, followed by China's later mass export of defective and misbranded personal protection equipment, has fueled American distrust and determination to act.

Looking forward, international opinion toward the global order will be shaped by how the world emerges from this COVID crisis. In particular, the way in which the United States, China, the European Union, Russia, and the United Kingdom behave in the race to produce a vaccine will be consequential.

"Vaccine nationalism"—the desire to acquire vaccines and to use them at home before allowing distribution abroad—is an obvious and understandable temptation. The United States, at the height of the lockdown, was losing 16,000 lives and $80 billion a week.[19] Yet if the winners in the vaccine race fail to include in the initial round of inoculations foreign frontline medical workers and others abroad in urgent need of protection, it will undermine their claims to be responsible stewards of, or stakeholders in, the global order.

The sharp, negative reaction around the world to reports of the Trump administration buying up virtually the entire summer supply of the anti-COVID drug remdesivir, coming on the back of its invocation of the Defense Production Act to block the export of medical goods, should be a warning shot.[20] If the United States succumbs to vaccine nationalism, it will become vastly more difficult for it to rally nations to its vision for future global economic structures. Generosity, in contrast, will afford it considerably more leverage in trying to reform the present One World model or to draw allies to its side for a shift to Two Worlds.

NOTES

1. Jacob M. Schlesinger, "How the Coronavirus Will Reshape World Trade," *Wall Street Journal*, June 19, 2020.

2. Francis Fukuyama, *The End of History and the Last Man* (New York: Free Press, 1992).

3. Matthew C. Klein and Michael Pettis, *Trade Wars Are Class Wars: How Rising Inequality Distorts the Global Economy and Threatens International Peace* (New Haven, CT: Yale University Press, 2020): 126.

4. See, for example, James Bacchus, Simon Lester, and Huan Zhu, "Disciplining China's Trade Practices at the WTO: How WTO Complaints Can Help Make China More Market-Oriented," *CATO Institute*, November 15, 2018.

5. "Isolationism," Dictionary.com.

6. Joseph S. Nye, Jr., "The Changing Nature of World Power," *Political Science Quarterly* 105, no. 2 (Summer 1990): 177–192.

7. The White House, *National Security Strategy of the United States of America*, December 2017, https://www.whitehouse.gov/wp-content/uploads/2017/12/NSS-Final-12-18-2017-0905.pdf.

8. Mira Rapp-Hooper, *Shields of the Republic* (Cambridge, MA: Harvard University Press, 2020): 63.

9. Noah Smith, "Don't Give Up on Bringing Manufacturing Back to the U.S.," *Bloomberg Opinion*, June 12, 2020; Ana Swanson and Peter Eavis, "Trump Expands Steel Tariffs, Saying They Are Short of Aim," *New York Times*, January 27, 2020; Aaron Flaaen and Justin Pierce, "Disentangling the Effects of the 2018–2019 Tariffs on a Globally Connected U.S. Manufacturing Sector," Finance and Economics Discussion Series 2019-086 (Washington, DC: Board of Governors of the Federal Reserve System), December 23, 2019; Reade Pickert, "US Pays Bulk of Tariff Costs as Levies Fail to Save Steel Jobs," *Bloomberg*, January 6, 2020; Chad P. Bown, "Trump's Steel and Aluminum Tariffs Are Cascading Out of Control," Peterson Institute for International Economics, February 4, 2020; Benn Steil and Benjamin Della Rocca, "China's 'Massive' Trade Offer Leaves U.S. Farmers \$7 Billion Worse Off," Council on Foreign Relations, October 29, 2019; Benn Steil and Benjamin Della Rocca, "Trump's Tariffs Are Killing American Steel," Council on Foreign Relations, January 18, 2019.

10. Chad P. Bown and Mary E. Lovely, "Trump's Phase One Deal Relies on China's State-Owned Enterprises," Peterson Institute for International Economics, March 3, 2020.

11. Financial Times Editorial Board, "Building Resilience Should Not Lead to Trade Barriers," *Financial Times*, June 12, 2020; Martin Wolf, "The Dangerous War on Supply Chains," *Financial Times*, June 23, 2020.

12. Douglas A. Irwin, "International Trade Agreements," in *The Library of Economics and Liberty: Economies Outside the United States,* 2nd ed. (Liberty Fund Inc., 2007).

13. Benn Steil, *The Marshall Plan: Dawn of the Cold War* (New York: Simon & Schuster, 2018): 86.

14. Hal Brands, "What Does China Really Want? To Dominate the World," *Bloomberg Opinion*, May 20, 2020.

15. Liza Lin, "China Pours Funds into Tech Push," *Wall Street Journal*, June 12, 2020.

16. Greg Ip, "United Front on China Starts to Take Shape," *Wall Street Journal*, June 18, 2020; Robert D. Atkinson and Clyde Prestowitz, "China's Reaction to the Pandemic Shows Why the U.S. and Its Allies Need a NATO for Trade," *Washington Post*, May 20, 2020.

17. Margaret Rouse and Gerry Christensen, "6G" SearchNetworking, TechTarget, October 7, 2019.

18. Valentina Pop, "EU to Boost Defenses against Foreign Firms," *Wall Street Journal*, June 18, 2020.

19. Lawrence H. Summers, "Given What We're Losing in GDP, We Should Be Spending Far More to Develop Tests," *Washington Post*, May 5, 2020.

20. Sarah Bosely, "US Secures World Stock of Key Covid-19 Drug Remdesivir," *The Guardian*, June 30, 2020.

Chapter Eleven

Prospects for the United States' Post-COVID-19 Policies

Strengthening the G20 Leaders Process

John Lipsky

The COVID-19 pandemic has confronted the international system with its second major challenge of the past fifteen years. The first challenge—the global financial crisis (GFC) of 2007–9—led to the creation of the Group of 20 Leaders Summit process.[1] The response of this new grouping to its first challenge appeared to be coherent, credible, and effective. The G20's contribution to the response to the current challenge—the coronavirus pandemic—has seemed much less so. Nonetheless, individual G20 countries' economic policy response to the pandemic has been rapid and massive, though not coordinated with other G20 partners.

What is the future of the G20 in a post-Covid-19 world? Ultimately, the US authorities, who played a critical role in the G20's formation, will have to decide whether to maintain support for the G20 leaders' self-definition as "the premier forum for international economic cooperation."[2] A critical consideration will be whether the emergence of China as a global economic power should and will influence US (and others') views regarding the future role for the exiting international institutions.

The thesis of this chapter is that the original—and unprecedented—formation of the post–World War II institutional structure was a success. Nonetheless, the system has been undergoing substantial evolution from its earliest days, in part

John Lipsky is the Peterson Distinguished Scholar at the Henry A. Kissinger Center for Global Affairs and a Senior Fellow at SAIS's Foreign Policy Institute.

reflecting problems with the institutions' original design and in part reflecting shifting challenges.

The forces that motivated formation of the G20 leaders remain relevant, and they are likely to heighten the need for international cooperation in the future. At the same time, specific adjustments are possible that would substantially enhance the G20 leaders' effectiveness, as well as that of the broader system of global governance. These include the short-term challenge of restoring global growth and the medium-term reforms to enhance the stability and effectiveness of the international financial system while avoiding new trade protection and improving the global trading system. There will be a longer-term task of coping with the unprecedented amount of debt, especially government debt, that is being accumulated in response to the pandemic as well as the unprecedented expansion of central bank balance sheets. In short, there is great need for a reinvigorated G20, but much will depend on US leadership.

Origins and Evolution of the Post–World War II Institutional Framework

The novel institutional framework of global governance established at the end of World War II was intended to prevent the factors that the framework's architects viewed as essential causes of the Great Depression and the subsequent world war. These included (1) lack of an effective forum for the discussion and adjudication of political and security issues; (2) lack of a multilateral forum for international trade, leading during the 1920s to the construction of beggar-thy-neighbor trade barriers; and (3) lack of effective international monetary and financial arrangements, beyond the fragile gold standard maintained by key central banks, which eventually collapsed.[3]

The critical post–World War II global institutions were the United Nations, to deal with political and security issues; the International Trade Organization, to be tasked with the reduction of trade barriers; and the International Monetary Fund, to insure the restoration of international financial markets that would support enlarged international trade flows. The IMF's Bretton Woods companion—the International Bank for Reconstruction and Development[4]—was intended to tap domestic financial markets, backed by member governments' guarantees, in order to provide capital to countries whose economies had been damaged in the war—this in the absence of anything resembling what are now called international capital markets. Each institution was both multilateral and treaty-based, with the goals that they would be recognized universally as legitimate and rules-based and that their decisions would carry the force of international law.

None of these institutions functioned exactly as intended. The principal flaw in the post–World War II institutional framework reflected the emergence of the Cold War. To begin with, the United Nations suffered, as it does to this day, from a congenital inability to reach decisions to act in controversial matters. As the Cold War intensified, the increasingly fraught relations between the Soviet Union and United States (and its allies) ensured that the UN could act decisively only on the relatively rare occasions of great-power consensus. Today, with the US-China relationship becoming increasingly difficult, the United Nations' effectiveness remains limited by its basic structure. By comparison, the Soviet Union's decision to create parallel economic institutions made the functioning of the General Agreement on Tariffs and Trade (GATT) and the Bretton Woods institutions smoother.

The GATT began with a relatively limited membership (twenty-three founding members). However, its key members shared a desire to lower trade barriers, especially tariffs, on a broad and sustained scale. As a result, by the end of the last multilateral agreement concluded under the GATT (the Uruguay Round that concluded in 1993), the average tariff among key members had fallen to 5%, from the initial post–World War II average rate of 22%. These liberalizations helped to produce virtually perpetual growth in international trade which outstripped the growth in domestic demand, at least until the GFC became virulent in 2008. In short, the liberalization of international trade for sixty years provided a reliable spur to world economic growth, despite organizational weaknesses of the GATT and its successor organization, the World Trade Organization (WTO).

Unlike the UN, the IMF was organized to facilitate action, even regarding controversial issues. Thus, the Executive Board's operational decisions are taken by majority vote.[5] The IMF's internal organization also promotes action, as the managing director chairs the Executive Board—and sets its agenda—as well as directs Fund staff. Voting power is apportioned according to "economic weight," leaving the members themselves to define this in negotiation. However, a quinquennial review of voting shares is mandatory under the Articles, providing the institution with a permanent mechanism that was intended to preserve the institution's legitimacy and representativeness. The organization of the World Bank is analogous to that of the IMF in that the World Bank similarly possesses a strong executive and its voting power mimics that of the Fund.

Collapse of the Bretton Woods "System"

The principal responsibility of the IMF, as stated in its constitutional Articles of Agreement, was "to promote exchange stability, to maintain orderly exchange arrangements among members and to avoid competitive exchange depreciation." In practice, the Fund was charged at the outset with maintaining the so-called dollar exchange standard, in which exchange rate stability was to be maintained by all members (except for the United States) by pegging their currencies to the US dollar, while the United States guaranteed the convertibility of the dollar to gold for official holders at a fixed dollar price. Critically, it also was "to assist in the establishment of a multilateral system of payments in respect of current transactions between members and in the elimination of foreign exchange restrictions." The Articles specify that "no member shall, without the approval of the Fund, impose restrictions on the making of payments and transfers for current international transactions."

This was revolutionary, in the sense that when the IMF began operations, such exchange restrictions were ubiquitous rather than exceptional. By actively and effectively promoting the dismantling of payments restrictions on trade and other current transactions, the Fund played a key role in creating a system that provided increasingly ample financing to support the trade opportunities that resulted from the ongoing reduction in tariffs and in other trade barriers.[6]

However, a fatal flaw in the IMF's dollar-exchange system emerged quickly in a potentially unresolvable tension between the United States' domestic policy goals and its systemic responsibilities. Such tension arose powerfully in the late 1960s, and by 1972, the dollar-exchange system had broken down irrevocably. This "collapse of the Bretton Woods system" was viewed widely as a historic systemic failure. However, the existence in many countries of liquid parallel foreign-exchange markets implied that the dollar-exchange standard of fixed rates actually operated with much more flexibility than is understood commonly.[7]

The collapse of the dollar-exchange standard ushered in a new "non-system" for exchange rates, with each IMF member allowed to choose their own policies, including floating their exchange rate. However, contrary to the conventional benign contemporaneous expectations of leading academics and other experts, the era of generalized floating among key currencies did not give rise to "stabilizing speculation." In fact, the post-1972 period was marked by an unexpected and largely unforeseen rise in inflationary pressures, especially in the United States, and the emergence of historically unprecedented payments imbalances.

By definition, current account imbalances imply the existence of capital flows as balancing items, but the Fund's Articles of Agreement did not give the institution any authority over international capital transactions. In fact, some of the architects of the Bretton Woods framework, including John Maynard Keynes, were opposed to the creation of international capital markets on the grounds that they led inevitably to destabilizing speculation. Thus, the financing capabilities of the IMF were intended to allow the institution to help reduce international financing strains deriving from what are by today's standards exceedingly modest-sized balance of payments deficits.

A Period of Systemic Crises and Systemic Improvisation

Three large themes emerged in the period between the collapse of the Bretton Woods dollar-exchange standard and the end of the beginning of the post–Cold War era. First, the large advanced economies effectively managed economic and financial relations among themselves in a separate format from that of the Bretton Woods institutions, although their actions in principle remained compatible with their obligations under the rules-based system that they had created. At the same time, the major economy authorities still pursued trade liberalization through multilateral negotiations within the framework of the GATT.

Second, it was established de facto that the IMF had primary responsibility for organizing crisis resolution measures for developing and emerging economies, through essentially ad hoc, tripartite negotiations involving debtor governments, official funding sources led by the IMF itself, and commercial lenders. Third, one outcome of the first generation of the tripartite crisis resolution agreements that would have a substantial future impact was the creation of an increasingly liquid market for dollar-denominated bonds issued by developing economies. In other words, capital markets became much more open to international investors and borrowers.

The key events of this period included the US Federal Reserve's dramatic interest rate increases that began in 1979 under Fed Chair Paul A. Volcker and peaked in 1982. The resulting sharp advanced economy recession—with sustained high US interest rates—produced a Latin American debt crisis. One result was an emerging critical role for the IMF as the architect of tripartite "rescue packages." The US dollar's subsequent rapid rise in the early 1980s boosted the United States' current account deficit, leading to the first convening in September 1985 of the "Group of 5" finance ministers—subsequently expanded to the Group of 7[8]—that met regularly as an informal "Executive Committee" of the global economic and financial system.

In this new setup, the IMF played only a minor role in discussions among the Group of 7 about their own policies. However, the Group of 7 itself failed to exercise firm control over financial markets. For example, a public dispute between the United States and the German authorities about appropriate policies inspired the "Black Monday" stock market crash in October 1987.

The Seismic Changes and Crises of the 1990s

The decade of the 1990s opened with a series of seismic events that dramatically altered the topography and challenges of the global system. The greatest impact was felt after the progressive collapse and late 1991 dissolution of the Soviet Union, ending the Cold War and permitting entry of the former Soviet Republics and the so-called "satellite" states (along with Russia) into the Bretton Woods institutions. The fall of the Berlin Wall in late 1989 led to German reunification during the following year and the historic 1992 Maastricht Treaty on European Monetary and Economic Union. In 1991, India began to implement a significant program of trade liberalization, and in 1992, China embarked on a program of privatizations that decisively accelerated its "opening up" policies. Finally, the GATT's multilateral Uruguay Round trade agreement was concluded successfully in 1993, and soon after, the World Trade Organization superseded the GATT.

Put another way, the process of globalization suddenly—and by and large unexpectedly—entered a new phase: the Bretton Woods institutions became universal, as had been intended by their architects. Trade flows accelerated, and the patterns of trade shifted toward Asia. At the same time, private sector capital flows expanded rapidly to take advantage of the new opportunities and grew to swamp official flows in scale.

As the architects of the IMF had never anticipated the emergence of large-scale cross-border capital flows and gave the Fund no direct responsibilities over such flows, the Fund was relatively unprepared for the initial crises in this new world of large-scale cross-border capital flows in the form of marketable securities. In particular—although it was assumed commonly that the Fund had responsibility for preventing economic and financial crises—it has no facilities that could be useful in this regard, rather than one dominated by traditional bank loans.

The inability of the existing institutional framework to deal smoothly with this expansive new phase of globalization quickly became evident. First was the

"Tequila Crisis" in 1994–95, involving Mexico and other Latin American countries. Spurred by sudden capital flight from Mexico, this was, in effect, the first crisis of confidence in a world of securitized finance. Halting the rapid withdrawal of funds from Mexico and elsewhere required the ad hoc organization of large-scale financial support, supplied mainly by the United States, the IMF, and the Bank for International Settlements (which is owned by central banks) in order to prevent the crisis from spreading further.

Recognizing that the growth of international capital markets presented a new, systemic challenge, the IMF's ministerial-level International Monetary and Financial Committee adopted in their September 1997 Hong Kong meeting a resolution recommending that the Funds' Articles of Agreement be amended to give the Fund authority over capital market arrangements. The ensuing "Asian Financial Crisis" that unfolded almost immediately demonstrated the inadequacy of the existing institutional arrangements, but it also precluded consideration of such an enlargement of the Fund's authority.

The Asian crisis itself ushered in a series of other financial crises, including the commercial bank–threatening 1998 collapse of the US hedge fund LTCM and the simultaneous Russian default, the Brazil crisis of early 1999, and the Turkish banking crisis of 2000. But it also led to two important institutional innovations. First of all, it was clear that the Group of 7 no longer served as an adequate "Executive Committee" for global economic institutions. A joint Canadian-US proposal resulted in the formation of the Group of 20 countries, which met at the level of finance ministers.[9] Although this grouping held regular meetings, it never assumed operational responsibilities, and it progressively devolved into more of a talking shop and a venue for bilateral side meetings between finance ministers.

Global Payments Imbalances and the Financial Crisis

Technological changes produced a mid-1990s US productivity burst, fueling the "dot.com" bubble. Even after this bubble burst, US growth outstripped that of other advanced economies. The result was the emergence of unprecedented—and to the architects of the postwar institutions, unimaginable—payment imbalances. The heart of the concerns regarding "global imbalances" was the record US current account deficit, which peaked in 2006 at 6% of gross domestic product, while China recorded a current account surplus of nearly 10% of its GDP.

The architects of the post–World War II system never could have envisioned such massive payments imbalances, as it would not have been possible previously to obtain the necessary finance in the amounts required. These imbalances were widely seen as inherently unstable, reflecting excessively expansionary policies on the part of the US authorities, together with massive one-sided currency market intervention by the Chinese authorities acting to maintain a massively undervalued exchange rate to promote their export industries.

After Tim Adams, the US under secretary of the Treasury for international affairs, famously admonished the IMF for having been "asleep at the wheel" while these imbalances built up, the IMF's managing director, Rodrigo de Rato, initiated in 2005–6 the innovative Multilateral Consultations on Global Imbalances.[10] With the authorization of the Fund's Executive Board, Fund management organized a series of confidential meetings involving five key authorities to seek agreement on a set of mutually consistent fiscal, monetary, and structural polices that could sustain global growth while reducing payments imbalances.[11] Although they reached agreement on a set of policy programs—which were made public at the April 2007 meeting of the IMF's International Monetary and Financial Committee—the lack of commitment of the US authorities to the process was signaled clearly by their refusal to contemplate any further meetings of the group to monitor compliance or to make any needed adjustments in their policy plans.

The perceived failure of the Multilateral Consultations had an important systemic implication. Despite the conclusion of Fund staff and management as early as August 2007 that a financial crisis had become inevitable, their warnings that dramatic policy action would be needed were not taken seriously by key advanced economy authorities.[12] As the global financial crisis exploded in September 2008 with the collapse of Lehman Brothers, it was concluded that a new institution— the Group of 20 Leaders Summit process—and not the IMF, would manage the international crisis response.

The G20 Leaders Summit process was proposed formally by President George W. Bush at the IMF annual meeting in October 2008, with the inaugural set for Washington in November 2008. Eventually, the G20 Leaders declared their new grouping to be the premier forum for US international economic cooperation. Thus, the G20 Leaders—who together represented 65% of global population, 75% of global trade, and 85% of global GDP—asserted their role as directing the activities of the pre-existing multilateral institutions, at least in the area of economic and financial policies.

From the outset, the G20 stated that their first priority was "to restore global growth and to achieve needed reforms in the world's financial systems." In their April 2009 London Summit, the G20 Leaders—with the strong support of newly elected US President Barack Obama—agreed on a consistent set of expansionary fiscal and monetary policies, mandated the creation of the Financial Stability Board to address financial sector reform,[13] pledged to avoid new protectionist measures and instead to complete the WTO's Doha Development Round of multilateral trade negotiations, and agreed to provide substantial new resources for the IMF and other international financial institutions.

Thus, although the advanced economies had been slow to react to the onset of the GFC, once it arrived they quickly reached substantive agreements on concrete policy actions. G20 Leaders proceeded as if their individual countries' interests were broadly consistent with those of their G20 partners. The coherence of the G20's initiatives subsequently was considered widely to have enhanced their effectiveness and boosted confidence in their eventual success.

In contrast, the response to the coronavirus pandemic in many ways has been paradoxical. Even before the G20 Leaders held their Extraordinary Summit in March 2020, virtually all members already had undertaken fiscal and monetary measures that were larger in scale and scope than those taken in the context of the entire GFC. Yet public coordination and consultation has been far less pronounced than that in 2008–9. The Leaders Statement issued in March 2020 following their virtual summit contained no concrete policy commitments. The subsequent Communique of G20 finance ministers and Central Bank governors issued in April mainly endorsed measures that had been announced previously. G20 economies appear to be facing distinct choices and prioritizing domestic considerations over global cooperation.[14]

Policy Challenges for the G20 Leaders

An obvious issue regarding the current institutional arrangement is whether the key G20 authorities continue to view the Leaders process as their "premier forum." For example, US President Donald J. Trump has not shown any particular interest in the G20 Leaders process nor has he suggested that he views the process as an important policy-making venue.

Even beyond the views of current Leaders, it remains to be seen whether the G20 Leaders' structure—which is partial and not universal, voluntary and not treaty-based—ultimately will prove to be effective. One obvious weakness is that the G20 Leaders' current decision-making practice requires consensus—it is not able to reach decisions on controversial matters if there is any disagreement. Similar to the Soviet role in limiting the possibility for UN action, an aggressive China increasingly out of step with others in the G20 casts doubt on the future effectiveness of the group.

Central banks have been exceptionally aggressive in response to the pandemic in their support for credit markets, acquiring vast amounts of debt instruments and loans while accumulating unprecedented totals of excess bank reserves. These actions by and large have been successful in maintaining the liquidity of financial markets, while no doubt introducing significant distortions. For example, the issuance of US corporate bonds has reached record highs, as corporations have taken advantage of historically low interest rates and exceptional market liquidity, despite the fraught fundamental outlook.

The path back to financial market normality (whatever that will prove to be) has no pre-existing roadmap but no doubt will require cooperation and coordination internationally to avoid creating destabilizing market volatility. While mechanisms for consultation among central banks exist already, they will not have been utilized previously in such potentially stressful conditions.

At the same time, the scale of government debt—and, in some cases, private sector debt—will be very much outsized relative to previous experience. For example, the IMF's latest *World Economic Outlook* update anticipates a US general government deficit in 2020 of nearly 24% of GDP, bringing gross debt to more than 140% of GDP. As a result, it is possible that new venues for consultation and cooperation will be required to avoid creating new uncertainties about the management of such huge amounts.

Already, the G20 Leaders—together with key nongovernmental actors—have attempted to address the debt challenges of the poorest countries through a temporary debt service moratorium, labeled the Debt Service Suspension Initiative, or DSSI. This effort is being closely watched, not only as a potential template for future measures if the economic recovery remains weak but also as an indication of the Chinese authorities' willingness to cooperate with G20 partners in this area.[15]

Since China did not object to the endorsement of the DSSI in the G20 Ministers' Communique, they may be willing to cooperate with its G20 partners to a greater degree than has been the case previously. At this point, however, the degree of their cooperation is not yet clear, nor is the success of even this limited effort assured.

The impact of the COVID-19 crisis, while not originating in the financial sector, no doubt will have a substantial impact over the near and even medium term on official liquidity support and when that should end and insolvencies begin, especially if business failures loom in a potentially sluggish post-pandemic recovery. In such a case, financial, monetary, and fiscal policies easily could become intertwined and give rise to conflicts over the implications of decisions on these issues for other G20 economies. But so far there is little indication of any willingness to cooperate on this issue by means of the G20 architecture.

The outlook for international trade also appears fraught. First of all, the pandemic already has resulted in a sharp drop in international trade, with an unprecedented pace of the decline. The two largest economies—the United States and China—are engaged in a dispute over trade policies that has resulted in the imposition of new trade barriers, and their bilateral negotiations so far have produced only a limited agreement.[16] At the same time, the United States and the European Union appear to be at loggerheads over the taxation of digital commerce, with each side threatening to impose new sanctions.

Finally, there is a broad consensus that the WTO's own organization and processes require substantial reform, but it can't be taken for granted in the current environment that this consensus will lead to action. In any case, many of the basic issues—especially those not involving simple tariff reductions—that would be addressed in new trade agreements are not likely to be reached successfully in a highly complex multilateral framework but rather only on a bilateral or plurilateral basis.[17]

The taxation of firms operating in multiple jurisdictions has become a source of friction, especially with regard to digital commerce. This is a difficult issue that will be highly relevant, even beyond the current US-EU dispute. Allied with the issue of taxation of such commerce is the application of competition law.

The final basic item on the G20 Leaders' agenda was the reform of the international financial institutions. The London G20 Summit agreed to provide substantial new resources for the IMF and the multilateral development banks (MDBs). In Seoul, the Leaders agreed to a new distribution of IMF voting shares, in which the ten largest quotas were apportioned to the G7 countries (minus Canada) plus the BRIC countries (Brazil, Russia, India, and China). Japan retained the second-largest quota overall, while the BRIC shares totaled more than 15%, which for the first time gave them joint veto power over any amendment to the Articles of Agreement.

Moreover, it was agreed that the new quotas would be ratified by the time of the 2012 IMF annual meeting, that there would be a review of the principles for determining "economic weight," and that there would be a new round of quota adjustments on the basis of the new calculations. In any event, the United States did not ratify the new quotas until December 2015.[18]

Some Possible Approaches to Strengthen the Post-COVID-19 World Order

A fundamental current issue is whether institutional changes are needed in order to best address the systemic weaknesses exposed by the COVID shock and to make new progress on the policy reforms first put in motion by the G20 Leaders in responding to the GFC.

It seems self-evident that an open, rules-based, nondiscriminatory international system of global governance requires the support of its members. It also has come to be considered conventional wisdom that the nature of the US-China relationship, whether one of competitors or adversaries, will prove to be pivotal in establishing the terms of global governance in the coming decades. The Chinese authorities, for their part, have declared repeatedly their support for the existing multilateral system and its key institutions. What is less clear at this time, however, is the practical implication of this expression of fealty. Also uncertain are the views of the US authorities, now and in the future.

At an operational level, US officials remain engaged actively in the existing institutions. Looking forward, the establishment of a productive and predictable US-China relationship is a *sine qua non* for strengthening the institutions of global governance. Beyond that, the engagement of the US government at the highest levels in support of the process is a second requirement for progress. At the same time, it is possible to envision a series of reforms to the G20 process and to the associated multilateral framework that could enhance the system's overall effectiveness, while maintaining the G20 Leaders process as a spur to new progress.

Finally, despite widespread talk of a future "de-globalization," intensified global engagement is virtually mandated by the pressure of such forces as technology advances and the digitalization of economic activity, climate change, demographic shifts, and the associated unprecedented force of cross-border immigration, together with growing concerns about inequality.

Aligning the G20 Leaders and the Bretton Woods Institutions

Some of the traits that hamper the decision-making ability of the United Nations are shared by the G20 Leaders, in that the designation of a chair rotates annually and decisions in practice are taken by consensus. In addition, the Leaders lack a permanent staff, and there is no legal basis for their decisions. Nonetheless, in those circumstances where there is consensus, the G20 Leaders can act effectively and powerfully, and they can command the actions of the Bretton Woods institutions. In contrast, the Bretton Woods institutions possess strong executives, highly capable staffs, and an ability to act credibly even when a consensus is lacking, reflecting the majority-rule structure of their voting.

Thus, a potential avenue to strengthen the framework of global governance would be to align the country composition of the G20 Leaders with that of the IMF's International Monetary and Financial Committee (IMFC) and that of the IMF's and World Bank's Executive Boards.[19] Already at present, when a consensus exists regarding needed actions or policy initiatives, as was the case during the GFC, the G20 Leaders can act with credibility and great effectiveness. In cases where a consensus is lacking, operational decisions still can be reached credibly at the level of the Bretton Woods institutions' Executive Boards, reflecting the majority-rule principle that governs normal decision-making in these institutions.

In short, if it is in the interest of the United States to strengthen the framework of global governance, this step would make sense, and it would not require any diminution of the relative role of the US in the Bretton Woods institutions. It also would heighten the likelihood that US alliances could prove more productive.

INTERNATIONAL MONETARY FUND

Over recent years, the Fund has substantially improved the variety of financial facilities that it can provide for crisis resolution. A challenge for the Fund is that it is widely held to be responsible for crisis prevention. Until now, however, it has not possessed any financing facility that could be useful in crisis prevention in the context of securitized cross-border finance.

During the GFC, the US interbank funding market was frozen temporarily, reflecting banks' uncertainties about the content of counterparty bank portfolios. Many foreign banks held US dollar assets that were financed with funds borrowed in the interbank market. When they were shut out of renewed dollar funding by the lack of interbank liquidity, the Federal Reserve provided unlimited dollar swap lines to the European Central Bank (ECB), which on-lent them to eurozone banks, thus preventing potential insolvencies.

Subsequently, the key advanced economy central banks—including the Federal Reserve, the ECB, the Bank of England, the Bank of Canada, the Swiss National Bank, and the Bank of Japan—created a network of permanent unlimited swap lines, thus limiting the illiquidity risk for their banks' international operations. The Federal Reserve also provided temporary swap lines to nine other countries' central banks, including those of Brazil, Mexico, South Korea, and Singapore.

These temporary lines were renewed in the spring of 2020, thus reducing the risks that there would be any market concerns about these banks' access to US dollar liquidity. By reducing the risks of sudden market volatility, these moves served to solidify the position of the US dollar as the dominant international reserve currency. But the question remains: What about the 174 Fund member countries that don't have access to Fed swap lines?

It has long been a principle in national financial markets that the central bank can act usefully as a lender of last resort, so long as its actions are prudent and do not give rise to unjustified moral hazard. The Fed has chosen to do so in these specific cases. The Fund, in turn, has been moving toward acting in this regard by making short-term credits available without ex post conditionality.

The newly approved Short-Term Liquidity Facility (SLF) marks the first time that the Fund has been authorized by its members to offer a true swap-like facility, although with limited eligibility. Nonetheless, with the Fund finally able to offer swap-like facilities, it should be allowed to expand the eligibility for this facility to all member countries. If so, the Fund would begin to gain credibility as being much more capable in crisis prevention.

FINANCIAL STABILITY BOARD

Like the G20 Leaders themselves, the Financial Stability Board (FSB) is a voluntary association of a rather disparate set of officials from finance ministries, central banks, regulators, supervisors, standard-setting bodies, and international institutions. Given the impetus for reform created by the global financial crisis, and given the conviction among financial market institutions themselves that reforms were needed following the GFC, the FSB has overseen significant progress in making the financial system more stable and resilient. Nonetheless, the work of the FSB is far from complete, and the G20 Leaders should make sure that it has the authority and motivation to make further progress.

The FSB relies on consensus agreement, and there are several areas where progress on reforms has been either partial, halting, or virtually nonexistent. Ultimately, the creation of the FSB (with the participation of twenty-four country authorities and thirteen institutions)—and, before it, the Financial Stability Forum (FSF)—is a reflection of the IMF's lack of authority over international capital transactions which implicitly leaves a vacuum.

If the G20 Leaders are serious about creating a level and effective playing field in financial markets, including capital markets, perhaps a long-term goal should be to develop the FSB into an international institution with broader membership, with a firm legal basis, and with independent surveillance responsibility (not just conducting peer reviews, as is its current practice).

WORLD TRADE ORGANIZATION

Just as there is a clear sense that the world trading system is at a crucial point—with serious disputes brewing amid a historic decline in trade volumes—the World Trade Organization itself is facing unprecedented difficulties. Each of the WTO's three basic functions—administering trade rules, providing a dispute settlement mechanism, and serving as a venue for trade negotiations—is either under pressure or not working at present.

The issues challenging the WTO, and the world trading system, are serious and varied. The searing experience of the pandemic, including the difficulty in obtaining medical supplies, has added to dissatisfaction with the status quo. China's renewed emphasis on the role of its state enterprises and its ongoing commitment to its Belt and Road Initiative also have raised concerns about the treatment of state subsidies and nondiscrimination in contracting.

At the same time, the United States has become a disruptive force within the trading system. The current US Special Trade Representative (USTR) states that he prefers bilateral negotiations, because the United States can get a better deal that way, as it is always the biggest participant in any such negotiation. The United States has failed to make appointments to fill vacancies on the WTO's appellate tribunal, thus crippling it through lack of a quorum. Similarly, the USTR complains about the excessively procedural nature of the WTO's practice, but the United States' authorities have not offered a detailed plan for reform. Finally, the United States' phase one trade agreement with China has aspects that represent the type of trade diversion that the post–World War II work of the GATT and the WTO were intended to overcome.

In short, a pre-pandemic consensus existed that the WTO, and the trading system in general, needed serious reform and modernization. So far, however, the United States' authorities have not been at all clear about their specific goals or vision of what should replace the status quo. Thus, the US position at present seems to be "we want a better deal, but we can't say clearly what that means." Perhaps post-pandemic, the United States could start to clarify what it hopes to accomplish in this sphere and how it hopes to do it.

Final Comments

The United States, like virtually the entire world, is faced with a set of difficult post-COVID-19 policy challenges. In the short run, the principal challenges are medical—controlling the pandemic—and restoring economic activity. There is no clear roadmap to success in either sphere, but a more cooperative approach, such as that in evidence in 2008–9, is likely to be more effective in boosting confidence than uncoordinated efforts. The medium term is filled with myriad challenges, as discussed above. In this regard, the G20 Leaders have substantial unfinished business. As with the short-term challenges, failure to follow through with efforts already under way would risk creating the sense of moving backward, undermining confidence. Finally, the legacy of the pandemic is going to be an unprecedented amount of debt—for governments, for businesses, and for individuals—and of historically large central bank balance sheets. Once again, the potential interactions in addressing these issues point to a need for effective international cooperation.

The avenues for progress are clear, if difficult. The history of the post–World War II period is one of broadly successful institutional innovation and adaptation. Hopefully, this period is far from over.

NOTES

1. Henceforth, for brevity, this grouping will be referred to interchangeably as the G20 Leaders or simply the G20.

2. G20 Leaders Statement: The Pittsburgh Summit, September 24–25, 2009.

3. Maurice Obstfield and Alan M. Taylor, "International Monetary Relations: Taking Finance Seriously," *Journal of Economic Perspectives* 31, no. 3 (Summer 2017): 3–28.

4. Subsequently expanded into the World Bank Group.

5. By tradition, the IMF's Executive Board decisions are taken by consensus, although the consensus is formed in the context of an explicit understanding of what actual voting would produce in the way of a decision.

6. The IMF continues to track the exchange rate and trade regimes, and it publishes an Annual Report on Exchange Arrangements and Exchange Restrictions.

7. Carmen M. Reinhart and Kenneth S. Rogoff, "The Modern History of Exchange Rates: A Reinterpretation," *Quarterly Journal of Economics* 119, no. 1 (February 2004): 1–48.

8. The seven countries include the United States, Japan, Germany, the United Kingdom, France, Italy, and Canada.

9. The Group of 20 includes the Group of 7 countries, plus Argentina, Australia, Brazil, China, India, Indonesia, Mexico, the Russian Federation, Saudi Arabia, South Africa, South Korea, Turkey, and the European Union.

10. A detailed description of the Multilateral Consultations on Global Imbalances can be found on the IMF website.

11. This included the United States, the eurozone, China, Japan, and Saudi Arabia.

12. In January 2008, the Fund's managing director called for 2% of GDP fiscal stimulus in the advanced economies. In March 2008, the Fund's first deputy managing director warned in a speech that fiscal support was going to be required for the financial system. Other, private, warnings also were waved off.

13. The Financial Stability Board includes the members of the Financial Stability Forum plus those G20 members who were not already a member of the FSF.

14. At the same time, the degree of international cooperation on developing treatments for COVID-19 is without historic parallel.

15. Since the GFC, Chinese entities have become by far the largest lenders to low-income countries. Heretofore, the Chinese authorities had insisted that their arrangements in these cases were bilateral and that they do not divulge the terms of such lending. Moreover, they are not members of the Paris Club of official lenders, which ensures equal treatment by Club members in cases of renegotiation.

16. Disturbingly, the specifics of their partial deal appear to be at variance with the underlying principles—such as nondiscrimination and the avoidance of measures that result in trade diversion—that guided the post–World War II process of trade liberalization.

17. For example, issues such as the definition of subsidies, the protection of intellectual property, and sanitary standards in agricultural trade all are unlikely to be resolved if the WTO's 164 members must reach a consensus agreement. Moreover, defining standards and rules for access to markets in services is increasingly important but exceedingly complex.

18. In their April 2020 meeting, G20 ministers reset the timing of the agreement on the next quota adjustment—which undoubtedly will award China the second-largest vote—to December 2023.

19. Of course, such a step would require alterations either in the size and/or the composition of the G20 or else of the IMF's and World Bank's Executive Boards (and potentially the conversion of the IMFC into the IMF Ministerial Council). Representation at the IMF and World Bank Board will still require the formation of constituencies in order to guarantee universal representation. With their structure directly aligned with the Bretton Woods institutions, the G20 Leaders process would fit much more logically and coherently into the structure of global governance. For example, this would eliminate the current awkwardness of the G20 ministers meeting only hours in advance of the IMFC, even though there already is a substantial overlap in the composition of the two groups.

PART V / Global Politics and Governance

Chapter Twelve

When the World Stumbled

COVID-19 and the Failure of the International System

Anne Applebaum

What Happened

In the first half of March 2020, the borders of the United States of America slammed shut. They had already begun to close in January, when President Donald Trump's administration announced restrictions on visitors from China, a "ban" that was late, chaotic, and incomplete. In fact, tens of thousands of travelers continued to arrive in the United States from China every day, including from Wuhan, where the novel coronavirus had originated.[1] Six weeks later, the closures were hardly much smoother. Without warning its European allies, the United States abruptly announced impending restrictions on travelers from Europe, producing a rush to get home that led to higher rates of coronavirus infection inside the United States.[2] Passengers who knew they were ill got on planes, afraid of being stranded. Many were stuck standing for hours in crowds at airports and at security checkpoints.

This same mistake was repeated in other countries. On March 14, Poland also shut its borders to all noncitizens. One of the side effects of this decision, taken without much forethought, was chaos on the German border. Baltic and Ukrainian tourists and truck drivers waited in their cars for days; the German Red Cross wound up bringing them food and water.[3] Abrupt travel decisions taken

Anne Applebaum is a staff writer for *The Atlantic* and a senior fellow at the Agora Institute and the School of Advanced International Studies, Johns Hopkins University.

inside some countries had equally catastrophic effects. On March 24, India announced a sudden lockdown that left migrant day-laborers without subsistence; many walked hundreds of miles to get back to their native villages, and some died along the way.[4] In the subsequent weeks, people all around the world scrambled to get home. Many countries eventually organized charter flights to help their citizens, but even so, many wound up stranded for weeks.

This chaos was unprecedented. In the past, countries dealing with pandemics had weighed travel and border decisions very carefully. At the time of the Ebola crisis in 2014–16, President Barack Obama's administration had considered closing borders to travelers from West Africa but decided against it.[5] This, one former White House official told me, was because border closures, without careful planning, can slow down movement of equipment and expertise. In practice, they also created clusters of infectious people at airports and other checkpoints. Closures also give the illusion of resolute action without changing the reality on the ground. Trump's announcements of a halt in travel, first from China and then from Europe, did not in fact halt the spread of the virus, which was already being transmitted from person to person inside the United States.

All of this could have been avoided. Had there been consultation, had the consequences been thought through jointly, had international organizations stepped in to manage the process, the closures might have gone off more smoothly, and the response might have been more fruitful. It was reasonable to put temporary brakes on international and even domestic travel. It was not reasonable to do so in a manner that made the virus spread more quickly.

But then, many international organizations were not ready for this task or, indeed, for any of the others that the worst pandemic since 1918 was about to present. Despite myriad international conferences going back many years, despite worthy scientific papers and statements of intent, international institutions were not only unprepared to cope with the travel issues; they could not help with the backlogs in personal protective equipment, with the need to coordinate communications, or with the sudden political and economic instability. The perception of failure immediately clung to European institutions, transatlantic institutions, and United Nations institutions alike. And yet these institutions were created for exactly this kind of moment. Precisely because this was a genuinely global crisis—a new disease, spreading quickly, with the potential to harm everyone in the world—the failure of global organizations seemed particularly acute.

Not all of the institutions failed in exactly the same way or for the same reasons. In some cases, the problem was directly to do with leadership. During the first phase of the pandemic, especially as it hit Italy very hard, the European Union (EU) suffered from what can only be described as a failure of imagination. Unlike Asian countries, European countries had no recent experience with pandemics, and almost everyone, from politicians to journalists and analysts, underestimated the risk. At major European meetings in January and February—the World Economic Forum in Davos, the Munich Security Conference—the virus was scarcely discussed. As late as March 9, when the Italian outbreak had already begun, Ursula von der Leyen, the president of the European Commission, referenced the coronavirus only glancingly at a press conference reviewing her first hundred days in office. The Italian government's initial calls for emergency measures were not heeded either.[6]

Later, as each country became engulfed in its own health crisis, the EU improved its response, but its actions were poorly explained and communicated. In the weeks following the initial moment of stasis and confusion, both Germany and France delivered large quantities of equipment to Italy—far more, in total, than China, despite enormous publicity around a Chinese transport plane that landed in Rome. The EU also activated large joint-purchasing mechanisms so that member states would not have to compete against one another. Still, EU leaders did not make their efforts clear, and the initial failures left a bad impression. In early March, 88% of Italians told pollsters that Europe was failing to support them.[7] In June, there was a slight recovery, but 63% of Italians still said the EU had failed its citizens. The numbers were not much higher in Germany, France, or much of the rest of Europe, where most people simply said that the EU had been irrelevant during the worst days of the crisis.[8]

Transatlantic Western clubs fared even worse, though here the fault was almost entirely American. Trump, who had spent much of his presidency railing against his allies—at one point he called the European Union a "foe"; at another point he said Europe was "worse than China"—not only failed to warn Europeans before shutting down transatlantic travel; he seems never to have consulted with them at all, not on the science nor on the borders. In the absence of the United States, the whole idea of transatlantic cooperation became moot. As recently as 2014, the G7 had served as an effective forum to push back against the Russian invasion of Ukraine and to agree upon sanctions. This time, even a virtual meeting of G7 foreign ministers ended in ludicrous rancor when the American secretary of state, Mike Pompeo, insisted on using the expression "Wuhan virus" and the others gave up in disgust.[9] Even when the EU eventually recovered its equilibrium and began to cope with the economic fallout of the pandemic, the transatlantic alliance did not.

To be fair, neither the EU nor the G7 was set up with pandemics in mind. The G7 has never been more than a talking shop, a club of rich countries that meet to resolve mostly economic problems; in Europe, health matters have historically been delegated to member states. But the World Health Organization (WHO) is a body explicitly created to cope with global pandemics. And although the institution has a decades-long record of success—among other things, the WHO is responsible for eliminating smallpox and for suppressing many other diseases—on this occasion it made a series of surprising mistakes. Because criticism of the WHO has now become part of US politics—the Trump administration has made the WHO a scapegoat for its own failures—it is important to remember that, despite some of the over-the-top rhetoric, the WHO failed the world in some important ways during the early days of the crisis. Certainly the organization adhered far too closely to the narrative of a Chinese government that initially sought to conceal the nature and spread of the coronavirus. As late as January 14, the organization's leadership ignored evidence from Taiwan—which is not, thanks to Chinese pressure, a WHO member—that the novel coronavirus could be transmitted from person to person. Yet Taiwan was a credible voice: the country had sent medical teams to Wuhan in December and had experienced the impact of Chinese cover-ups before. So had authorities in Hong Kong, who also believed by early January that the coronavirus could be transmitted between humans.[10] Even so, the WHO did not take their evidence seriously.

Other mistakes followed: the WHO's strange insistence that face masks were not necessary, for example, even as mounting evidence has shown that they can cut the transmission of the virus quite effectively, and the WHO's decision to wait until March 11 to declare the existence of a pandemic, even though the disease had already spread. The WHO's determination to compliment China in its public statements, and ignore Chinese mistakes, was equally strange. Following a fact-finding mission in February, the organization put out a report lauding China for having "rolled out perhaps the most ambitious agile and aggressive disease containment effort in history," not only ignoring the early suppression of information but also underplaying the psychological and economic costs of the Wuhan lockdown, as well as the violations of human rights.[11]

The precise dynamics that created the problems at the WHO and those that led the EU to stumble were of course different; the sources of dysfunction inside Western institutions differ from those inside the UN system. It is nevertheless important to look at all of them as a group, since their joint failure contributed to an overall perception that the system had failed, that nation-states were left by themselves, that complacent international bureaucracies were not up to the job. And although some aspects of this perception are unfair, it is not totally wrong either. The international system in its current state is plagued with deep problems, and now is the right time to solve them.

Why It Happened

Any analysis of the international institutions in the spring of 2020 has to begin with one central, salient failure: the Trump administration's abdication of leadership. The absence of an American voice was remarkable from the very beginning of the crisis, and indeed it was widely remarked upon. In April, Carl Bildt—a Swedish prime minister in the 1990s, a UN envoy during the Bosnian War, and a foreign minister for many years after that—told me that, looking back on his 30-year career, he could not remember a single international crisis in which the United States had no global presence at all. "Normally, when something happens"—a war, an earthquake—"everybody waits to see what the Americans are doing, for better or for worse, and then they calibrate their own response based on that." This time the Americans were doing nothing and talking to nobody, at least at the highest level.[12]

In part, the American absence was explained by the chaotic state of the Trump White House. The volatility and lack of process in the Trump administration have been well described elsewhere, including by former national security adviser John Bolton.[13] These were compounded in the spring of 2020 by the president's initial attempts to cover up the spread of the virus, because he feared it might harm his reelection prospects. But America's absence from the international stage during the subsequent weeks is also explained by broader changes in ideas and ideology. Trump's instinctive dislike of allies, alliances, and international institutions has some broader support and deeper roots.

Since the 1970s, most American presidents, Republicans and Democrats alike, have, when speaking about the international system, done so using the language of democracy and universal rights. By contrast, the Trump administration speaks about "sovereignty." Although this is a word with multiple meanings, some positive and some negative, in the context of the international system, "sovereignty" means something very specific. It's the word that nations use when they want to deny international institutions legitimacy of any kind. In 2019, Trump gave a UN speech in which he declared that "the future does not belong to globalists," using a word invented and popularized by the online alt-right: "The future belongs to patriots. The future belongs to sovereign and independent nations who protect their citizens, respect their neighbors, and honor the differences that make each country special and unique."[14]

Trump's subordinates have echoed this language, and it has been picked up by a large swath of foreign policy experts in Washington too. Rex Tillerson, Trump's first secretary of state, argued that the promotion of human rights was a distraction from America's "national security interests, economic interests."[15] The current secretary of state, Mike Pompeo, has created a commission to examine whether the United States might also redefine "human rights" in line with his conservative religious beliefs.[16]

There is support for these views in the United States. Although the majority of Americans disagree with them—and tell pollsters, for example, that the United States should strengthen the United Nations—a minority does not.[17] There is also a certain amount of cynicism associated with the long-standing American support for universal values. Even many of those affiliated with the Democratic Party or the Obama presidency will tacitly acknowledge, if only off the record, their own ambivalence about the promotion of democracy or human rights, the policies that the party advocated in the past. They might be uncomfortable with the open nationalism of the Trump administration, but they never liked the Bush administration's "democracy" agenda either. This absence of any sense of shared political values forms the background to the American lack of interest in the fate of its European allies during the coronavirus crisis, as well as the de facto disintegration of the G7. If national sovereignty is more important than shared values, after all, then why should the fates of other democracies be of any special concern to the United States?

This ideological change has had important consequences, for in fact it echoes and amplifies the language that authoritarian states also use inside the UN system. When anyone protests the Iranian regime's extrajudicial murders, for example, or the Chinese government's repression of the people of Hong Kong, those regimes shout "sovereignty." When anyone cites the phrase "all human beings are born free and equal in dignity and rights," advocates of "sovereignty" describe this as just another example of Western imperialism. *Respect neighbors*, to quote the language of Trump's UN speech, is what the Chinese say when they want to shut down international critics of their repressive policies toward their Uyghur Muslim minority population in Xinjiang. *Honor differences* is what the Iranians say when they do not want the UN or independent human rights groups to comment on their arrests of women who refuse to wear head scarves.

The phrase bleeds into other areas too. "Sovereignty" is the argument that the Chinese have deployed against any suggestion, from the WHO or anyone else, that they should launch an independent investigation of the origins of the coronavirus. Why should they do so, if they are sovereign?

If this argument has been gaining ground in recent years, that is because of the second important source of weakness in the international system: the Chinese effort, going back several years now, to dominate or direct international organizations, especially within the UN system, and to instill within them autocratic values. For American diplomats, a UN posting is a backwater. By contrast, the Chinese have been sending their best and brightest diplomats into the international system for many years. Chinese nationals now run four major UN agencies: the International Civil Aviation Organization, the International Telecommunication Union, the Food and Agriculture Organization, and the Industrial Development Organization.[18] Chinese leaders have run the UN Department of Economic and Social Affairs since 2007. Even as the United States withdraws money and troops, China has expanded the country's presence in UN peacekeeping operations. In 2015, President Xi Jinping promised to establish a $1 billion "peace fund," and offered to contribute 8,000 troops.[19]

Although the holders of jobs in these kinds of organizations are meant to be apolitical, some do not hide their national bias. In 2018, Wu Hongbo, former undersecretary general for the UN Department of Economic and Social Affairs, told a Chinese studio audience that although he was an "international civil servant" who cannot take orders directly from his own country's government, there are exceptions to that rule: "When it comes to Chinese national sovereignty and security, we will undoubtedly defend our country's interests." Among other things, he explained how he once prevailed upon the UN security police to expel an activist—a representative of the repressed Uyghur minority, and a critic of China—from a seminar in the UN building.[20]

The Trump administration has belatedly noticed this Chinese project, seeking, for example, to block a Chinese candidate from becoming the head of the World Intellectual Property Organization.[21] But the United States no longer provides an ideological alternative, a pole of thinking around which other countries can gather. "American national interests" is not a cause that even Europeans or America's traditional Asian allies can rally to, let alone Africans or Latin Americans. Without shared goals or values, there is no particular incentive for other countries to support the United States in the UN or anywhere else.

Nor, more importantly, is the United States willing to invest the same kinds of sums in the developing world as China. For it is not just talent that China throws at the system. China also uses financial tools—investments, loans, and, allegedly, bribes—to convince other autocracies to vote its way, in the UN and elsewhere, to confirm its candidates, and more generally to build a circle of friends. The main formal vehicle for the distribution of money is China's Belt and Road Initiative—China's plan to improve the Eurasian infrastructure, from Rome to Beijing. Belt and Road is famously untransparent; if large sums of money disappear into the pockets of local leaders, China doesn't mind. At the same time, China repeatedly seeks to give the impression that it is the world's most important development project. Liu Zhenmin, the current leader of the UN Department of Economic and Social Affairs—the body formerly run by Wu Hongbo—speaks of Belt and Road and the UN's own "Sustainable Development Goals" as almost interchangeable: "both of them serve the purposes and principles of the Charter of the United Nations," not least because they "aim to promote win-win cooperation," in a world where "sovereignty" is the ruling principle.[22]

The behavior of the WHO's leadership in early 2020 cannot be linked directly to this combination of Chinese ambition, personnel, and money. But it is true that, in advance of being named to the post in 2017, the current WHO director-general, Tedros Adhanom, publicly stated his support for the "One China" policy—rejecting, in effect, Taiwan's application for membership, a decision that had important consequences in 2020.[23] Consciously or otherwise, some of those who work for international institutions may now feel it is better to agree with China, lest it harm their career prospects; as US influence fades, what America thinks matters less. No wonder it has become so difficult for the WHO or any of the UN's other agencies to hold China to account in any important sense.

European governments continue to play important roles in the UN system, especially in the various UN bodies that deal with human rights, which the United States has mostly abandoned in disgust. Indeed, many European countries continue to put international cooperation, human rights, and democracy promotion at the heart of their foreign policy, considering these principles to be more critical to their national interest than the abstract concept of sovereignty. In the spring of 2020, for example, the Swedish foreign minister held a series of online meetings with activists and analysts to discuss the intersection of the coronavirus and authoritarianism, a topic that the government considered to be of vital interest.[24]

Yet these efforts are partial and uncoordinated, amounting to less than the sum total of effort. As a bloc, Europe is the world's largest economy, as well as an important and influential source of regulation and thinking about trade. But the failure of Europeans to form a common political front, either with one another or with the world's other democracies, is indeed the third important source of weakness in the international system. EU member states, plus Britain, could create stronger and more public links with Asian democracies—Japan, South Korea, Taiwan—as well as with Australia, New Zealand, and the democracies of Africa and Latin America. They could use their own money and international clout to influence appointments and policy, or to force UN institutions to hold countries accountable. But they still behave more like a regional block, both within and outside the UN, one that has now been substantially weakened by Brexit. As a result, Europe is not associated even with the ideas and principles that Europeans believe in—about democracy, about cooperation—and Europe has been largely unable to attract or influence other countries.

Strangely, given the amount of ink that is spilled describing the EU's supposedly overbearing ambition for control, most of its failures are in fact the result of its members' *refusal* to pool resources—their refusal, in other words, to share sovereignty. The eurozone crisis of a decade ago might have been avoided, for example, if the common currency's members had decided to require its members to coordinate their fiscal and banking policies before being allowed to join. The EU's refusal to place real penalties on member states that break the organization's own rules about judicial independence and press freedom has also weakened the overall institutional commitment to those issues, externally as well as internally. The same is even more true in security policy. In theory, Europe has an External Action Service, a "foreign ministry" with diplomats and embassies. In practice, the EU keeps choosing "foreign ministers" without influence or a strong international profile, whom its political leaders then ignore. Twenty years ago, when France and Britain still had real foreign policy ambitions (and real armies), this would not have mattered so much. But now France is distracted by its internal problems, Britain is consumed by Brexit, while Germany, for all of the obvious historical reasons, still finds it difficult to speak too loudly or forcefully.

At least a part of the bloc's current leadership understands this situation. Precisely because they are aware that their reaction was both slow and badly communicated, the COVID-19 crisis could be a turning point for European leaders. Both Angela Merkel and Emmanuel Macron are committed to a large-scale European recovery fund that some have described as a "Hamiltonian" deal that will finally knit the bloc together into a genuine federation.[25] But unless Europeans are also willing to commit to supporting a set of principles and ideas that can create unity and inspire others, the bloc will still have trouble acting as a coherent force in international politics.

Finally, there is a fourth and final source of weakness that applies to all of the institutions under discussion. In truth, all international bureaucracies, and indeed many national bureaucracies, share—at the moment—a set of critical faults. Conceived and built in the 20th century, and based on models created in the 19th century, many of them are simply unable to do their jobs with the speed and efficiency that modern citizens now demand. In an era when people can buy a pair of shoes with the click of a computer mouse or express an opinion by checking a box on their telephone, the unnecessarily drawn-out processes and procedures of modern bureaucracy, and indeed modern democracy, can seem cumbersome and out of date. Looking around the world, there are one or two countries—Taiwan and Estonia, for example—that have successfully digitalized their governments and their communications. But most nations have not done so, and international institutions are even farther behind.

The consequences of this failure to evolve could be grave. We have just learned, the hard way, that the world was unprepared to collaborate in the wake of a pandemic. But we are no better prepared to react to the next catastrophe. Increasingly, it is clear that the changes required, particularly to the agencies that belong to the UN system, are so profound that they require far more than mere "reform." They may require rethinking what these agencies do, and how they do it. Indeed, they may require rethinking the nature of international cooperation altogether.

How to Fix the System

Over the past several months, politicians and analysts alike have argued that the joint economic and medical crises created by the coronavirus constitute a breaking point: after this event, many aspects of daily life will be different. But in the world of international institutions, the opposite is more likely to be true. Inertia is built into the system, because so many that are part of it have no incentive to change.

There is a danger that this inertia will be enhanced by misplaced nostalgia, in both the United States and Europe, for a supposed golden age in international cooperation. Post-Trump—whether in 2021 or 2025—many will argue for a return to the status quo ante, for the United States to simply rejoin the UN institutions such as the Human Rights Council or the WHO that it has so recently criticized. Many will want to sign up once again to the Paris Climate Agreement, itself an ineffective half-measure, and to again pay lip service to the old language of universal rights. The temptation to make very few changes will be strong: "Go back to what we were doing before" is the easiest policy in the world for officials to follow, because it requires no special creativity or thought.

But the temptation should be resisted. Some of the UN's institutions, created for another era, cannot be saved. Authoritarian influence is too strong now, bureaucratic stasis too powerful, old ways of doing things impossible to change. There are real questions as to whether America can ever have the influence it once enjoyed. Once burned, many nations will be twice shy—and afraid of following American leadership. Even if the next American president chants the old mantras, everyone now knows that his successors might not.

Some of the all-Western institutions have outlived their usefulness as well. The G7, which started out as an informal club for private conversations between the leaders of the world's most important economies, has declined into a kind of public relations exercise, with statements, heavy symbolism, and an unnecessary media circus. NATO retains its central importance, but it too needs to change. In an era when "warfare" no longer means just tanks and bombs, the institution is long overdue for a major revival. NATO has facilitated cooperation on cybersecurity, but not enough. The West's most important security institution also needs a common strategy on disinformation and both military and nonmilitary propaganda. And, of course, it needs better plans for coordinated responses to health challenges, which next time could come from biowarfare.

There are some other models, some hints at what international cooperation could look like if we began to think about it differently. Paradoxically, even as politicians squabbled during the COVID-19 crisis, the scientific community has worked together with exceptional harmony. Andrew Pekosz, a virologist at Johns Hopkins University, told me that from the beginning, scientists in multiple countries have been sharing databases, genetic sequences, and more: "When it comes to basic research," he said, "networks of like-minded scientists develop quickly, and you can move forward."[26] All of the groups working on vaccines have been able to take advantage of this research; there has even been some low-key, off-the-record, successful grassroots collaboration between scientists and doctors in the United States and China.

Maybe these scientific networks offer a model for the future cooperation. Perhaps spontaneous coalitions of countries, with an interest in achieving a particular goal, might find it easier to cooperate within ad hoc networks. Instead of permanent bureaucracies meeting in stuffy conference rooms in New York or Geneva, maybe we need a floating pool of people who can manage online conferences, provide expertise, move from project to project. The transaction cost may be higher, but this is a price worth paying for the resulting flexibility. This notion is not entirely new. Before we had the International Criminal Court, we had ad hoc war crimes tribunals. The ICC is now a permanent institution; as a result, it has inspired a backlash. If tribunals were created only if and when they are needed— only when, in other words, there is sufficient regional or global consensus— they would not incur the same kind of reaction. Decentralizing the UN system could also help solve another looming conflict—between the need for democracies to confront China on some issues, such as human rights, and to cooperate on other issues, such as vaccines or climate. If the organizations that deal with these things are different, that might help.

We already have one example of how that might work. Back in May, at an online meeting convened by the European Union, representatives of more than three dozen countries and international organizations—Europe as well as South Africa, South Korea, Australia, Israel, Canada, and Japan—pledged nearly 8 billion euros to develop vaccines, treatments, and new ways of diagnosing coronavirus infection. More importantly, they also agreed to make these medical advances accessible not just to their citizens but to the entire world. The United States—the world's leading source of doctors and medical innovation—was not there. But perhaps some future American administration will once again see the point of joining or even leading the rest of the democratic world, the countries that share our values, in joint projects like this one. Institutions created to cope with a new problem may function better than existing institutions that are scrambling constantly to reform themselves in order to keep up with new problems.

The world's democracies also need to think more broadly about their cooperation strategy over the next decade. After two decades of putting counterterrorism at the center of national grand strategy, in 2017, the United States formally adopted a National Security Strategy that was focused, instead, on great-power competition, on the dual threat to US interests from Russia and China. But although investments have been made in building up American military power in order to meet this new challenge, little thought has been given to the battle of ideas. The coming contest between democracy and dictatorship will not be won by an America that trumpets "sovereignty" and "our national interest."

Europe has done no better. The European Union speaks often about the need to promote human rights or tolerance, but little time is spent on the real-world issues that could unite the international democratic camp as well as inspire those outside it who would like to join. A push to truly halt kleptocracy and corruption, for example, using new institutions that demand real financial transparency, would be genuinely popular. Deeper attention could be paid to internet regulation in democracies too. Both Russia and especially China have tried hard to embed autocratic values into internet and cyber governance. Democracies, so far, have only dealt with this subject piecemeal. This is a project that has advanced in some European countries, but it requires a commitment from the entire democratic camp. Decisions about what a truly democratic internet looks like—not an internet run by a few secretive companies—have yet to be made.

But these are just suggestions. Until now, the authority of many international institutions has come simply from the fact that every nation of the world belongs to them. The authority of new institutions, grounded in democratic values, would have to come from something else: the power of their language, the example of their members, the strength of their commitment, and, of course, thoughtful American leadership. A revival of our commitment to universal values is necessary, and a reform of the international system is possible. We just have to be led by people who want to do it.

NOTES

1. Dave Keating, "Italy Banned Flights from China before America—It Didn't Work," *Forbes*, March 12, 2020, https://www.forbes.com/sites/davekeating/2020/03/12/italy-ban ned-flights-from-china-before-americait-didnt-work/#409bc05a481b.

2. Greg Miller and Josh Dawse, "One Final Viral Infusion: Trump's Move to Block Travel from Europe Triggered Chaos and a Surge of Passengers from the Outbreak's Center," *Washington Post*, May 23, 2020, https://www.washingtonpost.com/world/national -security/one-final-viral-infusion-trumps-move-to-block-travel-from-europe-triggered-chaos -and-a-surge-of-passengers-from-the-outbreaks-center/2020/05/23/64836a00-962b-11ea-82b 4-c8db161ff6e5_story.html.

3. "Traffic Chaos at German-Polish Border a Threat to Local Supply Chains?" *Deutsche Welle*, March 19, 2020, https://www.dw.com/en/traffic-chaos-at-german-polish-border-a -threat-to-local-supply-chains/a-52834298.

4. Vikas Pandey, "Coronavirus Lockdown: The Indian Migrants Dying to Get Home," *BBC News*, May 20, 2020, https://www.bbc.com/news/world-asia-india-52672764.

5. Interview with Amy Pope, former National Security Council staffer, March 20, 2020.

6. Maurizio Massari, "Italian Ambassador to the EU: Italy Needs Europe's Help," *Politico*, March 11, 2020, https://www.politico.eu/article/coronavirus-italy-needs-europe-help/.

7. Michel Rose, "Europe Failing to Communicate Its Response to Coronavirus Crisis, France Says," *Reuters*, March 25, 2020, https://www.reuters.com/article/us-health-corona virus-europe-france/europe-failing-to-communicate-its-response-to-coronavirus-crisis -france-says-idUSKBN21C3DT.

8. Katherine Butler, "Coronavirus: Europeans Say EU Was 'Irrelevant' during Pandemic," *The Guardian*, June 24, 2020, https://www.theguardian.com/world/2020/jun/23/europeans-believe-in-more-cohesion-despite-eus-covid-19-failings.

9. Alex Marquardt and Jennifer Hansler, "US Push to Include 'Wuhan Virus' Language in G7 Joint Statement Fractures Alliance," CNN, March 26, 2020, https://www.cnn.com/2020/03/25/politics/g7-coronavirus-statement/index.html.

10. Zeynep Tufekci, "The WHO Shouldn't Be a Plaything for Great Powers," *The Atlantic*, April 16, 2020, https://www.theatlantic.com/health/archive/2020/04/why-world-health-organization-failed/610063/.

11. "Report of the WHO-China Joint Mission on Coronavirus Disease 2019 (COVID-19)," World Health Organization, February 24, 2020, https://www.who.int/docs/default-source/coronaviruse/who-china-joint-mission-on-covid-19-final-report.pdf.

12. Interview with Carl Bildt, former prime minister of Sweden and Sweden's former minister for foreign affairs, April 25, 2020.

13. John Bolton, *The Room Where It Happened: A White House Memoir* (New York: Simon & Schuster, 2020).

14. "Remarks by President Trump to the 74th Session of the United Nations General Assembly," Whitehouse.gov, September 24, 2019, https://www.whitehouse.gov/briefings-statements/remarks-president-trump-74th-session-united-nations-general-assembly/.

15. Yeganeh Torbati, "U.S. Needs to Balance Foreign Alliances: Tillerson," *Reuters*, May 4, 2017, https://www.reuters.com/article/us-usa-diplomacy-tillerson-idUSKBN17Z2BJ.

16. Robin Wright, "The Unbelievable Hypocrisy of Trump's New 'Unalienable Rights' Panel," *New Yorker*, June 19, 2020, https://www.newyorker.com/news/our-columnists/the-unbelievable-hypocrisy-of-trumps-new-unalienable-rights-panel.

17. Dina Smeltz, Ivo Daalder, Karl Friedhoff, and Craig Kafura, "America Divided: Political Partisanship and American Foreign Policy, Results of the 2015 Chicago Council Survey of American Public Opinion and US Foreign Policy," Chicago Council on Global Affairs, 2015, https://www.thechicagocouncil.org/sites/default/files/CCGA_PublicSurvey2015.pdf.

18. Courtney J. Fung and Shing-Hon Lam, "Analysis: China Already Leads 4 of the 15 U.N. Specialized Agencies—and Is Aiming for a 5th," *Washington Post*, March 3, 2020, https://www.washingtonpost.com/politics/2020/03/03/china-already-leads-4-15-un-specialized-agencies-is-aiming-5th/.

19. Michael Martina and David Brunnstrom, "China's Xi Says to Commit 8,000 Troops for U.N. Peacekeeping Force," *Reuters*, September 29, 2015, https://www.reuters.com/article/us-un-assembly-china/chinas-xi-says-to-commit-8000-troops-for-u-n-peacekeeping-force-idUSKCN0RS1Z120150929.

20. "《开讲啦》我的时代答卷·前联合国副秘书长吴红波：优秀的外交官要有强烈的爱国心和进取精神 20181222 | CCTV 《开讲啦》官方频道," YouTube, December 22, 2018, https://www.youtube.com/watch?v=pmrI2n6d6VU&t=24m56s.

21. Emma Farge and Stephanie Nebehay, "Singaporean Defeats Chinese Candidate to Head U.N. Patent Office," *Reuters*, March 4, 2020, https://www.reuters.com/article/us-un-election-wipo/singaporean-defeats-chinese-candidate-to-head-u-n-patent-office-idUSKBN20R17F.

22. Kristine Lee and Alexander Sullivan, "People's Republic of the United Nations: China's Emerging Revisionism in International Organizations," Center for a New American Security, May 14, 2019, https://www.cnas.org/publications/reports/peoples-republic-of-the-united-nations.

23. Yanzhong Huang, "Tedros, Taiwan, and Trump: What They Tell Us about China's Growing Clout in Global Health," Council on Foreign Relations, June 7, 2017, https://www.cfr.org/blog/tedros-taiwan-and-trump-what-they-tell-us-about-chinas-growing-clout-global-health.

24. I attended one of these meetings on June 4, 2020.

25. Anatole Kaletsky, "Europe's Hamiltonian Moment," *Project Syndicate,* May 21, 2020, https://www.project-syndicate.org/commentary/french-german-european-recovery-plan-proposal-by-anatole-kaletsky-2020-05?barrier=accesspaylog.

26. Interview with Andrew Pekosz, professor of molecular microbiology and immunology, Bloomberg School of Public Health, Johns Hopkins University, April 28, 2020.

Chapter Thirteen

Public Governance and Global Politics after COVID-19

Henry Farrell and Hahrie Han

The COVID-19 crisis is a major shock to the existing complex of global rules sometimes described as the "liberal international order." This order heavily emphasized global openness in trade and information flows, and it favored the presumptive liberalization of non-democratic societies that would naturally emerge from it. Yet the liberal order fell short of its promise to create enduring liberal governments in countries such as Egypt during the Arab Spring and China. The long-standing liberal democracies at the core of the order have become less enamored of openness than they used to be.

The limitations of the current version of the liberal international order had begun to emerge even before the COVID-19 pandemic. In part, these fractures resulted from a mismatch between the international order's objectives and its assumptions about democratic publics. While policy makers assumed that international rule systems were in the interests of democratic publics,[1] in practice those systems were insulated from them and sometimes even forcibly repressed them.[2] This constrained democracy at the national level, as controversial decisions were kicked upstairs to less directly responsive global institutions. The rules gov-

Henry Farrell is the Stavros Niarchos Foundation Agora Institute Professor of International Affairs at Johns Hopkins School of Advanced International Studies and editor in chief of the Monkey Cage blog at the *Washington Post*. Hahrie Han is the Inaugural Director of the Stavros Niarchos Foundation Agora Institute, a professor of political science, and faculty director of the P3 Research Lab at Johns Hopkins University

erning areas such as trade and intellectual property were strong, while those for issues such as global health were weak, even if, as Janice Stein observes, the strong rules on trade required buy-in from powers such as the United States to function properly.

Even though the international liberal order was not constructed to be at odds with the interests of democratic publics, in practice it evolved in that way because of three misguided assumptions. Proponents assumed that the interests of democratic citizens were consonant with and/or subsumed by their interests as consumers, that domestic and international political institutions were naturally reasonable reflections of those interests, and that all this meant that international institutions were democratically justifiable, even if they were not really democratically accountable. The first two assumptions misconceived both what citizens' interests are and how they are reflected in the political system, effectively undermining the third assumption. Putting aside questions of whether democratic responsiveness is necessary in principle, history has revealed the limitations of globalized institutions that operate without public accountability. In the end, a global system based on openness at the expense of democracy has generated forces that undermine its own logic. The coronavirus has accelerated this process of breakdown and forced a reckoning with possible alternatives.

In what follows we examine a different model of globalization, grounded in global institutions that are more directly or indirectly accountable to publics. Rather than simply criticizing, we begin from a question asked by Dani Rodrik.[3] If we were to start from scratch after the COVID-19 pandemic and imagine what globalization ought to look like, what would we want? Like Rodrik, we believe that a globalization based on public well-being (one that in the area of health, for example, accepted the benefits of intellectual property and the advantages of trade, but subordinated them as necessary to broader public needs) would be better than what we have today and better address the minimum shared needs of a broader global public across both democratic and non-democratic regimes. It would neither reject openness nor treat the assumed benefits of openness as sufficient reason for insulating global institutions from democratic publics.

We note two important provisos to the above. First, these arguments mark our first efforts to think through a crisis that is still unfolding and that may still throw up unexpected surprises. In a dynamic world, our insights and understandings may well evolve as circumstances change. Second, any proposal for a different approach to global institutions has to recognize that any new arrangements will be built on the foundations of the old. It is useful to ask what we would write on a blank slate so that we are not trapped by the standard answers to old questions, but that is a quite different thing from imagining that we *will* have a blank slate.

The Crisis of International Politics

Global institutions were on shaky ground before the COVID-19 pandemic hit. The existing international system was undermining its own foundations of support, especially in liberal democracies. Emergent changes to economic and information policy had already exploded the theory that guided US international economic policy for thirty years: that expanding openness on the international level will necessarily transform illiberal states into liberal ones. Many policy makers now fear that global openness is self-undermining rather than self-sustaining, so that open economic and informational flows will enable rising adversaries such as China and erode domestic support for global liberalism by enabling populism and allowing disinformation to spread.[4] These fears are exaggerated, and it is possible that the system may adapt to changed circumstances. Nonetheless, they highlight key weaknesses in our previous understanding of globalization.

Such weaknesses explain why policy makers were surprised when challenges to international liberalism arose in the two states most closely associated with global rules-based liberalism over the last 150 years: the United Kingdom and the United States. Even though the phenomena of Brexit and the election of Donald J. Trump were driven by specific national concerns, they both signal public discontent with an elite-driven model of globalization that increased support for populism.[5] There is still political support for rules-based openness in both countries. Many of the architects of Brexit wanted to move to a World Trade Organization–based order of free trade, without other restrictions, while public support in the United States for free trade is quite high. However, the coalitions through which diffuse public opinion is translated into policy have shifted away from the status quo in both countries, as elsewhere. A possible Joe Biden administration in 2020 will take an attitude toward trade very different even from what a Hillary Clinton administration might have done in 2016. The relationship between international economic openness, inequality, and populism dominates policy discussion to an extent that would have been unimaginable in the heyday of globalization.

The same is true for information policy, where the United States advocated open information flows and business self-regulation as the best approach both for global liberalism and for the interests of US firms. Now, both the Trump administration and the Biden campaign want to unravel Section 230 of the Communications Decency Act, the cornerstone of platform self-regulation. Both believe that the existing self-regulatory system is being weaponized, whether by foreign adversaries such as Russia (Biden's fear), or by platforms run by Silicon Valley liberals (the Trump administration's complaint). For their own reasons, the European Union, India, and other powers are similarly moving decisively against self-regulation with little US pushback. The United States is seeking to strangle intellectual exchange with China, which it sees as enabling a strategic competitor and even an adversary, cutting off the access of key Chinese universities to US technology and perhaps preventing Chinese graduate students from studying in the United States.

The coronavirus pandemic has further strained the system. The pandemic's most notable effect has been to highlight the vulnerabilities of the transnational supply chains enabled by global openness. The fall of trade barriers and the creation of global networks had radically transformed the global production system, allowing businesses to source components and supplies from across the world. In many sectors, production had become truly internationalized, so that products were built from components made by hundreds of suppliers in dozens of countries. The pandemic has sharply illustrated the fragilities of this system. When a pandemic means that manufacturers in one part of the world are no longer able to produce components (say, manufacturers of car parts in Lombardy), then entire production systems may be shut down. These problems reinforce other problems, such as a sudden rapid increase in demand for key medical supplies across many countries, at a time when supply is constrained. The consequence is not only economic stress but political contention, as countries quarrel over a limited quantity of crucial medical supplies, seeking to seize what they can while holding what they already have.

This means that the pandemic is feeding back into the existing stresses of the system and exacerbating them further. The global trade system was already in trouble, as the Trump administration sought to invoke security "exceptions" to justify protectionist limits on steel imports. As states begin to think about global supply chains as strategic sources of vulnerability, there is a high likelihood that the exception will become the rule, so that states stop thinking of global trade in terms of general benefits, but rather in terms of particular advantages. Equally, existing trends toward blocking open flows of information are likely to accelerate. The United States is fighting not only with China over who produces a vaccine (and hence plausibly has access to its benefits) but with its European allies. Apparent

US efforts to secure exclusive access to a possible vaccine produced by a European company have led to the German government taking a controlling stake in the company in question.

The Existing Understanding of Democracy and the International Order

Secular changes like the ones described above have multiple causes and complex consequences. In this essay, we focus on one crucial relationship: that between international institutions and democracy. The architects of the existing global order often assumed that the various aspects of liberalism would reinforce each other. Free trade and open information flows would strengthen existing democracies and gradually and peacefully liberalize societies that were ruled by autocrats, leading to the spread of democracy—or, at least, in the short to medium term, to more responsive and benign forms of rule. This justified a largely hands-off approach to democratic legitimacy. It was not necessary to make international institutions properly democratically accountable; indeed, trying to do so would make them less responsive to the actual wants of citizens.

This is not a feature of the current open-flows version of international liberalism, but it was present in its predecessor system, which John Ruggie drew on Karl Polanyi to dub "embedded liberalism."[6] In that system, states had greater room to manage their own economies, perhaps allowing more democratic control at the national level. However, the international institutions that governed that world of financial controls and more limited trade were no more open to democratic voice than their modern successors, and the advocates of Keynesian capitalism typically preferred the aristocracy of expertise to the vulgar opinions of the crowd. The transition from managed global capitalism to open flows was not a transition from international democracy to non-democracy, but from one form of international non-democracy to another.

Now the limits of openness alone have become more apparent, including within the democratic countries that were supposed to be the bulwark and mainstay of the liberal order. Furthermore, openness is far from the only desirable characteristic for a global liberal order, and it brings other problems in its wake. For example, pandemics are a predictable by-product of international interdependence: since at least the beginnings of the Black Death in Asia, they have crept along trade routes (although processes of contagion that used to take decades now take weeks). Yet our current model of globalization focuses on maintaining economic openness rather than on solving the problems that openness brings with it. US pressure and the WTO-associated regime known as the Trade-Related Aspects of Intellectual Property Rights (TRIPS) greatly complicated efforts to provide cheap antiviral drugs to the Global South during the AIDS epidemic.[7] Similar problems plague international cooperation over vaccine production for the novel coronavirus today. Who will own it? Who gets first access? Will there be restrictions on production and availability? The absence of any comprehensive framework to settle these questions is the outcome of multiple global causes, including the current intellectual property regime, strategic distrust among states, and the absence of binding rules for information sharing, research cooperation, and distribution in the global health regime. In the absence of such rules, informal cooperation can be beneficial, but it also has clear limits.

To better understand the relationship between democracy and the institutions of the global order, we need to understand both the underlying assumptions of the guiding orthodoxy and the possible alternatives. Three basic ideas guide the present debate. The first is that the interests of democratic citizens can be derived from their interests as consumers. The second is that domestic and international institutions are reasonably faithful reflections of those interests. The final assumption is that, because the first two hold, insulated international institutions are democratically justifiable, even if they are not directly democratically accountable. To the extent that these assumptions hold, democracy and an international order that emphasizes economic openness are mutually reinforcing. If they do not, however, the current order rests on shakier democratic foundations than are currently recognized.

The first assumption unites trade economics, international political economy, and the broad political consensus to which they contribute—that the interests of citizens can be readily identified with their interests as consumers. Under this argument, it is not necessary that citizens themselves understand these interests properly; as former head of the Council of Economic Advisers Gregory Mankiw described it, "No issue divides economists and mere Muggles more than the debate over globalization and international trade. Where the high priests of the dismal science see opportunity through the magic of the market's invisible hand, Joe Sixpack sees a threat to his livelihood."[8] All that is necessary is that elite "policy makers, observers and other participants"[9] grasp the logic of comparative advantage, as they do. This assumption tends to transform international economic policy disagreements into a fantasized battle between the forces of light (an assumed general public interest in increased openness) and darkness (various special interests that want to protect themselves from foreign competition). It led scholars of "open economy politics" to assume that citizens would vote in favor of openness if it were ever put to a free vote, since the "median voter" would benefit from it.[10] Furthermore, such scholars expected that protectionism would wither away over time, as increased international openness undermined the influence of protectionist interests, allowing for further international openness in an upwards ratchet.[11]

Second, both scholars and policy makers tended to think about domestic and international institutions in largely functionalist terms. Liberal scholars explained international institutions such as the WTO, the World Health Organization, and the International Monetary Fund as generally beneficial tools that states built to allow them to cooperate in addressing shared problems in a world where no state existed.[12]

This functionalist justification of international institutions often seemed a better alternative to the messy compromises of democratic politics. Policy makers, for example, wanted to remove the process of trade negotiation from control by Congress, where they feared that hundreds of legislators, each with his or her own special interest to protect, would make it impossible to reach consensus, and hence created "fast track" procedures under which Congress would agree to limit its own authority.[13] While economic openness was in everyone's interest, it was politically difficult to achieve at the national level. Hence, a combination of specialized international institutions and domestic negotiation arrangements that were insulated from ordinary politics would allow for greater openness than would otherwise have been possible.

Such arguments supported the claim that the international order supporting economic openness was democratically accountable, even if its arrangements were not subject to direct democratic control. Scholars like Andrew Moravcsik argued that this insulation prevented "the capture of government policy by narrow but powerful interest groups opposed to the interests of majorities with diffuse, longer-term, less self-conscious concerns," while fast-track authority allowed government to "override powerful particularistic interests in the name of the national (or median) interest."[14]

The problems with these assumptions have become increasingly clear in recent years. Democratic citizens certainly have an interest in economic prosperity, which has increased substantially on average as a result of global openness. Yet this interest is not exhaustive of their more general wants and desires. They equally have an interest in good health and an environment that will not be degraded by global warming, pollution, and short-term exploitation. Furthermore, the economic benefits of globalization have not been shared evenly. Some forms of inequality at the national level have been substantially exacerbated by the global economic order, whether it be the continuing racial disparities and increasing differences in life outcomes between rural and metropolitan America,[15] or the differences in prosperity between industrial and post-industrial regions in countries such as Germany, Italy, and the United Kingdom.

The institutional structures that underpinned the open economic order did not function as their defenders assumed and lacked accountability mechanisms grounded in a broad public interest. Procedures such as fast-track authority were captured by business interests, which used them to cement their own particular advantage with respect to international competitors.[16] Free-trade agreements became increasingly larded with intellectual property rules that cemented the advantage of producers in wealthy jurisdictions such as the United States and European Union, and they were frequently imported back into these jurisdictions as laws implementing those agreements.[17] Robert Keohane, who played a crucial role in justifying international institutions, came later to acknowledge, "Those of us who have celebrated as well as analyzed globalization . . . demonstrated that an institutional infrastructure was needed to facilitate globalization, but this infrastructure was constructed by and for economic elites. They [built] multilateral institutions to promote cooperation, but they built these institutions in a biased way. Global finance and global business had a privileged status, and there was little regard for the interests of ordinary workers."[18]

These inequalities have had stark consequences for the global health regime. As Susan Sell and Owain Williams note in a survey article published just before the pandemic, the market-based international system has been associated with higher inequality within countries, leading to substantial differences in morbidity[19] even before questions of different levels of access to healthcare.[20] While Sell and Williams acknowledge the benefits of trade and market expansion, they emphasize that the WTO trade regime makes it more difficult for states to take public health actions by banning unhealthy commodities. Haley Sweetland Edwards documents how investor-state dispute settlement (ISDS) treaties have had similar consequences, quoting one lawyer who pioneered lawsuits against toxic polluters as saying, "It wouldn't matter if a substance was liquid plutonium destined for a child's breakfast cereal. If the government bans a product and a U.S.-based company loses profits, the company can claim damages."[21] The WTO's 1994 TRIPS Agreement allowed US pharmaceutical manufacturers to launch a campaign against South Africa's efforts to produce cheap antiviral drugs to fight AIDS in the 1990s, with the support of Bill Clinton's administration.[22] Efforts by developing countries and activists to push back against such measures have led the United States and the European Union to press for more stringent "TRIPS-plus" rules in bilateral and small-group multilateral trade negotiations.

Plausible counterarguments can be made against many of these criticisms. Open trade arrangements have produced a general increase in prosperity and substantial reductions in global inequality, even as they have increased inequality within many countries. Patent protection obviously offers incentives to pharmaceutical manufacturers to develop and test new drugs. Yet these counterarguments would also have to deal with the fact that the attachment of stringent intellectual property rules to international trade agreements, and the transformation of the ISDS system into a means of targeting general regulations that may hurt some individual business, happened without much public debate. It is possible that the "global finance and global business" interests that Keohane describes were driven by the public interest, but you would not want to bet on it.

Such problems weaken claims that current international institutions are democratically justified: these institutions only reflect a narrow range of the interests that people have, and they are dominated by powerful economic actors rather than ordinary people. This is not to say that they are not useful or that they have no benefits. But the claim that trade negotiation arrangements and international institutions are democratic despite the fact that they are insulated from democratic publics (or in strong versions of the argument, *because* they are insulated from national democracies) is hard to maintain.

Equally, they narrow our democratic imagination. As Danielle Allen has argued, "the move to treat material gain, money, as a proxy for utility permits universalization," but it also turns "our attention away from the underlying demographic and institutional arrangements of a society. . . . Who has power and on account of what sorts of institutional structures and according to what sorts of allocations of resources and opportunities?"[23] This is true not only of domestic arrangements within given societies, but also the relationships between societies and the world economy and global institutional structures within which they are embedded.

The COVID-19 pandemic exacerbated these problems, accentuating preexisting patterns of domestic inequality. While good data are still emerging, what data there are suggest that substantial differences in coronavirus survival reinforce existing patterns of inequality.[24] In the blunt description of researchers, "black workers face two of the most lethal preexisting conditions for coronavirus—racism and economic inequality."[25] While general data are unavailable, there is good reason to believe that undocumented migrant workers have faced an unusually high toll. Production facilities such as meatpacking plants that rely heavily on migrant labor have been particularly hard hit.[26] Coronavirus has devastated migrant workers in Singapore, who labor under harsh conditions and live together in crowded dormitories.[27]

The political inequality of influence has reinforced these economic disparities. Politicians came under intense pressure not to impose controls that would protect workers in meatpacking plants, many of whom are undocumented immigrants. When Smithfield Foods' chief executive, Kenneth Sullivan, complained to Nebraska's governor about stay-at-home-order "hysteria," he suggested that "social distancing . . . is a nicety that makes sense only for people with laptops."[28] The same company was also the first to warn of an urgent risk of a meat shortage in the United States, while sending a record-breaking amount of pork to China in the month of April.[29] While reliable cross-national data are even scarcer, there is good reason to expect that the pandemic will greatly exacerbate global inequality. Initial estimates suggest that the pandemic will push hundreds of millions into poverty in South Asia and sub-Saharan Africa.[30]

Existing global institutions have not acted effectively to solve global problems. On the one hand, the institutions that underpinned global openness in trade were not designed to deal with unexpected shortages in essential goods. Commitments to international trade have been nearly universally ignored as states rushed to hoard supplies of critically needed personal protective equipment, ventilators, and medicine, or alternatively to seize what they could in a global scramble.[31] On the other hand, specialized multilateral organizations such as the WHO have been incapable of coordinating a global response to the pandemic. They cannot maintain information flows in situations where states do not want them to. While its rules mandate that states provide information to help prevent the outbreak of epidemics, the WHO is in general fearful of naming states that break rules, let alone recommending actions against them.[32] These difficulties are likely to get worse in the future. The lack of global rules around vaccines is giving rise to fears of a brutal scramble for access if and when an effective vaccine becomes available.[33] Equally, the present intellectual property regime is likely to make it far harder for poor countries to gain timely access to any vaccine, especially when powerful developed countries decline to pool patents.[34]

A Pragmatist Alternative

These are both the worst and the best of times to start thinking about reshaping the relationship between democracy and the international system. The world is in the grips of a massive crisis that has exposed the disadvantages of the present system. At the same time, the historical moment demands a reckoning with the fundamental structures that underlie our political world order and a consideration of a wide range of possibilities for change. We thus take Rodrik's challenge to reimagine globalization from first principles, with the notion not of profit but public well-being at the center. We start from the argument that the existing approach of insulating key decisions about global politics from democratic publics delegitimizes global politics and weakens democratic publics. So what would we do differently?

We start from a pragmatist perspective.[35] John Dewey's *The Public and Its Problems* is regarded as a classic of American democratic thought.[36] Yet it is only incidentally about American democracy. Instead, it starts from a straightforward set of intuitions: that democracy starts from the need to solve the problems of an interdependent public; that institutions need to be connected to those publics; and that the nature of the public changes as global interdependence increases. What this means is that we ought to evaluate existing institutional arrangements—whether at the level of the nation-state, international organizations, or other levels—according to whether they are indeed connected to publics and whether they solve the problems of interdependence. Dewey's understanding of democracy stresses the accountability of institutions to publics. For Dewey, the "state" (by which he means something like our notion of "institution") is the means through which the public organizes itself; when it is not responsive, it becomes corrupt.

Generating this kind of accountability raises two key questions: first, can publics themselves articulate their needs? Second, how do institutions become connected to those public needs, and what are the governance structures that hold the institutions accountable? Unfortunately, most nations currently fall badly short on both dimensions, and the problems grow worse when we move to international institutions.

We can see this in countries such as the United States and the United Kingdom that were supposed to be shining democratic cities on the hill for the global world order but failed to solve the most basic problems in people's lives. In neither country did the democratic system respond well to crisis. The pandemic forced millions of people to make untenable choices between feeding their families and protecting their health. The political system provided few opportunities for them to express their dissatisfaction, obliging the public to turn to networks of self-created mutual aid or to labyrinthine lines snaking through the parking lots of food banks across the country, while elected politicians such as Donald Trump blamed China and the WHO for the pandemic.

It is tempting to treat such limitations of public accountability as demand-side problems, reflecting weaknesses in publics themselves. There is plenty of evidence that most people fall far short of the informed, tolerant, engaged democratic citizen imagined in idealized conceptualizations of democracy.[37] As political scientist Philip Converse famously wrote in the mid-20th century, "most people do not know most things about politics."[38] Political scientist Robert Dahl may have put it best when he wrote that "politics is a sideshow in the great circus of life."[39] Yet the recent wave of protests unfurling around the world in response to the killing of George Floyd highlights the pent-up demand people have for political change. These protests are not isolated but build on previous waves across many democracies to suggest deep and widespread unrest.[40]

Instead of focusing on the demand side, we can examine the supply-side question: what opportunities do people have to articulate a collective public interest in a global world? Instead of stipulating the interests of citizens, we can create opportunities that help them articulate these interests better and build institutions that are more genuinely responsive to these interests. Doing so can contribute to a more democratically legitimate global order in two ways. First, providing the public with opportunities that layer from the local to the national level to experience democracy and exercise the democratic voice creates a generalized public accountability that is currently absent in most democratic regimes but could be a cushion in times of crises like the coronavirus pandemic. Had governments been more accountable to broad publics, there might have been checks that could have mitigated the worst impacts of the pandemic and greater public trust for the measures that governments did take. Second, to the extent that such mechanisms of accountability can be laddered up to international institutions, such institutions themselves can become more directly accountable.

Even creating opportunities for the collective articulation of public interest is hard under modern conditions. Dewey's arguments suggest that people need real opportunities to join with others to build collectivities of sufficient size to press against inept governments. Scholars such as Theda Skocpol, Marshall Ganz, and Ziad Munson point to how the United States did this in the past: at the turn of the 20th century, approximately forty organizations nationwide could claim 1% or more of all American adults, the equivalent of 2.1 million people today, as dues-paying members (suggesting that the equivalent of perhaps 50 million to 85 million adults paid to be part of these organizations).[41] Most of these organizations were federated, creating laddered spaces through which the public engaged in civic and political activity on the local, state, regional, and national levels, and allowing them to realize their interests in the public sphere. Some federated organizations were directly concerned with foreign policy. David John Allen's recent dissertation documents how international affairs councils and similar organizations sought to introduce ordinary citizens to the discussion of international affairs and how the arguments of Converse and his peers helped persuade funders to abandon these efforts in the 1960s.[42]

Such opportunities are now sparse. Surveys find that in the modern era, approximately 78 million American adults spend time volunteering,[43] but most of this volunteer work is not connected to a larger project of creating shared political communities or structures that articulate common interests and channel political power. The result is a public space that emphasizes Albert Hirschman's mechanism of "exit" rather than democratic voice and advocacy, minimizing the experiences people have with collective accountability.[44]

Alongside civil society, political parties can play a crucial role in redressing this lack of opportunity. In the United States and other modern democracies, political parties used to be engines of articulation and accountability. Parties are structured to work in every community across a nation. They have majoritarian incentives to be inclusive in order to build the majorities they need, and the scale to connect local communities with national voices. When political scientist V. O. Key was studying early 20th-century American political parties, he described the precinct captain as a "buffer between governmental agencies and the voters." These captains did everything from "distributing food" to "obtaining employment" to "see[ing] the judge and attempt[ing] to mix mercy with justice." As such, the precinct captains acted as a "guide" to the community for residents.[45] Historians still debate the nature of the work these precinct captains undertook, but one thing is clear: they had a public to which they were actually accountable. Nowadays, scholars describe political parties as "hollow," arguing that beyond their ability to raise money, they lack any tangible or meaningful presence in the lives of voters or even party activists.[46] Even in the most hotly contested American battleground states, the Democratic Party lacks a meaningful presence. During an election year in North Carolina, thirteen out of a hundred county parties provide no contact information for the public to reach party leaders. An additional fourteen provide only a link to intermittently updated Facebook pages. In Wisconsin, twelve out of seventy-one county parties provide no scheduling information about public meetings. In Arizona, two out of fifteen lack any contact information.

Comparative research shows that parties are being hollowed out in many countries, precipitating democratic decline as key decisions are delegated to international institutions.[47] The late Peter Mair has shown that in Europe "the development of [the European Union] has clearly played a major role in the hollowing out of policy competition between political parties at the national level."[48] Parties came to depend less on mass membership than on elite resources, while common EU economic policies narrowed the "policy space," so that parties' policy positions became increasingly indistinguishable, while difficult decisions were farmed out to international institutions. This in turn provided the opportunity for populist anti-system parties to challenge them and win voters, especially on the right.

Some parties, such as the Frente Amplio in Uruguay, are exceptions to the rule. They have maintained their organizational strength, providing insight into what a renewed system of democratic globalization might look like.[49] Verónica Pérez Bentancur, Rafael Piñeiro Rodríguez, and Fernando Rosenblatt argue that the Frente Amplio sustained its organizational strength thanks not to activists nor leaders but to organizational rules and structures that created appropriate incentives not only for activists to stay engaged but also for party leaders to remain accountable to them. Such organizations create the venues through which people can learn to be part of a community debating and developing a range of ideas to solve its problems.

Even if people have opportunities to articulate a collective interest, the second problem is ensuring that institutions can discern the articulated interests of the public and be held accountable. New technologies and efforts to increase government accountability through participatory budgeting processes, for example, have created pockets of engagement in both the Global South and the Global North.[50] However, opportunities for input are not the same thing as accountability unless citizens are given the opportunity to actually negotiate with decision makers on behalf of their interests.

The ideal would be to design institutional arrangements that create feedback effects which both incentivize and enable collective public engagement and allow those who are engaged to have seats at the decision-making table. Localized examples of such institutions exist, for instance, through programs such as the Community Reinvestment Act (CRA) and the Home Mortgage Data Act (HMDA) in the United States, federal laws created to outlaw "red-lining," or identifying neighborhoods in poor communities of color where banks refused to make loans.[51] The CRA required banks to create public oversight boards that would hold them accountable for failing to lend equitably, while the HMDA mandated that banks make sufficiently detailed local lending data available so that the public could see whether they were engaged in fair lending practices. These laws gave local communities the opportunity not only to provide oversight but to organize around the data and skills they needed to be effective advocates in that process. Organizing happened not because it was mandated but because the design of the policy allowed for particular policy feedbacks.[52] Banks, then, were subject to review by these publics that organized around the problem and the information.

The problem, however, is that doing this at the international level is extremely hard. The communities that are affected by international trade policy, for example, tend to be diffuse and hard to organize. The ways in which policy affects them are complicated and hard to understand. Most citizens have neither the resources nor the time nor the expertise to pay sufficient attention, making capture by narrow interest groups likely, and leading to more repetition of the oscillation between elite capture, public resentment, and ineffective populism.

However, important experiments suggest that we can usefully bring the public into complex and fraught debates. For example, much research has focused recently on sortition, in which a group of randomly selected citizens are assembled to consider the different sides of a policy question. Experts from a variety of perspectives present both information and different perspectives to the randomly chosen citizens, who then reach a collective recommendation. These approaches have not, to our knowledge, been applied to questions of international politics, but they have set the stage for popular votes on other complicated and divisive questions. For example, in Ireland, two successful recent constitutional amendments—on marriage equality and abortion rights—resulted from recommendations made by a group of randomly selected citizens, the Irish Citizens' Assembly, on divisive social issues on which politicians were unwilling to legislate.[53] The recommendations enjoyed a high degree of democratic legitimacy because ordinary citizens knew that people like them had listened, deliberated, and come up with options that reflected their understanding of the best way forward.

Such approaches could be applied to difficult international policy choices, such as trade agreements, as an alternative to standard legislation and fast-track procedures, both of which are more vulnerable to capture. As with anti-redlining measures, such arrangements might in turn reshape into party and organizational politics, creating the kinds of feedback loops that democracy requires. Equally, such groups could help to evaluate different proposals to deal with complex problems such as the coronavirus pandemic, which require trade-offs between global openness, international cooperation, and domestic security.

Of course, such institutions would only go so far. They would only indirectly reflect the genuinely global public interests that are being produced by international emergencies such as climate change and pandemics. Building genuinely representative global institutions is a far harder challenge. Still, arrangements like these could help to build domestic legitimacy for complex and sometimes costly international policies, while helping ensure that these policies stuck closer to what the public actually wanted.

Conclusions

As do most proposals for change, we focus on the positive rather than the negative. It is important to acknowledge that democracy has problems too, as the response to coronavirus has amply demonstrated. However, the current global order is increasingly unsustainable, and it is likely to become ever more so as problems such as global warming and pandemics proliferate. An approach that is based on deliberately insulated international policy making and global institutions will be simply unable to make the hard trade-offs that are needed, let alone to justify them to domestic publics. The populist alternative—withdrawing from a global order that is perceived as inherently corrupt—will have even worse consequences. We have little choice but to figure out how to make the global order more democratically responsive.

There are many other problems that we do not have space to address properly. One is very obvious: that many powerful states are non-democratic, or only very imperfectly democratic, and that this is not likely to change any time soon. This too will limit the forms that global cooperation can take and prevent deep democratization. International politics will never be a truly democratic space so long as powerful states are non-democratic, and it would be very hard to build such a space even were democracy to spread more generally throughout the world. Democratic theorists argue about whether a "demos" is needed for democracy to work; even if it is not, the potential conflicts and disagreements between people are more vexing, by several orders of magnitude, on the international level than on the national level.

Still, even in the absence of utopian transformation, it is possible to make international politics friendlier to the needs of democratic publics. After all, autocratic states have to be minimally responsible to their citizens' needs too, which means that there is some shared ground where democracies and non-democracies may negotiate over providing global goods such as health or an environment in which people can live. It is possible, even likely, that bringing public interests to bear will make negotiation over some issues more difficult and create a global order that is less focused on openness. This may be a problem for some. but such an order is more likely to be politically robust, at least against internal dissent arising within core democracies. Moreover, by starting with concrete problems that concern publics, it may be easier to cooperate over shared interests in urgent problems that also concern non-democratic countries than if we frame cooperation in terms of abstract principles that are more likely to give rise to conflict.

There is a final point. In the summer of 2020, the United States saw protests that were historically unprecedented in their scale, penetration, and persistence over time. They also have had an international component. It is striking that Black Lives Matter protests have diffused to other democracies such as the United Kingdom and France. Here, there is a loose analogy to the cross-national waves of protests that toppled authoritarian regimes during the Arab Spring, in that one movement's symbols and organizing techniques can provide a template that can readily be adopted by others. However, in contrast to the Arab Spring, the current protests build on a broader wave of domestic mobilization, which has been gaining strength for the better part of a decade. Scholars such as Lara Putnam, Erica Chenoweth, and Jeremy Pressman are documenting how young Black Lives Matter activists have been quietly organizing in post-industrial areas like Beaver County, Pennsylvania, for years, creating political alliances that may now reshape American electoral politics.[54]

In short, the question may no longer focus on elite concerns of how best to integrate the public to keep the system working. The frustrations of the COVID-19 pandemic, and of government failure to deal with the pandemic, may lead to a new wave of public unrest, which may then be channeled into existing frustrations and will surely spill over into international politics. These frustrations are likely to be especially strong in democracies such as the United States, Brazil, and Mexico, where inept right-wing or left-wing populist leaders are in charge and clearly utterly unprepared to deal with the challenges that they confront. Ready or not, the public is coming.

NOTES

1. Robert O. Keohane, Stephen Macedo, and Andrew Moravcsik, "Democracy-Enhancing Multilateralism," *International Organization* 63, no. 1 (2009): 1–31.

2. Adam Dean, "Arresting the Opposition: Labor Repression and Trade Liberalization in Developing Countries" (unpublished manuscript, 2019).

3. Dani Rodrik, "Globalisation after Covid-19: My Plan for a Rewired Planet," *Prospect*, May 4, 2020, https://www.prospectmagazine.co.uk/magazine/dani-rodrik-globalisation -trade-coronavirus-who-imf-world-bank.

4. Henry Farrell and Abraham Newman, "The Janus Face of the Liberal International Information Order: When Institutions are Self-Undermining," *International Organization* (forthcoming).

5. See Dani Rodrik, "Why Does Globalization Fuel Populism?" (unpublished manuscript, June 2020); and J. Lawrence Broz, Jeffry Frieden, and Stephen Weymouth, "Populism in Place: The Economic Geography of the Globalization Backlash," *International Organization* (forthcoming).

6. John Ruggie, "International Regimes, Transactions, and Change: Embedded Liberalism in the Postwar Economic Order," *International Organization* 36, no. 2 (1982): 379–415.

7. Christopher May and Susan K. Sell, *Intellectual Property Rights: A Critical History* (Boulder, CO: Lynne Rienner, 2006).

8. N. Gregory Mankiw, "Beyond the Noise on Free Trade," *New York Times*, March 16, 2008, https://www.nytimes.com/2008/03/16/business/16view.html.

9. Jeffry A. Frieden and David A. Lake, "International Relations as a Social Science: Rigor and Relevance," *Annals of the American Academy of Political and Social Science* 600 (July 2005): 136–56.

10. David A. Lake, "Open Economy Politics: A Critical Review," *Review of International Organizations* 4, no. 3 (September 2009): 219–44.

11. Lake, "Open Economy Politics."

12. Robert O. Keohane and Lisa L. Martin, "The Promise of Institutionalist Theory," *International Security* 20, no. 1 (1995): 39–51.

13. Todd Tucker and Lori Wallach, "The Rise and Fall of Fast Track Authority" (Washington, DC: Public Citizen, 2008), https://www.citizen.org/wp-content/uploads/rise_and _fall_fast_track_trade_authority.pdf.

14. Andrew Moravcsik, "Is There a 'Democratic Deficit' in World Politics? A Framework for Analysis," *Government and Opposition* 39, no. 2 (2004): 336–63.

15. Danielle Allen, "Political Equality and Empowering Economies—Toward a New Political Economy" (unpublished manuscript). See also Anne Case and Angus Deaton, *Deaths of Despair and the Future of Capitalism* (Princeton, NJ: Princeton University Press, 2020).

16. Dani Rodrik, "What Do Trade Agreements Really Do?" *Journal of Economic Perspectives* 32, no. 2 (2018): 73–90.

17. Susan K. Sell, "The Rise and Rule of a Trade-Based Strategy: Historical Institutionalism and the International Regulation of Intellectual Property," *Review of International Political Economy* 17, no. 4 (2010): 762–90.

18. Robert O. Keohane, "International Institutions in an Era of Populism, Nationalism, and Diffusion of Power," The Warren and Anita Manshel Lecture in American Foreign Policy presented at Harvard University, Cambridge, MA, December 12, 2016, https://wcfia .harvard.edu/lectureships/manshel/2016/transcript.

19. Susan K. Sell and Owain Williams, "Health under Capitalism: A Global Political Economy of Structural Pathogenesis," *Review of International Political Economy* 27, no. 1 (2020): 1–25.

20. Case and Deaton, *Deaths of Despair.*

21. Haley Sweetland Edwards, *Shadow Courts: The Tribunals That Rule Global Trade* (New York: Columbia Global Reports, 2016).

22. Meredith Wadman, "Gore under Fire in Controversy over South Africa AIDS Drug Law," *Nature* 399 (1999): 717–18, https://doi.org/10.1038/21472.

23. Allen, "Political Equality and Empowering Economies."

24. Richard V. Reeves, Tiffany Ford, and Sarah Reber, "Race Gaps in COVID-19 Deaths Are Even Bigger than They Appear," Brookings Institution, June 16, 2020, https://www .brookings.edu/blog/up-front/2020/06/16/race-gaps-in-covid-19-deaths-are-even-bigge r-than-they-appear/.

25. Elise Gould and Valerie Wilson, "Black Workers Face Two of the Most Lethal Pre-existing Conditions for Coronavirus—Racism and Economic Inequality" (Washington, DC: Economic Policy Institute, June 1, 2020), https://www.epi.org/publication/black -workers-covid/.

26. Koen Swinkels, "Covid-19 Superspreading Events Database," *Medium*, June 12, 2020, https://medium.com/@codecodekoen/covid-19-superspreading-events-database-4c0a7 aa2342b.

27. Shibani Mahtani, "Singapore Lost Control of Its Coronavirus Outbreak, and Migrant Workers Are the Victims," *Washington Post*, April 21, 2020, https://www.washington post.com/world/2020/04/21/singapore-lost-control-its-coronavirus-outbreak-migrant-wo rkers-are-victims/?arc404=true.

28. Michael Grabell, Claire Perlman, and Bernice Yeung, "Emails Reveal Chaos as Meatpacking Companies Fought Health Agencies Over COVID-19 Outbreaks in Their Plants," *ProPublica*, June 12, 2020.

29. Michael Corkery and David Yaffe-Bellany, "As Meat Plants Stayed Open to Feed Americans, Exports to China Surged," *New York Times*, June 16, 2020, https://www.ny times.com/2020/06/16/business/meat-industry-china-pork.html?smid=tw-share.

30. Daniel G. Mahler et al., "Updated Estimates of the Impact of COVID-19 on Global Poverty," World Bank, June 8, 2020, https://blogs.worldbank.org/opendata/updated-es timates-impact-covid-19-global-poverty; see also Davide Furceri et al., "COVID-19 Will Raise Inequality If Past Pandemics Are a Guide," VoxEU, May 8, 2020, https://voxeu.org /article/covid-19-will-raise-inequality-if-past-pandemics-are-guide.

31. Henry Farrell and Abraham Newman, "This Is What the Future of Globalization Will Look Like," *Foreign Policy* (summer 2020).

32. Helen Branswell, "Trump Faulted the WHO's Coronavirus Response, but It's Guided by Rules the U.S. Helped Write," *STAT*, April 8, 2020, https://www.statnews .com/2020/04/08/trump-faulted-who-coronavirus-response-guided-by-rules-u-s-helped -write/.

33. Richard Milne and David Crow, "Why Vaccine 'Nationalism' Could Slow the Coronavirus Fight," *Financial Times*, May 14, 2020, https://www.ft.com/content/6d542894 -6483-446c-87b0-96c65e89bb2c.

34. "Coronavirus: Everyone Wins When Patents Are Pooled," *Nature* 581 (May 2020): 240, https://doi.org/10.1038/d41586-020-01441-2.

35. Some of what we say here recapitulates arguments made in Henry Farrell and Jack Knight, "Reconstructing International Political Economy: A Deweyan Approach" (unpublished manuscript), and Hahrie Han, Elizabeth McKenna, and Michelle Oyakawa, *Prisms of the People: Power and Democracy in 21st-Century America* (Chicago: University of Chicago Press, forthcoming).

36. John Dewey, *The Public and Its Problems: An Essay in Political Inquiry* (New York: Henry Holt, 1927).

37. Christopher H. Achen and Larry M. Bartels, *Democracy for Realists: Why Elections Do Not Produce Responsive Government* (Princeton, NJ: Princeton University Press, 2017).

38. Philip E. Converse. "The Nature of Belief Systems in Mass Publics [1964]," *Critical Review* 18, nos. 1–3 (March 2006): 1–74.

39. Robert A. Dahl, *Who Governs? Democracy and Power in an American City* (New Haven, CT: Yale University Press, 1961).

40. Lara Putnam, Erica Chenoweth, and Jeremy Pressman, "The Floyd Protests Are the Broadest in U.S. History and Are Spreading to White, Small-Town America," *Washington Post*, June 6, 2020; Max Fisher and Amanda Taub, "The Global Protest Wave, Explained," *New York Times*, June 28, 2020, https://messaging-custom-newsletters.nytimes .com/template/oakv2?uri=nyt://newsletter/375eeb8b-49fd-4a0f-933c-9ef2ed0a10d8.

41. Theda Skocpol, Marshall Ganz, and Ziad Munson, "A Nation of Organizers: The Institutional Origins of Civic Voluntarism in the United States," *American Political Science Review* 94, no. 3 (2000): 527–46.

42. David John Allen, "Every Citizen a Statesman: Building a Democracy for Foreign Policy in the American Century" (PhD diss., Columbia University, 2019), https://academic commons.columbia.edu/doi/10.7916/d8-3hqc-4p16.

43. "Volunteering in U.S. Hits Record High; Worth $167 Billion," Corporation for National and Community Service, November 13, 2018, https://www.nationalservice.gov /newsroom/press-releases/2018/volunteering-us-hits-record-high-worth-167-billion.

44. Albert O. Hirschman, *Exit, Voice, and Loyalty: Responses to Decline in Firms, Organizations, and States* (Cambridge, MA: Harvard University Press, 1970).

45. V. O. Key Jr., *Politics, Parties, and Pressure Groups*, 3rd ed. (New York: Crowell, 1952).

46. Daniel Schlozman and Sam Rosenfeld, "The Hollow Parties," in *Can America Govern Itself?*, ed. Frances E. Lee and Nolan McCarty, 120–52 (Cambridge: Cambridge University Press, 2019).

47. Steven Levitsky and Daniel Ziblatt, *How Democracies Die* (New York: Crown, 2018).

48. Peter Mair, *Ruling the Void: The Hollowing of Western Democracy* (London: Verso, 2013).

49. Verónica Pérez Bentancur, Rafael Piñeiro Rodríguez, and Fernando Rosenblatt, *How Party Activism Survives: Uruguay's Frente Amplio* (New York: Cambridge University Press, 2019); see also Rafael Piñeiro Rodríguez and Fernando Rosenblatt, "Stability and

Incorporation: Toward a New Concept of Party System Institutionalization," *Party Politics* 26, no. 2 (2020): 249–60.

50. See, for example, Archon Fung, Mary Graham, David Weil, *Full Disclosure: The Perils and Promise of Transparency* (New York: Cambridge University Press, 2008); Sanjeev Khagram, Archon Fung, and Paolo de Renzio, *Open Budgets: The Political Economy of Transparency, Participation, and Accountability* (Washington, DC: Brookings Institution Press, 2013); Hollie Russon Gilman, *Democracy Reinvented: Participatory Budgeting and Civic Innovation in America* (Washington, DC: Brookings Institution Press, 2106); and K. Sabeel Rahman and Hollie Russon Gilman, *Civic Power: Rebuilding American Democracy in an Era of Democratic Crisis* (New York: Cambridge University Press, 2019).

51. Peter Dreier, "The Future of Community Reinvestment: Challenges and Opportunities in a Changing Environment," *Journal of the American Planning Association* 69, no. 4 (December 2003): 341–53.

52. For a synthesis, see Andrea Louise Campbell, "Policy Makes Mass Politics," *Annual Review of Political Science* 15, no. 1 (2012): 333–51.

53. David Farrell and Jane Suiter, *Reimagining Democracy: Lessons in Democracy from the Irish Front Line* (Ithaca, NY: Cornell University Press, 2019).

54. Erica Chenoweth, Lara Putnam, and Jeremy Pressman, "Black Lives Matter beyond America's Big Cities: Here's the New Geography of Youth Activism," *Washington Post,* July 8, 2020, https://www.washingtonpost.com/politics/2020/07/08/black-lives -matter-beyond-americas-big-cities/.

Take It Off-Site

World Order and International Institutions after COVID-19

Janice Gross Stein

COVID-19 changes everything, we are told. We know, almost certainly, that it does not. COVID-19 is an accelerator of global changes that were already under way, much more than it is a generator of sharp shifts in direction. The cumulative impact of these trends that preceded the pandemic was to begin the transition away from American hegemony toward a world order framed by the relationship between China and the United States. The pandemic will accelerate these processes of world order change. Whether that relationship will become one of all-out rivalry or collaborative competition will be determined by the policy choices leaders in both capitals make.

I make three arguments. First, the pandemic has quickened and deepened changes in patterns of global digital-communications infrastructure, trade, and finance that began more than a decade ago. These changes are consistent with a broader pattern of what I call "the rebordering of the world" in the larger context of the framing impact of the deepening conflict between the United States and China and the retreat from globalization and push toward regionalization.

Second, I look briefly at two international institutions—the World Trade Organization (WTO) and the World Health Organization (WHO)—and show why, in

Janice Gross Stein is the Belzberg Professor of Conflict Management in the Department of Political Science and was the founding director of the Munk School of Global Affairs and Public Policy at the University of Toronto (serving from 1998 to the end of 2014).

the context of an increasingly polarized world order, they are less able to fulfill the two critical functions of coordination and control. Dysfunctionality in established international institutions is the lagging indicator of a world order in transition. They are performing poorly not because of bugs in their systems but because their design features are a poor fit with the evolving world order.

Third, I look off-site for innovation in international governance and pay special attention to three different patterns of hybrid governance that have the potential to scale. The first is a scientific network that leapt across borders to share data and then worked with the WHO to purposely build a network of globally connected laboratories. This is a story of governance innovation that begins off-site and scales to include on-site and create a nimble hybrid institution. The second moves from on-site to off-site. When the United States deliberately paralyzed dispute resolution within the WTO, a group of like-minded states developed a work-around that built on WTO processes but moved it off-site. Finally, off-site, international standards-setting bodies that are populated by private companies but work in the shadow of states are making rules for next-generation technologies that will rewire global infrastructure.

A World Order Fractured and Rebordered

THE DEEPENING CONFLICT BETWEEN THE UNITED STATES AND CHINA

The immediate national responses to the pandemic took place within the larger framework of escalating hostility between the United States and China. Although the rhetoric of today focuses on management by China of the virus and worry about overwhelming dependence on Chinese manufacturers of essential health care equipment, that conflict began long before COVID and is playing out in an intense competition for leadership across multiple dimensions. Prominent among these is a fierce struggle for leadership in technology.[1] Years before the coronavirus began to spread, the United States moved to deny China first-mover advantage in building the next-generation digital infrastructure (5G) that will serve as the platform for the Internet of Things.

Why does it matter who builds the next generation of digital infrastructure, and what does this competition for leadership in technology tell us about the characteristics of the evolving world order and governance? Control of communications infrastructure has always been central to great-power dominance and world order.[2] "Leadership in 5G is a useful proxy," Eric Schmidt said at the conference that preceded this volume, "because advantage in platform technologies is a strong indicator of global advantage. When we fragment the technology stack, we split the world."[3]

The next-generation technology will be the platform for the rapidly expanding digital economy and digital health platforms, and it will be critical to the development and scaling of artificial intelligence, robotics, cyberwarfare, and autonomous weapons that will reshape national and international security. Digital networks are becoming increasingly fused with economic advantage and national security as commerce, public health, and warfare move online. The competition between China and the United States over 5G is of course about technology, but it is also about manufacturing, finance, scale, and the institutions of the next generation that will shape coordination, competition, and collaboration as well as exchange and control. Mapping 5G infrastructure is one way of estimating the parameters of the world order to come.

China's leaders recognized the importance of leadership in technology in the shaping of the global order and invested in the development of 5G networks as a strategic priority. Huawei, China's leading telecommunications company and national champion, has developed a substantial lead in 5G technology. Its costs are lower than those of its three competitors—Nokia, Ericsson, and Samsung—and the quality of its technology is widely, although not universally, regarded as high.[4]

As it became apparent that Huawei was moving to build the next-generation communications infrastructure and reap the benefits of the global first mover, the United States moved to constrain Huawei. It was the Obama administration that in 2016 instructed the Federal Communications Commission to ensure that all 5G technologies met a stringent set of security standards. The Trump administration at first rescinded those instructions but then banned Huawei products from the US government and its contractors, put Huawei on the Entity List, and prohibited the export, either directly or indirectly, of technology by American companies to Huawei.[5] The Trump administration also put enormous pressure on friends and allies, particularly the "five eyes" that have special intelligence sharing arrangements with the United States, to follow.[6]

The pandemic has accelerated the swing against Huawei in Europe and Canada. Even before the pandemic, Australia had banned Huawei, and New Zealand had imposed increasingly stringent conditions. As the pandemic gathered steam, Britain announced a review of its earlier decision to allow Huawei to build parts of the periphery of its network. Canada has still not yet announced its decision, but it seems increasingly unlikely that, amid a national conversation about shorter supply chains to bolster security, it will permit Huawei to build a significant part of even the periphery of its next-generation network.

The map looks very different across Africa, the Middle East, and Latin America. Even before the pandemic, Huawei had a commanding position in most of Africa, enabled by China's significant investment through the digital Belt and Road Initiative. America's two closest allies in the Gulf, Saudi Arabia and the United Arab Emirates, had both announced partnerships with Huawei. In Asia, Japan has banned Huawei, and India is now considering doing so, but Malaysia, Vietnam, and Thailand are all considering allowing Huawei to build significant parts of their networks.

The emerging pattern of the next-generation global communications infrastructure, already clear before the outbreak of the pandemic, shows a world divided and demarcated by the growing competition between the United States and China for leadership in next-generation technology.[7] The line of division is fuzzier at times than the map suggests, because networks in some countries are agglomerations built on combinations of suppliers, including Huawei as well as Nokia, Ericsson, and Cisco, that are building backbone. Especially in Europe, foreshadowing arguments that would be made forcefully during the pandemic, governments chose to use a multiplicity of suppliers, hoping to reduce their dependence on any one supplier in the marketplace.

COVID-19 has only deepened and sharpened that fuzzy line that was already running across the global map, creating sharp strategic dilemmas for smaller powers and challenging the way international institutions function.[8] The decisions governments make about Huawei in the next few years will foreshadow the way they navigate a world order that is increasingly framed by deepening competition between the two great powers, each weakened in different ways by the pandemic.

The Rebordering of the World

Layered on top of the fissure created by the broad competition between China and the United States is a process that I call "rebordering." As the pandemic spread, rebordering became visible to the naked eye as governments embargoed the export of critical health equipment and closed their borders to travel. Even the United States and Canada, in a decision that is unprecedented in their history, closed their border to all but essential goods and services. In Europe, where until 2016 borders had largely disappeared, borders thickened quickly in response to the spread of the coronavirus.

This process of rebordering, along with the newly heightened importance of geography and place, also predates the pandemic. China, of course, led the way in rebordering by creating its Great Firewall to block citizens' access to outside information in the name of "digital sovereignty." In 2019, Russia passed a law that allows the Kremlin to cut Russia off from the internet by requiring providers to install special filters and routers controlled by Roskomnadzor, the state communications agency. That equipment can block access to information that the Kremlin considers harmful and, in a crisis, redirect or cut off traffic completely. Russia also plans to create its own domain names, separate from the Internet Corporation for Assigned Names and Numbers, challenging the governance institution that assigns names through its domain name system. Iran has already built its own national intranet, known as the "halal net," which has a separate hardware backbone of cables, servers, and data centers. Tehran can close off access to the World Wide Web but still provide a suite of digital services inside the country. Cuba also has a national intranet as does North Korea.[9]

Rebordering was also visible in the growing chorus of demands from governments in open societies that data that their citizens generated be "localized." As societies become increasingly digital, citizens have become more concerned about who controls their data. The push for data localization, where governments are insisting that their citizens' data be stored on servers physically located in their own country, reinforces the importance of place. The visual imagery of "clouds" notwithstanding, geography and borders, which never really went away, were back with a vengeance even before COVID-19.

The pandemic will give a substantial push forward to localization. National borders will become even more prominent in the integrated physical-digital world that we are moving toward and pose new challenges for governance.

Retreat from Globalization toward Regionalization

Reinforcing the impact of the deepening conflict between China and the United States and rebordering has been the retreat of globalization and the growth of regionalization. These three trends have converged to amplify their effects.

The pandemic swept through large parts of the world when globalization was already in retreat. In the last two decades of the 20th century, the pursuit of efficiency and just-in-time delivery accelerated the development of integrated global supply chains. The ratio of trade in goods to world gross domestic product reached 39% in 1990 and then rose steeply to a peak of 61% in 2008. By 2019, trade as a share of output in the global economy was lower than it was before the financial crisis, as were cross-border financial flows, which peaked in 2007.[10] The picture, however, is not uniform. Trade in services is up, as are flows of data across borders. International travel and migration were at all-time highs before the pandemic. The multiple dimensions of what we have packaged together under the loose label of "globalization" do not run in the same direction and are difficult to aggregate.

The regionalization of trade began long before the pandemic and is likely to accelerate in its wake. Global trade negotiations that gave rise to the international institution that governed world trade, the World Trade Organization, had lost momentum by the end of the last century. Governments moved increasingly to regional and bilateral agreements to accelerate trade. Within regions, trade grew in the three regions that account for the bulk of world trade—Asia, led by China; Europe, led by the European Union; and North America, led by the United States. In the last few years, as the Trump administration began weaponizing trade and imposing tariffs, trade between the United States and China has also declined dramatically. And automation, robotics, and 3D printing are all accelerating regionalization and the shortening of supply chains.

COVID-19 will very likely accelerate these trends even further. The pandemic led to heightened awareness of the importance of secure supply chains and strategic reserves that can meet the needs of vulnerable populations. The language of shortened supply chains and "onshoring" is hardly new, but it is now used more widely and with added urgency by political coalitions that seek at a minimum to diversify supply chains so that no government is hostage to a single manufacturer or a single country.

These changes in trade patterns map onto divisions that were becoming clear to analysts whose focus is technology. Writing before the pandemic, Steven Weber argued that there will soon be several regional economies defined not principally by geography but by technological boundaries written in standards and data flow practices, both institutions of informal governance. He suggests that the emergence of friction at the borders of these regions is intentional on the part of governments and is unwillingly and grudgingly accepted by global firms.[11]

There is a lively debate about how far regionalization and rebordering can go. The tensions run in multiple ways. It is not clear, for example, that regional supply chains will provide the security governments and publics are currently seeking through rebordering. In the early days of the pandemic, governments slapped export bans on face masks and personal protective equipment. A global black market running on cash drove purchases of scarce supplies, often through third-party intermediaries. The immediate response to COVID-19 has been overwhelmingly national. Regional and international institutions were largely out of sight, especially at the beginning of the pandemic.

This argument questions how well regionalization will withstand pressures from national governments. Yet governments have historically experienced difficulty in maintaining short supply chains in areas of strategic focus. These are likely to be shorter-term concerns, restricted to the acute phase of the epidemic. A second quite different argument questions how far rebordering can go in a world economy that runs on global supply chains. Rebordering imposes economic consequences and, consequently, governments, Henry Farrell and Abraham Newman claim, are "chained to globalization."[12] Even China and the United States, now competing across multiple dimensions, are aware of the significant economic and commercial consequences and are anxious to pursue the increasing returns to connection.

There is always friction between firms that seek economies of scale and governments that seek to assert control over their borders and provide security to their citizens. The two tendencies coexist and one constrains the actions of the other, but it is the relative balance and the directional trend that matter and give shape and texture to world orders. In the last decade, after more than twenty-five years of hyper-globalization, control and rebordering have become relatively more important. The pandemic can only accelerate that trend. As appreciation by governments of the political risks of efficiency and the value of resiliency grow, the incentive to pay a higher premium for some resilience and to decouple, at least in part, from globalization in strategic areas can only increase.[13]

Institutions and Governance in a Precarious World Order: The Spaces in Between

International Institutions in Health and Trade

International institutions that provide critical functions of control and coordination evolve, disappear, or adapt to the world order in which they live.[14] The Concert of Europe, a loosely constituted intergovernmental institution, shaped the expectations and beliefs of European leaders and governance in a 19th-century balance-of-power system. It did not survive the outbreak of major war and was replaced by the League of Nations.[15] The league disappeared not only because of its institutional deficiencies but also because it was nested in a world order with few shared beliefs, contested norms, and big powers that sought to disrupt the system.

After World War II, the United States created a set of international institutions, anchored within a framework of openness and liberalism, through the exercise of its hegemonic power. A tradition of liberal institutional scholarship reflected these norms and focused on solving information and coordination problems among states in a world where states wished to cooperate and were constrained only by their fear of cheating.[16] It is these institutions that now find themselves under pressure as the international order becomes increasingly precarious.

COVID-19 has shone the spotlight on two institutions within that broader network, the World Health Organization and the World Trade Organization. The WHO was created in 1948 in the rush of international institution building that followed the war. The WTO evolved almost forty years later out of an earlier looser agreement on trade and tariffs. Both these institutions are intergovernmental, depend on member states for their budgets and for agreement on norms and rules, work by consensus, and are effective only when they are able to provide meaningful control and coordination in the spaces that go beyond the state.

The two institutions play very different roles in their respective domains. The WHO broadly promotes, protects, and coordinates work on public health globally. The WTO grew out of the need for effective dispute resolution mechanisms as global trade deepened. It works far more within the shadow of the law than does the WHO. Both of these institutions have come under sustained attack in the last few years by the United States. The Trump administration has weaponized its funding for the first and the legal system in the second, claiming that these institutions do not serve US interests.

Much ink has been spilled on proposals to "reform" these institutions to improve their effectiveness, but reform is largely beside the point. The future of these institutions depends on the larger beliefs that are evolving as the United States loses its hegemonic status and on the "goodness of fit" with a world order that is in transition and generating forces that undermine these institutions.[17]

President Donald Trump, alleging that the WHO was overly deferential to China in the early stages of the pandemic, blocked a joint commitment by the G20 to strengthen the mandate of the WHO and give it additional resources to coordinate the response globally to the pandemic, threatened to withdraw the United States from membership, and withheld its annual funding contribution.

In response to widespread concern that the WHO was overly deferential to China in the very early phase of the pandemic, an overwhelming majority of its members voted in favor of a review of the WHO's management of the pandemic at some future date. This is not the first time members have pushed for an independent review of the performance of the organization. In the wake of SARS in 2003, the World Health Assembly, the governing body of the WHO, strengthened the International Health Regulations, the core legal requirements for state conduct in health emergencies. The revisions strengthened the WHO's surveillance capabilities, gave the director-general the power to declare an international emergency, and required member states to develop the capacity to detect and respond to outbreaks of disease. In the wake of Ebola, independent experts assessed the WHO's performance and made recommendations that led to the Health Emergencies Program that is today supplying masks and test kits to low-income countries upon request.[18] New agencies—the World Bank's Pandemic Emergency Financing Facility and the Africa Centres for Disease Control and Prevention—deepened the ecosystem of global health management. Nevertheless, as Steven Hoffman observed, the WHO can "advise but never direct; guide but never govern; lead but never advocate; evaluate but never judge."[19] Its members deliberately reject intrusive surveillance and actively keep the WHO weak.

The reforms did not give the WHO an independent intelligence capability, the power to conduct investigations, or to enforce compliance. Like all other intergovernmental institutions, it is reliant on what member states do and on the information that they provide. The politicization of the WHO was predictable in the context of an already tense relationship between China, where the disease began, and a president in Washington who managed the pandemic in such a shambolic way.

Although the WTO could not be more different than the WHO, politicization played a similar role in paralyzing that institution. The WTO, created in 1995, systematized international trade governance and provided for binding dispute resolution that provided some predictability in trade disputes. It also made it easier for members to lose trade disputes as it enabled elected officials to deflect blame and to comply. As one long-time analyst of the WTO observed, "winning is great, but sometimes losing is better."[20]

Over the next twenty-five years, the WTO evolved in two important ways that made it both more effective and more vulnerable. First, it expanded its remit to deal with issues like government procurement and trade facilitation and in so doing embedded norms in international trade governance that were increasingly contested over time. Second, judicial conflict management became more important as almost three-quarters of panel reports were cross-appealed. The Appellate Body (AB) became the core of dispute resolution, evolving toward a fully independent trade court.[21]

As the AB became more important, it became an obvious target for politicization by a dissatisfied United States. Since 2017, the Trump administration, angered by a ruling that it claimed "filled in new content" and amounted to judicial activism, refused to join in the consensus process of appointing AB members to replace those who were finishing their terms. The AB only has one remaining member and is unable to function. The conventional view of the WTO as the victory of law over politics misses the point. The Trump administration's capacity to weaponize dispute resolution is the victory of politics over law and governance.

GOVERNANCE MOVES OFF-SITE

Both these institutions mirror great-power tensions, contested norms, and evolution away from the liberal international order in which they were created. That one is ineffective and the other paralyzed should be no surprise. Yet governance is vital in both trade and health, even more so as the world order shifts, trade patterns change, and the spread of infectious diseases accelerates. Where are sites of governance beyond formal international institutions that may be nimbler? The dysfunctional institutions linger on, but new governance grows up off-site in their shadow and new hybrids evolve.

I look at three different paths to innovation: the first moves from on-site to off-site; the second begins off-site and scales to include on-site to create hybrid governance; and the third is largely off-site in the private sector.

A coalition of WTO members have moved governance off-site but build on on-site processes. Canada and the European Union have led a process to conclude an interim agreement that replicates as closely as possible the appellate process of the WTO. Provided that both parties agree, they can resort to Article 25—an existing mechanism to resolve trade disagreements—as an interim appeal arbitration procedure for any future disputes.[22]

Members have also turned increasingly to plurilateral deals among coalitions of the willing, to preferential trade agreements, and to regional trade agreements. Many of these agreements, however, are written with WTO text "incorporated," freeing up negotiators to work on "WTO plus" provisions. And some agreements like the United States–Mexico–Canada Agreement, which the United States has ratified, provide that any disputes over incorporated text must go to the WTO for resolution. Governance is now hybrid, working in and out of as well as around the WTO.[23]

Innovation in the governance of global health, less constrained by the need for law and precedent, began off-site but scaled to include the WHO. The signature form of governance are agile arms-length networks that operate within the shadow of the WHO. Like in the WTO, the move long predates the outbreak of COVID-19.

The Global Influence Surveillance and Response Network, known as the flu network, was established in 1952. The network began informally among scientists who worked with a model of open science to share data across borders. Over time it evolved to become a hybrid model of governance and now includes more than 140 national labs that are networked together through six WHO Collaborating Centers. Governments and foundations support the network, and scientists, participating without direct compensation, make horizontal peer-to-peer decisions about which strains of the flu virus to include in seasonal vaccines.

After a five-year negotiation, the network formalized its status and practices inside the WHO to ensure the global supply of vaccines. In 2011, the Pandemic Influence Preparedness Framework replaced the informal virus exchanges with a formal system requiring licenses to accompany the transfer of potential pandemic strains. Manufacturers of vaccines that benefit from the flu network must share benefits in return and disputes are referred to binding international arbitration. The informal network and the international organization needed each other and evolved together to create a hybrid pattern of governance. As Amy Kapczynski concludes, "[the flu network] . . . has characteristics of both significant openness—its information products are almost all freely shared with the public—and significant governance."[24]

The flu network played a critical role in the early management of COVID-19. Kapczynski estimates that 85% of the national public health laboratories that are now testing for COVID-19 are associated with the flu network. This was a network-in-waiting for scientists who early on recognized the severity of the threat. And the platform on which Chinese scientists first posted the COVID-19 virus sequences was the Global Initiative on Sharing All Influenza Data, a site created to share virus data.[25]

The flu network is only one example of a network that operates within the shadow of an international organization. Another is Gavi, the Global Alliance for Vaccines and Immunizations founded by the Bill & Melinda Gates Foundation that works closely with the United Nations in a somewhat different hybrid model. With COVID-19 now reported in almost all GAVI-eligible countries, the alliance is providing immediate funding to enable countries to protect health care workers, perform vital surveillance and training, and purchase diagnostic tests. The Global Health Security Agenda, another hybrid model, brings together states, international organizations, and a private-sector roundtable that commit to elevating global health security as a national priority. It organizes technical experts and task forces to surge capacity when needed. It seeks advice from the WHO but operates independently of it in an effort to move in a more focused and nimble way.

Also part of the ecosystem of informal governance are the networks of scientists that share information freely across borders in real time on platforms that are committed to open science and recognized by peers as clearinghouses for new research. Infectious disease specialists and virologists collaborate on websites and email chains to exchange information and sound alarms. An email chain developed among scientists by January 2020 was peppered with alarms that the novel coronavirus was highly infectious and serious. Virologists also come together for a weekly podcast series, *This Week in Virology*, to discuss the latest research.[26] By January, most were sounding an alarm about the severity of a virus that was circulating in Wuhan. By early February, scientists from Oxford and Tsinghua University led the creation of the Open COVID-19 Data Working Group that assembled detailed records for over 10,000 cases.[27] These informal exchanges in a broad variety of networks are critical sites of information sharing, early warning, and policy proposals for prevention and mitigation. They were generally far ahead of formal institutions that lagged emerging patterns in the data and strategic response.

How can this rich pool of information and expertise be better tapped in the future to provide better prevention, warning, and rules for disease management? Creative ideas for arms-length institutions are already being floated. One is to create an arms-length health stability board that would work in the shadow of the WHO just as the international Financial Stability Board, created in 2009 in the wake of the global financial crisis, played a significant role in deepening the resilience of the large banks in systemically important global financial markets.[28] A health stability board would focus only on preparedness, management, and response to threats to global health. Similarly, a Johns Hopkins University epidemiologist, Caitlin Rivers, has proposed the creation of a center for epidemic forecasting, similar to the National Weather Service.[29]

Analogous to the plurilateral agreements that are reshaping trade are coalitions of willing states that are coming together to finance and push the WHO forward. Costa Rica and Chile launched the COVID-19 Technology Access Pool with the WHO to make vaccines, tests, and treatments accessible to all. Almost forty states have signed on. Austria is leading a group of first movers, or countries that quickly flattened the curve of infection, to support the WHO and will likely be joined by the European Union, especially Germany, and by India and the African Union; all seeking a way through the US-China competition.[30] These new networks and institutions will be useful sites of innovation in governance only if they remain open to accepting new members so that they can scale.

Finally, the extraordinary role played by standard-development organizations in setting policies, making rules, and establishing norms is worthy of attention. Standard-setting processes appear to be "neutral," yet it has long been recognized that these processes are far more than technical.[31]

Governance of critical digital infrastructure for the next generation is happening off-site in several ongoing standard-setting processes for 5G. Standards shape information flows and innovation policy, influence competitiveness, and advantage some companies at the expense of others. Some of these processes are industry led and have multiple stakeholders, while others are government led and multilateral.[32] The United States prefers industry-led processes, but it does not enable and coordinate the participation of engineers from its private-sector companies the way China does in these processes.[33] China also actively steers the government-led multilateral processes. On-site and off-site, Huawei, enabled directly or indirectly by China, is playing an outsized role in shaping the standards for 5G, deepening its role as the preeminent builder of the hardware and firmware for the next-generation networks and its role as a rule maker in the next iteration of digital governance.[34]

The Advantage of Interdependence

Henry Farrell and Abraham Newman have argued that the cross-national layering of international institutions and "rule overlap" help to create new power asymmetries that cannot be reduced to measures of state power. Two implications follow from this analysis. First, international institutions contribute to reshaping the power of states and transnational actors and, indirectly, world order. In this sense, international institutions are far more important than what they do. Second, centrality in these international networks allows states to weaponize interdependence to their advantage.[35]

Centrality remains as important in the off-site and hybrid networks that I have described as it is in formal institutions. Indeed, it may be more important as formal institutions do less work, and rule making, norm setting, and governance increasingly move into hybrid networks that can scale.

States that are central to these hybrid networks will continue to have an advantage. To win, however, these states must play. China, for example, has used its centrality in multilateral standard-setting bodies to advance international standards on 5G that advantage Huawei, and it has coordinated participation of engineers from Chinese companies in industry standard-setting bodies to give Huawei first-mover advantage with all its benefits. It has deepened its involvement in the

International Telecommunication Union and its commitments to the WHO. Other governments are taking governance off-site and designing institutional work-arounds or add-ons to the institutions that Washington paralyzes. They are also creating plurilateral coalitions of the willing that include the private sector, foundations, and nongovernmental organizations as well as governments to engage in policy development, norm setting, and rule making.

Not so the United States. Under President Trump, the United States is leaving the field. It has announced its intention to withdraw from the WHO, has paralyzed dispute resolution in the WTO, and remains outside the new network for dispute resolution that is being created. Recently, it has sent confusing signals to engineers from its big companies about their participation in standard-setting bodies.

If the United States continues to self-isolate in the wake of COVID-19 and paralyze formal institutions, it will have given up the advantages of centrality that it enjoys in formal international institutions that are now moving into the background. Even more important, the United States risks finding itself alone as others accelerate their move to take governance off-site and create hybrid institutions.

NOTES

1. Graham T. Allison, "The Clash of AI Superpowers," *National Interest* (January–February 2020), https://www.questia.com/magazine/1G1-610852268/the-clash-of-ai-superpowers.

2. Heidi J. S. Tworek, *News from Germany: The Competition to Control World Communications, 1900–1945* (Cambridge, MA: Harvard Historical Studies, 2019); Heidi Tworek, "Information Warfare is Here to Stay: States Have Always Fought for the Means of Communication," *Foreign Affairs*, April 25, 2019, https://www.foreignaffairs.com/articles/germany/2019-04-25/information-warfare-here-stay; Simone M. Müller and Heidi J. S. Tworek, "'The telegraph and the bank': On the Interdependence of Global Communications and Capitalism, 1866–1914," *Journal of Global History* 10, no. 2 (June 2015): 259–283; Laura DeNardis, *The Internet in Everything: Freedom and Security in a World with No Off Switch* (New Haven, CT: Yale University Press, 2020).

3. Eric Schmidt, Keynote address at the World Order after COVID-19 Forum, June 30, 2020.

4. Governments and private-sector telecommunications companies think differently about quality. The private sector thinks about quality in a competitive marketplace largely as features and uptime while governments pay attention to vulnerability. The Huawei Cyber Security Evaluation Centre in Britain, set up by the government but paid for by Huawei, reported in March 2019 that the code in Huawei's products was replete with bugs and claimed that the company had made "no material progress" in fixing vulnerabilities that had been identified the year before. See British Cabinet Office, *Huawei Cyber Security Eval-*

uation Centre Oversight Board: Annual Report 2019, March 28, 2019, https://www.gov.uk
/government/publications/huawei-cyber-security-evaluation-centre-oversight-board-ann
ual-report-2019.

5. On May 5, 2020, the Bureau of Industry and Security in the Department of Commerce amended its foreign-produced direct product rule and the Entity List to target Huawei's acquisition of semiconductors that are the direct product of certain US software and technology. See US Department of Commerce, *Department of Commerce Adds Dozens of New Huawei Affiliates to the New Entity List and Maintains Narrow Exemptions through the Temporary General License*, https://www.commerce.gov/news/press-releases/2019/08/department -commerce-adds-dozens-new-huawei-affiliates-entity-list-and; and US Department of Commerce, *Commerce Addresses Huawei's Efforts to Undermine Entity List, Restricts Products Designed and Produced with U.S. Technologies*, https://www.commerce.gov/news/press-releases /2020/05/commerce-addresses-huaweis-efforts-undermine-entity-list-restricts.

6. Federal Communications Commission, *In the Matter of Fifth Generation Wireless Network and Device Security*, PS Docket 16-353, 2016, accessed March 3, 2020, https://apps .fcc.gov/edocs_public/attachment/DA-16-1282A1Rcd.pdf; Timothy B. Lee, "New Law Bans US Gov't from Buying Tech from Chinese Giants ZTE and Huawei," *Ars Technica*, August 14, 2018, https://arstechnica.com/tech-policy/2018/trump-signs-bill-banning-feds-fr om-using-huawei-zte-technology.

7. The line on the map is thin at the hardware level. Standards are designed to ensure interoperability, and endpoint modems will include multiple radio frequencies, as they do now. Border crossings would become more important, however, if the new 5G digital platforms were not fully interoperable and it becomes clunky to move across the frontier. There is an unexpected wrinkle that may create a frontier in what is supposed to be an interoperable system. The 3GHz and 4GHz spectrum (known as sub-6) that is being used for 5G in most of the rest of the world are exclusive federal bands in the United States that the Department of Defense uses actively. US carriers, unlike their counterparts around the world, turned to mmWave spectrum. This pattern, if it continues, will sharply divide the global market, putting US carriers at a distinct disadvantage. See Milo Medin and Gilman Louie, "The 5G Ecosystem: Risks & Opportunities for DOD," *Defense Innovation Board*, April 2019, https://media.defense.gov/2019/Apr/03/2002109302/-1/-1/0/DIB_5G _STUDY_04.03.19.PDF; and Paul Triolo, Kevin Allison, and Clarise Brown, *Eurasia Group White Paper: The Geopolitics of 5G* (New York: Eurasia Group, 2018), 18, https://www.eur asiagroup.net/siteFiles/Media/files/1811-14%205G%20special%20report%20public(1).pdf.

8. That fuzzy line may well become sharper as the Internet of Things that runs on 5G networks grows and challenges to interoperability deepen. Already, DeNardis concludes, interoperability is diminishing. DeNardis, *The Internet in Everything*, 135.

9. Until very recently, North Koreans could only access the countrywide *Kwangmyong* intranet; they can now access a small number of internet sites under tight government scrutiny. See Michael Grothaus, "Get Ready for the 'Splinternet': The Web Might Not Be Worldwide Much Longer," *Fast Company*, September 7, 2018, https://www.fastcompany .com/90229453/get-ready-for-the-splinternet-the-web-might-not-be-worldwide-much -longer; Oleg Matsnev, "Kremlin Moves toward Control of Internet, Raising Censorship Fears," *New York Times*, April 11, 2019, https://www.nytimes.com/2019/04/11/world/europe /russia-internet-censorship.html?searchResultPosition=1; and Andrei Soldatov, "Why

Russia Might Shut off the Internet: The Kremlin's Long Obsession with Central Control," *Foreign Affairs*, March 29, 2019, https://www.foreignaffairs.com/articles/russian-federa tion/2019-03-29/why-russia-might-shut-internet.

10. Anna Kantrup, Christoph Sprich, Nikolas Kessels, and Stormy Annika Mildner, "COVID-19 and Trade: Not the End of Globalization but Changes in Value Chains to Be Expected," American Institute for Contemporary Germany Studies (AICGS) at Johns Hopkins University, May 6, 2020, https://www.aicgs.org/2020/05/covid-19-and-trade-not-the-end-of-globalization-but-changes-in-value-chains-to-be-expected/; Richard Fontaine, "Globalization Will Look Very Different after the Coronavirus Epidemic," *Foreign Policy*, April 17 2020, https://foreignpolicy.com/2020/04/17/globalization-trade-war-after-coronaviru s-pandemic/.

11. Steven Weber, *Bloc by Bloc: How to Build a Global Enterprise for the New Regional Order* (Cambridge, MA: Harvard University Press, 2019).

12. Henry Farrell and Abraham L. Neuman, "Chained to Globalization: Why It's Too Late to Decouple," *Foreign Affairs* (January–February 2020), https://www.foreignaffairs .com/articles/united-states/2019-12-10/chained-globalization; Jon Lindsay, "Correspondence: Debating the Chinese Cyber Threat," *International Security* 40, no. 1 (Summer 2015): 191–195; Jeffrey S. Lantis and Daniel J. Bloomberg, "Changing the Code? Norm Contestation and US Antipreneurism in Cyberspace," *International Relations* 32, no. 2 (June 2018), 158, https://doi.org/10.1177/0047117818763006.

13. Janice Gross Stein, *The Cult of Efficiency* (Toronto: Anansi Press, 2002).

14. Danielle Allen, Henry Farrell, and Cosma Rohilla Shalizi, in "Evolutionary Theory and Endogenous Institutional Change," unpublished manuscript, use biological and epidemiological models to analyse the evolution of international institutions over time. Political scientists tend to think of institutions as shared beliefs and expectations that permit coordination and control. Economists think of institutions as patterned information processing that reduces the costliness of transactions. See also Douglas C. North, *Institutions, Institutional Change, and Economic Performance* (New York: Cambridge University Press, 1990); and Eleanor Ostrom, *Governing the Commons: The Evolution of Institutions for Collective Action* (New York: Cambridge University Press, 1990).

15. Henry Kissinger, *World Order* (New York: Penguin Books, 2015).

16. Liberal institutionalists argue that international institutions can increase transparency, provide authoritative and credible information, create opportunities for communication, and provide solutions to coordination problems to reduce the fear of cheating. See Robert E. Keohane, *After Hegemony: Cooperation and Discord in the World Political Economy* (Princeton, NJ: Princeton University Press, 1984); John Gerard Ruggie, "International Regimes, Transactions, and Change: Embedded Liberalism and the Postwar Economic Order," *International Organization* 36, no. 2 (1982): 379–415; G. John Ikenberry, *After Victory: Institutions, Strategic Restraint, and the Rebuilding of Order after Major Wars* (Princeton, NJ: Princeton University Press, 2001); G. John Ikenberry, "Liberal Internationalism 3.0: America and the Dilemmas of Liberal World Order," *Perspectives on Politics* 7, no. 1 (2009): 71–87; and Daniel Deudney and G. John Ikenberry, "The Nature and Sources of International Liberal Order," *Review of International Studies* 25, no. 2 (1999): 179–196.

17. Historical institutionalists who traditionally pay attention to path dependency and "stickiness," would expect these institutions to linger long past their best-before date. Far-

rell and Newman explore the endogenous forces that drive institutional change and decay through self-undermining feedback effects. See Henry Farrell and Abraham L. Neuman, "The Janus Face of the Liberal International Information Order: When Global Institutions are Self-Undermining," *International Organization*, forthcoming.

18. Thomas J. Bollyky and David P. Fidler, "It's Time for an Independent Coronavirus Review: The World Health Organization and Its Member States Must Learn from Their Mistakes," *Foreign Affairs*, April 24, 2020, https://www.foreign affairs.com/print/node /1125983.

19. Cited by Nathan Vanderklippe, "Chan Reshaped the WHO and Its Ties to China," *Globe and Mail*, June 13, 2020, A14.

20. Marc Busch, email message to author, June 7, 2020.

21. Rohinton P. Medhora, "The WTO: Ever Mutating, Planned Obsolescence or Unplanned Obsolescence," *CIGI*, May 11, 2020, https://www.cigionline.org/articles/wto-ever -mutating-planned-obsolescence-or-unplanned-obsolescence; Thomas Cottier, "Recalibrating the WTO Dispute Settlement System: Strengthening the Panel Stage," *CIGI*, April 20, 2020, https://www.cigionline.org/articles/recalibrating-wto-dispute-settleme nt-system-strengthening-panel-stage.

22. Canada now works with other WTO members under Article 25, including Australia, Brazil, China, the European Union, South Korea, and Mexico. Approximately thirty members have agreed to the interim procedure. See Valerie Hughes, "Approaches to Modernizing the Dispute Settlement Understanding," *CIGI*, April 20, 2020, https://www.cigion line.org/articles/approaches-modernizing-dispute-settlement-understanding.

23. At present there are some 303 preferential trade agreements in force and another 300 notified. This movement off-site is not without cost. As Marc Busch observes, design features are everything when thinking about new governance arrangements, but the big picture is predictability. "Too many separate bodies of rules," he concludes, "could be as bad as no rules at all." Marc Busch, email message to author, June 7, 2020.

24. Amy Kapczynski, "Order without Intellectual Property Law: Open Science in Influenza," *Cornell Law Review* 102, no. 6 (2017): 1539–1615. I draw heavily on her analysis of the flu network.

25. Amy Kapczynski, interviewed by Henry Farrell, email message to author, May 23, 2020.

26. *This Week in Virology* was started in September 2008 by Vincent Racaniello and Dick Despommier, two virologists at Columbia University Medical Center, to have regular informal conversations about viruses. See Vincent Rocaniello and Dick Despommier, "This Week in Virology," American Society for Microbiology, https://www.asm.org/Pod casts/Twiv.

27. Steven Johnson, "Vital Statistics: How Data Became One of the Most Powerful Tools to Fight an Epidemic," *New York Times Magazine* (June 2020): 45–49, https://www .nytimes.com/interactive/2020/06/10/magazine/covid-data.html?searchResultPosition=1.

28. Anita McGahan, "We Need a Financial Stability Board for Health," *Financial Times*, May 14, 2020.

29. Caitlin Rivers and Dylan George, "How to Forecast Outbreaks and Pandemics," *Foreign Affairs*, June 29, 2020, https://www.foreignaffairs.com/articles/united-states /2020-06-29/how-forecast-outbreaks-and-pandemics.

30. Ilona Kickbusch, "No 'Back to Normal' for the WHO," *CIGI*, June 15, 2020, https://www.cigionline.org/articles/no-back-normal-who?utm_source=cigi_newsletter&utm_medium=email&utm_campaign=maria-ressa.

31. Janet Abbate, *Inventing the Internet* (Cambridge, MA: MIT Press, 1999); Ken Alder, *The Measure of All Things: The Seven-Year Odyssey and Hidden Error That Transformed the World* (New York: Free Press, 2002); Laura DeNardis, *Protocol Politics: The Globalization of Internet Governance* (Cambridge, MA: MIT Press, 2009).

32. The primary industry bodies involved in setting standards for 5G are the 3rd Generation Partnership Project, which includes some 500 representatives that develop standards based on performance and interoperability criteria; the European Telecommunications Standards Institute, which is developing standards for network-function virtualization and multi-access edge computing; and GSM Association, which is developing best practices on important 5G topics. Governments are also negotiating technical specifications and radio spectrum allocation for 5G in the Radiocommunication Sector of the International Telecommunications Union. See Mike Dano, "Another Set of 5G Standards Was Just Released, but No One Really Cares," *Light Reading: 5G*, April 5, 2019, https://www.lightreading.com/5g/another-set-of-5g-standards-was-just-released-but-no-one-really-cares/d/d-id/750681; Stacie Hoffman, Samantha Bradshaw, and Emily Taylor, "Great Power Rivalries in 5G Technology Markets," in *Concert or Clash among Nations? The Future of Peace and Conflict Diplomacy*, ed. Chester A. Crocker, Fen Osler Hampson, and Pamela R. All (Washington, DC: Georgetown University Press, forthcoming).

33. In 2013, China's Ministry of Industry and Information Technology, the National Development and Reform Commission, and the Ministry of Science and Technology established the IMT-2020 5G Promotion Group to coordinate the contributions of China's telecom operators, research institutes, universities, infrastructure equipment manufacturers, and mobile device makers to the international standard setting process for 5G and to plan and execute strategy for standing up standalone 5G networks at scale. See Paul Trilio and Kevin Allison, *The Geopolitics of 5G* (New York: Eurasia Group, 2018): 14, https://www.eurasiagroup.net/live-post/the-geopolitics-of-5g.

34. Keith Johnson and Elias Groll, "The Improbable Rise of Huawei," *Foreign Policy*, April 3, 2019, https://foreignpolicy.com/2019/04/03/the-improbable-rise-of-huawei-5g-global-network-china. Farrell and Newman, "The Janus Face of the Liberal International Information Order," conclude that of the three large firms, Huawei has been the most active in setting the technical standards for 5G networks. See also Christine Fox and Thayer Scott's chapter in this volume, where they refer to the growing concern in the US Senate that China is systematically coordinating its companies in standard-setting bodies to make the rules for next-generation technologies.

35. Henry Farrell and Abraham L. Newman, "The New Interdependence Approach: Theoretical Development and Empirical Demonstration," *Review of International Political Economy* 23, no. 5 (2016): 736–756; Henry Farrell and Abraham L. Newman, *Of Privacy and Power: The Transatlantic Fight over Freedom and Security* (Princeton, NJ: Princeton University Press, 2019); Henry Farrell and Abraham L. Newman, "Weaponized Interdependence: How Global Economic Networks Shape State Coercion," *International Security* 44, no. 1 (2019): 42–79.

Chapter Fifteen

A "Good Enough" World Order

A Gardener's Manual

James B. Steinberg

The Nature of the Challenge

We stand at an extraordinary and challenging moment in world history. The twin, interrelated crises of COVID-19 and the breakdown of economic globalization have demonstrated both the weakness of current "world order" (or perhaps the lack of world order) and the urgent need for some kind of framework to manage these and future challenges going forward. Put another way, the most pressing issues facing us—to include the looming potential calamity from human-induced climate change and pandemic disease, technological transformation brought on by revolutions in information and biotechnology, and global economic insecurity—seem to require ever more international cooperation, at the very time that existing arrangements seem less likely than ever to produce this cooperation. Growing rivalry between major powers, coupled with increasing nationalism and popular distrust of political institutions, severely complicate any effort to facilitate the transnational efforts needed to address these challenges. Existing international institutions and arrangements have fallen short in rising to the task.

It is tempting in the face of this bleak picture to recall John F. Kennedy's aphorism that "[w]hen written in Chinese, the word 'crisis' is composed of two characters. One represents danger and the other represents opportunity"[1]—an obser-

The Honorable James B. Steinberg is University Professor of Social Science, International Affairs and Law at Syracuse University.

vation that Rahm Emanuel, President Barack Obama's first chief of staff, was wont to invoke ("a crisis is a terrible thing to waste").[2] It is true that many of the "world orders" of the past emerged from major crises, typically war and conquest: the Thirty Years' War and the Westphalian system, the Napoleonic Wars and the Concert, the US-led post–World War II era, and so on. The scale of death and destruction from COVID-19 and its consequences may not match those in magnitude (yet), but in its global reach it mirrors these world-shaking events of the past. Yet not all "crises" of global scale produce durable or even partially effective global responses, as the recent 100th anniversary of World War I has led us to recall. Crises may contain within them opportunity, but opportunities must be seized; successful outcomes are not inevitable.

So what kind of order might emerge from the current crisis, and what would it take to bring it about? My premise is that a future world order is not predetermined (à la Hegel or Marx), but at the same time it is constrained by what has come before. There is room for statecraft ("agency"), but not all options are on the table. As we think about possible world orders, it is important to be modest about the aspiration; even the most celebrated world orders of the past have been far less successful, comprehensive, or durable than the idealized versions sketched by some. The challenge is to develop a plausible construct that in some, albeit limited, ways meets the exigencies of our time.

If "world order" is the answer, what is the question? Much of the attention in recent debates has focused on interstate relations, and in particular "great power competition." No doubt, managing changing power relations and aspirations among states is important, but the most consequential challenges of our time—from climate change to pandemic disease, to economic prosperity, to managing the disruptive effects of technological innovation (particularly artificial intelligence and biology)—lie outside this framework (although state rivalry certainly complicates the ability to find solutions). The current preoccupation with managing state-to-state relations among politicians and pundits in Washington has distracted attention from the far more pressing set of issues that will dominate the coming decades.

What would a "reasonably successful" world order look like? It is helpful at the outset to consider some basic "design criteria" by which a desirable world order should be judged.

1. It should facilitate sufficient international cooperation to meet the major transnational challenges that no one state alone can manage, with an

emphasis on the existential and near existential challenges such as climate change and pandemic disease (including the possibility of human-manufactured pathogens).

2. It should facilitate efforts to reap the beneficial effects and mitigate the disruptive/dangerous security and economic risks of transformative information technologies and biotechnologies.

3. It should be able to manage (though not end) conflict among states and reduce the risk of catastrophic actions by non-state spoilers

4. It should take into account the diversity of perspectives (religious and secular) on what constitutes an acceptable form of governance (both domestic and transnational).

5. It should accommodate both nation-state and non-state actors in rule setting and enforcement.

6. It should command sufficient domestic political support within a broad range of nations to sustain the policies needed to maintain the order.

This is a tall order, with deep tensions among the criteria themselves, particularly between effective international action to meet transnational threats and the requirement for broad-based political support (legitimacy). "World Federalism" may have technocratic appeal but little popular support.

What Possible Models?

Since the end of the Cold War, both academics and practitioners have advanced a variety of concepts for a new "world order." These include a brief flirtation with a unipolar world / American Empire[3] (more recently, a Pax Sinica); a G2 "directorate" run by China and the United States;[4] major power "spheres of influence";[5] balance of power approaches;[6] a multipolar arrangement of the world's larger powers; an ideological consortium of like-minded states ("concert of democracies");[7] and transnational networks led by non-state actors.[8]

Each of these models faces substantial limitations. Most of them focus on managing interstate relations with little attention to how any of these arrangements might address the key transnational issues we face today. Of course, effective hegemony (by the United States, or China, or whomever) could in principle lead to a unilaterally imposed international coordination, but as we have seen, no state today or in the foreseeable future will have such predominance. At the same time, many contain elements that reflect the current international reality, which any new world order must accommodate: the diffusion of power among states and to non-state actors and civil society, but in the context of continued disproportionate influence of the world's two leading powers.

Despite the yearning for simplicity, there is reason to doubt whether any single, parsimonious, overarching model is either appropriate or achievable—the illusive search for the "next Kennan" bumper sticker. The fact is that today we face a diverse range of challenges, and the range of actors relevant to, or necessary for, effective action differs depending on the specific problem at hand; world-class sprinters fare poorly in marathons; to switch sports metaphors, what is needed are "horses for courses"—a collection of arrangements tailored to specific problems.

Even with respect to these "partial" world orders, the tensions among the various design criteria (particularly between efficacy, legitimacy, and political acceptability) means that we should be prepared to be satisfied with "second-best solutions" and avoid making the best the enemy of the good. Put differently, there are trade-offs among these various design criteria; it is not possible to maximize against all of them simultaneously. To take one prominent example (elaborated further below), the Paris Climate Agreement of 2015 was a pragmatic effort to reconcile the substantive challenge posed by carbon emissions with the political constraints of gaining nations' buy-in. In terms of what is required to mitigate the risk of human-induced global warming, the Paris Agreement clearly falls short, but compared with earlier, more top-down approaches, it was able to command broader public support.

Perhaps the central question is the degree to which a new world order can or should be based on shared values, or whether it should be premised on a fundamental acceptance of value and ideological diversity. The tension between the two approaches was a core feature of the post–World War II order in which two types of institutions uneasily existed side by side: the values-based institutions that grew out of the Atlantic Charter (NATO, CoCOM, OECD, the G7) and universal institutions characterized by the principles of the United Nations charter (sovereign equality, non-interference in internal affairs). There is considerable appeal to the former: arrangements based on shared values among like-minded states are easier to form, sustain, and enforce and are likely to aspire to more ambitious objectives. At the same time, more universal institutions have broader reach and reflect the international reality of cultural, historic, and religious diversity. This need not be an either/or choice; a blend of approaches is both possible and, as a practical matter, necessary. Despite the ongoing debate about the future of the "liberal international order," the reality is that LIO itself was part of a more complex of set of international arrangements even at the height of US power and influence. The question is not whether to abandon the goals and ideals of the liberal international order but rather how to embed them in a world where cooperation and conflict management requires the involvement of others who, at least for the moment, have different views.

The Pillars of a New World Order: What Might the New World Order Look Like?

Reasonably Effective International Arrangements

The most urgent challenge facing the current international order is the "underproduction" of international cooperation. There are many critical areas where everyone in principle would be better off if states cooperated—in economists' jargon, there are "positive-sum gains" to be had. The idea that interstate cooperation can produce positive benefits is hardly new, but globalization and the emergence of transformative technologies have dramatically increased the potential benefits of cooperation and the associated costs of autarky.

Why then has cooperation failed to emerge? There are a number of familiar explanations, from free riding and the absence of effective transnational enforcement mechanisms to prevent defection, to a preoccupation with the way the gains of cooperation are distributed ("relative gains"), to public mistrust of institutions (witness Brexit and President Donald J. Trump's critique of "globalists"). There is a rich academic literature on both the barriers to international cooperation and how these barriers can be overcome.[9]

What would it take to foster greater international cooperation? One of the most important insights, from both practice and theory—especially where the problem of cooperation involves more than two actors—is that there are considerable advantages to having some kind of structure (formal or informal), such as transnational organizations and arrangements to sustain cooperation. Over the years, there have been many efforts to develop effective strategies to achieve this goal. From the Central Commission for Navigation of the Rhine (established in 1816 and still functioning today) to the United Nations Alliance of Civilizations (founded in 2004 in response to the 9/11 attacks), states and civil society have adopted a range of approaches: single- versus multiple-purpose organizations, universal versus criteria-based membership, regional versus global, legally binding versus voluntary, to name just a few. In the aftermath of World War II and the advent of decolonization, these efforts focused on the UN and "universal" organizations, open to all states on the basis of "sovereign equality" (with important exceptions, most notably the UN Security Council).

Although the UN system has had its share of successes, it seems fair to say that the approach suffered from substantial weaknesses. Too often, these types of organizations are slow to act and face great difficulty in reaching consensus beyond "lowest common denominator" responses. From the UN Framework Convention on Climate Change to the World Health Organization (WHO) to the World Trade Organization (WTO), the limits of these broad-based arrangements have become increasing clear. Moreover, in a world in which civil society plays a more active role, the inherent "legitimacy" of one country–one vote decision making—irrespective of the country's size, stake in the problem, or form of government—is increasingly in question.

What can be done to ameliorate these limitations—to foster timely and effective international cooperation?

The past several decades have seen a movement toward a more pragmatic approach to international cooperation. From the creation of the G20 in the wake of the Asian Financial Crisis to the Major Economies Forum (established in 2009 to try to generate new momentum in the stalled UN-based climate talks), states have sought to develop arrangements that balance the value of inclusion with the necessity of timely and effective action to avoid the paralysis and lowest-common-denominator outcomes of more broad-based approaches.

A new international order will need to draw on the success of some of the more promising innovations of recent years. The first, building on the UN Security Council, the role of the "Quad" in NATO, and more recently the G20, is to establish an ongoing forum of systemically important countries that can provide leadership and momentum to efforts to foster cooperation—a kind of "directorate" that can in some cases take on the effort to promote cooperation directly or to spin off new groups and arrangements to tackle particular challenges. The success of the G20 in providing leadership during the 2007–9 financial crisis demonstrates the value of such a group; it might well have played the same role in response to the health and the economic consequences of COVID-19.

The advantage of a "directorate" is both smaller size (making agreement easier to reach and limiting the role of "spoilers") and the fact that there is a well-established, previously agreed upon place to turn as new crises and challenges develop. There are two principal difficulties: the problem of legitimacy (who is in and who is out) and (depending on who is "in") the difficulty of reaching agreement if there are deeply rooted divisions among the members. The UN Security Council's recurring inability to address contemporary problems reflects these limitations.

In the past, the G7 proved a powerful mechanism for spinning off institutions and regimes to address pressing transnational issues. The Financial Action Task Force (FATF) is a valuable example of this approach. Launched by the G7 after a decade of largely inconclusive negotiations within the UN Framework, the FATF evolved both in scope (from an initial focus on drug trafficking to include terrorist financing, transnational crime, and weapons of mass destruction proliferation) and membership (from the original eleven members to thirty-seven today, including China, Russia, and Saudi Arabia).[10] Although the initial group was small, it was systemically significant, comprising most of the major financial centers. Given the importance of these countries to the global banking system, their decisions, although technically binding only on its own members, became de facto global standards, since smaller states had little choice but to comply or risk financial isolation. By contrast, if the effort to address money laundering had been pursued through a consensus, one country–one vote approach, outliers that benefited from shadowy finance could have blocked or weakened meaningful actions—as so vividly illustrated by the ten-year effort to address money laundering through the UN-based Vienna Convention against Illicit Traffic in Narcotic Drugs and Psychotropic Substances.[11]

The experience of the FATF is particularly valuable in thinking about how 21st-century institutions can be effective in bringing about cooperation in the absence of binding transnational enforcement authority. The effectiveness of FATF stems in part from its norm-setting role and in part from its members' ability to impose costs on those who fail to comply. The two features are mutually reinforcing; the norms give legitimacy to the enforcement, while the enforcement gives teeth to the norms.

Similarly, the Missile Technology Control Regime (MTCR) was created by the G7 in 1987. Its impact has grown through expansion (it now includes thirty-five members, including, most recently, India) and because several significant nonmember states (including China, Israel, Romania, and Slovakia) have agreed to respect at least some of the MTCR rules.

More recently, the G20 has played a similar role, for example, in launching the Financial Stability Board in response to the 2008–9 financial crisis. Notably, the FSB succeeded an earlier, G7-led arrangement, the Financial Stability Forum.

A second approach is to constitute an ad hoc club or grouping to respond to specific challenges. Recent examples range across the most pressing transnational challenges, such as the Major Economies Forum (for climate change), the Nuclear Suppliers Group (NSG), and the Proliferation Security Initiative (PSI) (for nuclear and missile proliferation), to name just a few. Membership can be more specifically tailored to the countries that "matter" for a particular problem (which can vary from case to case.) The membership need not be fixed. It can be expanded over time to include others who meet membership criteria or performance commitments.

The ad hoc approach typically works best when a group of like-minded states seeks to fill a vacuum in transnational cooperation and raise the level of ambition. In the best case, the core group becomes a pole of attraction for other states. The Nuclear Suppliers Group, for example, began with just seven members (Canada, West Germany, France, Japan, the USSR, the UK, and the US) and now has forty-eight members. The virtue of the ad hoc approach is that members need be "like minded" only with respect to one particular issue rather than broadly aligned ideologically. Thus the US and the USSR were able to cooperate in founding the NSG despite the Cold War divisions. The Open Government Partnership, launched by President Obama in 2011, included as its founding members Brazil, Indonesia, and South Africa, despite the many differences between the members on issues ranging from trade to security (the Brazilian Workers' Party, under Presidents Lula and Rousseff, had been highly critical of the United States, and just one year before, Brazil had defied the US in seeking to reach a nuclear deal with Iran).

These kinds of ad hoc arrangements need not be limited to states; they can include substate actors and civil society (the Open Government Partnership includes civil society groups on its steering committee). Because such a group is self-constituted, there may be greater prospect for agreement. The principal difficulty is the "startup" problem: the practical difficulties of launching a new arrangement may make it less effective to respond to fast-moving developments. It is notable that after 9/11, countries turned to the FATF, an existing institution, to deal with terrorist financing, rather than pursue the time-consuming and fraught effort to launch a new organization.

A third approach is to rely on regional organizations. Because they are smaller and may be somewhat more homogeneous than a universal grouping, agreement may be easier, and they offer similar advantages of being an ongoing organization that can tackle emerging problems. Legitimacy is less problematic since the membership criteria are relatively "neutral" on key indicia (size, wealth, form of government, etc.). The potential value of regional organizations was one of the reasons the Obama administration prioritized joining the East Asia summit.

A final strategy to overcome the limits of large organizations is the use of "weighted voting," as, for example, in the International Monetary Fund and World Bank, or for some issues in the European Union. This hybrid gives all relevant states a voice, while limiting the ability of outliers to block broadly agreed upon action.

One key feature of these successful innovations is a high-level political dimension to give heft to the group's work and to foster domestic buy-in. Although there is an important role for bureaucratic structures in carrying out the day-to-day work of facilitating cooperation, absent high-level political leadership and engagement, these efforts can easily founder. The example of the WHO is indicative; the work is nominally guided by a "political" grouping (the World Health Assembly), but in practice this involves mid-level representatives with little engagement from national leaders.

SETTING RULES AND NORMS FOR EMERGING TECHNOLOGIES

These kinds of partial approaches are particularly well suited to grapple with the second key challenge facing any new world order: the urgent need to develop transnational norms and rules to govern the development and use of transformative new technologies. States acting alone have some, but limited, capacity to address these challenges. At best, the result of nation-centric approaches will lead to a proliferation of overlapping and conflicting rules that will create great waste and inefficiency and lead to deepening tensions between states over whose rules should prevail. More consequentially this approach can lead to a competitive "race to the bottom" and safe havens for malevolent actors to cause significant harm.

To take just one example, in the 1990s the Clinton administration began to explore rules governing the export of strong encryption, to limit the terrorist and criminal organizations' abilities to evade law enforcement. The experience demonstrated that acting alone, the principal impact of national action would simply harm US software firms, who could not access global markets compared with competitors in states that imposed no restrictions, while doing little to limit malevolent use. Today we see a movement toward a similar strategy to restrict export of artificial intelligence–related technologies, with—as many commentators have noted—similar risks of a "lose-lose" outcome: disadvantaging US firms, alienating US partners, and doing little to prevent the harms the controls are supposed to curb. To be effective in dealing with these new technologies, solutions must seek to go beyond national regulation.

International cooperation is needed not simply to manage the risks of these new technologies but also to reap the benefits. The value of international scientific collaboration in pushing the boundaries of discovery is well established; the gains of trying to reap national advantage in most cases are at best short term and come at the cost of delay and increased cost in achieving the potential benefits of breakthroughs in areas such as biomedical research, renewable energy, and the like. Hyper-national approaches will particularly harm the poorest nations, who lack the capacity for indigenous innovation, as the global digital divide well illustrates. Even more harmful is the looming danger of biological divide between have and have-not countries.[12]

Universal organizations are particularly ill-suited for developing rules to address these emerging problems. By their nature, large consensus-based organizations tend to follow the development of widely accepted rules rather than lead the process, particularly where the problems are new and there are deep divisions (often ideologically based) about how to proceed. The abortive effort in the Conference on Disarmament to establish rules governing the use of Lethal Autonomous Weapon Systems (LAWS) is an important illustration of the problem.[13] Similarly, UNESCO's decades-long effort to address human cloning has led to a search for alternative approaches.[14]

As with the problem of international cooperation more generally, here, too, there are two alternative models on how to elaborate internationally agreed rules. Rules are established that are open to others to adhere to by (1) a small group of diverse states with differing perspectives that broadly reflect the range of international views or (2) a group of like-minded states with similar outlooks. There are obvious advantages to the first option if there is substantial common ground among these states. But as we have seen in recent years, in areas such as cyber-crime, ideological and political differences among key states may make agreement difficult.

The alternative—elaboration of norms by like-minded groups—has made some progress possible. In the field of cyber, for example, the development of the Budapest Convention offers a valuable example. A relatively small group of fairly like-minded states developed a set of rules governing cybercrime; over time, additional states outside of Europe have joined. In a similar vein, the EU's elaboration of the General Data Protection Regulation has become a benchmark for other countries' regulatory efforts; even where, as with the United States, nations differ about the appropriate rules and standards, they have had to modify their "first choice" and move toward standards harmonization.

These partial solutions have obvious limitations, particularly if systemically important states refuse to join and can gain significant advantage over states that do join and comply. But this problem is really not different in kind from the challenges faced by universally agreed upon rules in the absence of effective enforcement. In both cases the "defector" can gain a potential advantage. Arguably, in the case of broadly agreed norms, states face some greater pressure to conform to a norm or rule they have formally embraced, but the cases of Russia (with respect to the UN Charter's ban on aggression) and China (on human rights included in the Universal Declaration) show that there are limits to this constraint. The like-minded approach also risks exacerbating tensions with states that are excluded from the initial rule setting and who, for substantive or political reasons, will simply resist adhering to rules set by others. If the states outside the like-minded bloc are strong enough and have a sufficient stake in an alternative normative regime, this approach could lead to competing "like-minded" blocs (à la Cold War), thus contributing to conflict.

There is no hard-and-fast rule as to which approach should be pursued; the most fruitful approach will vary with subject matter (another example of horses for courses). In the best of cases, over time those norms and rules elaborated under either of these "partial" processes will become widely accepted and states will face increasing pressure from other states and civil society to join (witness the experience with the Ottawa Treaty on landmines). But what is important is to recognize that even partial solutions can have benefits and waiting for broad international consensus to emerge is a recipe for inaction. For two decades, the United States has failed to ratify the Biological Weapons Convention, in part out of concerns over the efficacy of compliance mechanisms and the advantages that might accrue to states that fail to comply. These problems are real; cheating cannot be totally precluded and some states will remain outside. But as the experience of the Non-Proliferation Treaty (NPT) suggests, there are substantial benefits, even when some states remain outside the regime and some nominally inside fail to comply.

Engaging the Public and Civil Society

A new world order must recognize that while states remain a central element of the international landscape, the experience of the last decades has demonstrated that legitimacy and acceptability cannot be taken for granted, even when governments can agree among themselves. The backlash against deepening integration in the EU, the grassroots movement against landmines, and the protests against free trade have all demonstrated the fundamental need to include non-state voices and perspectives in order to sustain effective international action. In recent years there has been a growing trend to give civil society a significant role in international negotiations and the operations of international organizations.[15] In the 1999 Kyoto Climate Change negotiations, for example, nongovernmental organizations and business groups were included in the US delegation. More recently, the UN relied heavily on stakeholder input in the development of the Sustainable Development Goals, responding to a criticism that the predecessor Millennium Development Goals were largely a product of insider experts with little public input.

The WTO experience demonstrates the fundamental importance of including civil society in shaping the rules. The breakdown of the Seattle WTO negotiations in the face of protests over the secret "green room" negotiations was a harbinger of a broader trend; despite greater engagement with civil society in connection with the recent Trans-Pacific Partnership trade talks, concerns about openness and transparency contributed to the Obama administration's failure to gain ratification.

Engaging civil society can be especially valuable in developing norms and standards governing new and emerging technologies, particularly where scientific and technical expertise is critical to effective action. From the International Engineering Task Force (IETF), which helped set standards governing the operation of the internet, to the Intergovernmental Panel on Climate Change (IPCC), groups of experts can help contribute to consensus building, although the IPCC experience demonstrates the limits of civil society in rule setting without political backing.

There is no doubt that broadening civil society participation and increasing transparency will complicate being able to reach agreements; the familiar tactics of horse-trading and informal exploration of compromises are much harder if exposed to constant public scrutiny by affected constituencies. But the ultimate test of efficacy is not having reached an agreement but rather implementing it, and the difficulties associated with including civil society are increasingly the necessary price for adequate public support.

Involving civil society can also help address the problem of enforcement, in part because the enhanced legitimacy that comes from stakeholder involvement makes voluntary compliance more likely, and in part because civil society can have an important role in monitoring and publicizing compliance/noncompliance, which can contribute directly to enforcement.

Sino-US Relations

Addressing the dramatic deterioration in Sino-US relations is essential to constructing a reasonably good new world order—not only because there is a real danger that the growing rivalry could turn into real conflict with devastating consequences not just for the two countries. Absent some basic joint understanding about managing these bilateral relations, there is little prospect to build the needed global cooperation necessary to meet the most pressing transnational challenges. Put another way, a new Sino-US understanding is the necessary underpinning to meaningful progress on the three key objectives of a new world order: enhanced global cooperation, addressing the impact of new technologies, and avoiding major-power conflict.

The need for such an understanding to avoid a major interstate conflict is self-evident; we should constantly be mindful that while the "Cold War" stayed largely cold, we lived in the shadow of a global holocaust for decades. It would be foolhardy to assume that some invisible hand will save us from that same danger should Sino-US relations continue to deteriorate.

But a new understanding is vital not simply to avoid a third world war. Absent Sino-US cooperation, efforts to address the key transnational threats will be limited at best. Because both countries have such a consequential role in most of the major issues of our time—from sustaining global growth, to climate change, to technological innovation—partial solutions that include only one will at best have limited impact. In part this is a question of efficacy: consider a climate agreement that does not include the two largest emitters of greenhouse gases.

In addition, neither side is likely to move unilaterally to address a global problem if it believes the other will gain an advantage by failing to reciprocate. The recent US decision to walk away from the Intermediate-Range Nuclear Forces Treaty (because it leaves China free to develop missiles that threaten the US and its allies) and growing dissatisfaction (among Democrats and Republicans) with the WTO (driven by doubts about China's commitment to fair and open trade) are motivated by a legitimate concern about whether China is seeking unilateral advantage. Similarly, the US decision to withdraw from the Paris Climate Agreement can undermine the likelihood that China will effectively rein in its greenhouse gas emissions.

In the past, the United States was able to join with like-minded states to develop international organizations and regimes with the hope or expectation that China would simply accede to them—witness the experience of the NPT and related regimes (nuclear supplier group, MTCR) as well as the WTO and the FATF. There may still be some circumstances under which China might be willing to join a regime established by others. For example, there was some reason to believe that had the United States ratified the TPP, China might have been open to joining. But increasingly, China is unlikely to become part of arrangements in which it had no voice in shaping and is increasingly willing to offer alternative arrangements to compete with US-centric institutions (Shanghai Cooperation Organization, Asian Infrastructure Investment Bank, the Belt and Road Initiative, the Conference on International Confidence Building in Asia). China has enough clout to make it costly for many states to join US-centric institutions and has offered states a variety of inducements to join the China-centric camp. Thus the danger of the United States or China pursuing a "like-minded" strategy that deliberately excludes the other, as it risks further dividing the world into competing camps rather than promoting needed cooperation.

Taken together, these factors make a powerful case for the centrality of Sino-US cooperation as the most promising avenue to broader international cooperation, as the Obama-Xi agreement on climate illustrates. But reaching these bilateral agreements will be increasingly difficult if the overall context is an adversarial relationship between the two. The United States and the Soviet Union did find areas of cooperation during the Cold War (smallpox eradication, space exploration); perhaps more important, during the era of détente, the United States and the Soviet Union set bounds to the areas of competition (through arms control agreements and the Helsinki Accords). But even that model will be insufficient to create the context for meaningful Sino-US cooperation on the most important but challenging transnational tasks of our time. So long as both sides are preoccupied with relative gains, reaching agreement on issues of the global economy and environment as well as on emerging transformational technologies will be difficult. The case of COVID-19 has proved painfully instructive. Rather than providing global leadership in cooperative measures to mitigate and ultimate prevent the disease, both sides are focused on how the other is seeking to use the crisis for national advantage. COVID has proved that it is nearly impossible to insulate areas where cooperation would benefit both countries from the political rivalry.[16]

As I have written in more detail elsewhere, the "golden period" of Sino-US cooperation (from the Nixon visit to the mid-2000s) was characterized by a more or less explicit view that the relationship was not zero-sum.[17] Unless the two sides develop a new form of understanding that takes into account both China's rise as a near peer of the United States and the United States' legitimate determination not to simply cede global dominance to China, the prospect that the two countries will provide global leadership for cooperation is dim. On the contrary, by focusing on relative gains, the stage really is set for a new cold war in which both sides seek to line up countries to oppose the other; a recipe for friction and stalemate rather than global cooperation.

What can be done to create a context to limit the rivalry and create space for cooperation? During the Cold War, the framework that helped limit US-USSR rivalry revolved around formal treaty and negotiations, from the Anti-Ballistic Missile Treaty through the Helsinki Final Act. This approach has failed in the context of post–Cold War US-Russian relations and is even less likely to be successful in transforming Sino-US relations. A new understanding will need to be based on a willingness by each side to demonstrate through its actions; that is, in making choices about how each pursues its national interests, it will, where possible, seek to do so in ways that do not directly threaten the other's concept of its national interest. At its core, this means abjuring strategies that are inherently zero-sum, particularly the pursuit of primacy and emphasizing sufficiency.

Achieving and implementing such an understanding will not be easy. There may be cases, perhaps fundamental, where the conflict between the two sides' conceptions are ultimately irreconcilable. But difficult does not mean hopeless: for nearly fifty years the United States and China have managed the uniquely sensitive issue of Taiwan by each not directly challenging the other's bottom line (for the US, no reunification by force; for China, no de jure independence for Taiwan). Many areas of dispute today can be managed in a similar fashion. For example, the United States could achieve its fundamental interest in freedom of navigation in the South China Sea by agreeing with China to voluntary limits on each side's use of the waters and islands in the region. Each side could evolve its military doctrine away from offensive-oriented strategies that seem threatening to the other (A2D for China; long-range precision strategic strike by the US) toward less destabilizing postures. The agreements reached between the United States and China during the Obama administration on commercial espionage[18] and nonmilitarization of the South China Sea islands,[19] if implemented transparently by China, offer another example of ways to put a break on the growing rivalry and demonstrate the possibility of a positive-sum outcome.

The values agenda represents an especially difficult and important test. The United States must find ways to remain true to its conviction on the universality of human rights and democracy without pursuing actions that will be seen by China as an effort to weaken China or force regime change. Each side must accept that efforts to pursue its "first best" choice (supremacy) is unachievable and ultimately counterproductive.

This in turn would open up the space for pursuing positive-sum outcomes. A good place to start would be biomedical research and public health. Rather than focus on the competitive aspects, both sides could agree to lead an international and open collaboration, along the lines of the International Space Station or small-pox eradication.

Conclusion

Many discussions of world order labor heavily under the shadow of the biblical image of creation: a short burst of concentrated activity leading to a fully formed new world. From Westphalia to Vienna to Paris 1919, Bretton Woods and San Francisco 1946, there was yearning for a constitutive moment that would guide the next era. We all long to be "present at the creation." Whatever merit the metaphor may have in describing the establishment of previous world orders, it seems implausible today. Instead, we should draw inspiration from Max Weber's "slow boring of hard boards" or George F. Kennan's metaphor of policy planning as gardening. By focusing on the building blocks and trial-and-error implementation guided by the design criteria outlined above, we can reasonably hope to bring some modest order to the current chaos. This is ambition enough.

The United States is uniquely well positioned and capable of leading this effort, for three reasons. First, the US remains by far the preeminent economic, military, and technological power in the world and, as a result, has an outsized influence on the choices that others will make. Second, the habit of leadership and the tradition of pragmatic problem solving fit the needs of the moment. Cooperation is rarely self-organizing; although many or all can benefit, it takes a first mover to galvanize the effort. Pragmatism has been the American way; the US is rarely prone to the reflections of the alleged French diplomat who is said to have asked, "Yes, I know it works in practice, but can it work in theory?" Third, the United States has much to gain; by taking the lead, the new arrangements and norms are more likely to reflect US values and interests.

Progress, if only partial, is possible. To succeed, US strategy must reject two great temptations. The first is an illusory belief that the US can thrive and be secure by going it alone; our historical experience cautions against such an approach, which is even more likely to fail in a world where borders and oceans are little protection against dangers, even from faraway places. The second is a premature decision that the United States and China are fated to be rivals in an all-out competition in which only one side can prevail. The US must be prepared to do what is necessary to protect ourselves and our friends' security, prosperity, and way of life against all challengers (state and non-state actors); if China is determined to achieve global or regional dominance and pursue its interests at the expense of the United States and our allies, we should resolutely meet that threat, even if it means a new cold war. But such an outcome should come as a result of China's choice, not ours; the United States should continue to make clear that we are prepared to work hard and creatively to pursue a different path if China, too, is ready in deed and not just rhetoric. Following this course could open the small window that remains for the US and China to work together and with others to build new structures of cooperation. If it fails, others are more likely to rally to our side in a rivalry that was not our choice.

NOTES

1. John F. Kennedy, "Remarks of Senator John F. Kennedy at University of New Hampshire: India and China," Durham, New Hampshire, March 7, 1960, John F. Kennedy Presidential Library & Museum, https://www.jfklibrary.org/archives/other-resources/john-f-kennedy-speeches/university-of-new-hampshire-19600307.

2. The original expression has been attributed to Stanford economist Paul Romer. See Jack Rosenthal, "A Terrible Thing to Waste," On Language, *New York Times Magazine*, July 31, 2019, https://www.nytimes.com/2009/08/02/magazine/02FOB-onlanguage-t.html.

3. William Wohlforth, "The Stability of a Unipolar World" *International Security* 24, no. 1 (Summer 1999): 5–41.

4. Edward Wong, "Former Carter Advisor Calls for a 'G-2' between US and China," *New York Times*, January 2, 2009, https://www.nytimes.com/2009/01/12/world/asia/12iht-beijing.3.19283773.html.

5. Ted Galen Carpenter, "Accepting Spheres of Influence in the 21st Century," Cato Institute, May 7, 2014, https://www.cato.org/publications/commentary/accepting-spheres-influence-21st-century.

6. Barry R. Posen, *Restraint: A New Foundation for US Grand Strategy* (Ithaca, NY: Cornell University Press, 2014).

7. James M. Lindsay, "The Case for a Concert of Democracies," *Ethics and International Affairs* 23, no. 1 (April 2009): 5–11.

8. Anne-Marie Slaughter, *The Chessboard and the Web: Strategies of Connection in a Networked World* (New Haven, CT: Yale University Press, 2017).

9. For a survey of the literature, see Duncan Snidal and Michael Sampson, "Interstate Cooperation Theory and International Institutions," *Oxford Bibliographies*, last modified November 25, 2014, https://www.oxfordbibliographies.com/view/document/obo-9780199743292/obo-9780199743292-0093.xml?rskey=UA9tNS&result=132; and in some cases, for example, where there is repeated interactions among parties, cooperation can emerge even without formal or informal agreements; see, generally, Kenneth A. Oye, "Explaining Cooperation under Anarchy: Hypothesis and Strategies," *World Politics* 38, no. 1 (October 1985) 1–24.

10. See Mark T. Nance, "The Regime That FATF Built: An Introduction to the Financial Action Task Force," *Crime, Law and Social Change* 69, no. 2 (March 2018): 109–129, https://doi.org/10.1007/s10611-017-9747-6.

11. One participant in the Vienna negotiations colorfully observed, "I would rather have my teeth pulled out than to sit through another one of those negotiations." Nance, "The Regime That FATF Built," 114.

12. David P. Clark and Nanette J. Pazdemik, "Bioethics in Biotechnology," in *Biotechnology: Applying the Genetic Revolution* (London: Elsevier Academic Press, 2009), 665–694.

13. See "Decision on Autonomous Weapons Talks Eludes CCW," *Arms Control Today,* no. 49 (December 2019), https://www.armscontrol.org/act/2019-12/news-briefs/decision -autonomous-weapons-talks-eludes-ccw.

14. Adèle Langlois, "The Global Governance of Human Cloning: The Case of UNESCO," *Palgrave Communications* 3, no. 17019 (2017), https://doi.org/10.1057/palcomms.2017.19.

15. My own first experience with civil society participation was as part of a nongovernmental organization observer group in the 1985 Treaty on the Non-Proliferation of Nuclear Weapons Review conference.

16. We have seen this in the past. Despite the positive model of US-USSR space cooperation, in 2011 Congress restricted space-related cooperation between the US and China.

17. See James B. Steinberg, "What Went Wrong: US-China Relations from Tiananmen to Trump," *Texas National Security Review* 3, no. 1 (Winter 2019–20), https://tnsr.org/2020 /01/what-went-wrong-u-s-china-relations-from-tiananmen-to-trump/.

18. Kim Zetter, "US and China Reach Historic Agreement on Economic Espionage," *Wired*, September 25, 2015, https://www.wired.com/2015/09/us-china-reach-historic-agree ment-economic-espionage/.

19. Jeremy Page, Carol Lee, and Gordon Lubold, "China's President Pledges No Militarization in Disputed Islands," *Wall Street Journal*, September 25, 2015, https://www.wsj .com/articles/china-completes-runway-on-artificial-island-in-south-china-sea-1443184818.

PART VI / Grand Strategy and American Statecraft

Chapter Sixteen

Maybe It Won't Be So Bad

A Modestly Optimistic Take on COVID and World Order

Hal Brands, Peter Feaver, and William Inboden

E very crisis seems epochal in the moment, when normal patterns of behavior are profoundly disrupted and normal patterns of policy are profoundly inadequate. Yet determining, in real time, which crises will indeed have seismic effects—sweeping away one era and ushering in another—is uncertain. The tremendous flux that crises create can make it hard to remember that the international system has more inertia than we realize. It also means that the most confident predictions can prove to be wrong.

So what effect will COVID-19 have on the international system? At this point, no one knows, because no one knows how much damage, over how much time, the pandemic will inflict. It is possible to imagine a scenario in which nationwide lockdowns are lifted, governments muddle through with basic precautionary measures, a vaccine becomes available, and the existing system survives mostly intact. It is just as easy to imagine a scenario in which a far more lethal second wave hits, neither vaccines nor herd immunity provide rescue, and COVID leaves a shock every bit as profound as World War I or World War II.

Hal Brands is the Henry A. Kissinger Distinguished Professor at the Johns Hopkins School of Advanced International Studies. Peter Feaver is the director of the Duke Program in American Grand Strategy and professor of political science and public policy at Duke University. William Inboden is the William Powers, Jr. Executive Director of the Clements Center for National Security and associate professor at the Lyndon B. Johnson School of Public Affairs at the University of Texas at Austin.

At this relatively early stage, the bulk of informed opinion leans toward a maximalist—and deeply pessimistic—appraisal. COVID-19 is causing "the end of the liberal world order," writes G. John Ikenberry. A recent Council on Foreign Relations report offers a similarly bleak assessment.[1] Other observers argue that the crisis may shift the global ideological balance toward autocracy; that it may be America's "Suez moment" and accelerate China's ascent; that it may end or dramatically roll back globalization; and that it will, or should, cause Washington to fundamentally reorder its approach to national security.[2] COVID-19, the early consensus holds, will be a hinge in history, akin to the assassination of Archduke Franz Ferdinand in 1914—or perhaps even the crises of the 1930s and 1940s.[3]

Maybe, but maybe not. Precisely because there is so much uncertainty today, we must consider a range of futures. To be clear, COVID-19 is *not* a geopolitical blip of little consequence. It has already taken a ghastly human toll and caused disastrous dislocations. It is sharpening the key rivalry of the 21st century and highlighting strains that were already disordering the world. The post-COVID landscape will be different than the landscape of December 2019.

But it will not necessarily be a fundamental altering of the global system on par with what happened when World War II destroyed two leading great powers, Germany and Japan; catalyzed the collapse of the great European colonial empires; and propelled the United States to international primacy. And it need not be a dramatically more menacing landscape. Yes, there is one scenario in which COVID-19 ends the US-led international system—and the most extreme version of that scenario might begin to approximate a World War II level of change. There is also another scenario in which the pandemic weakens autocracy and populism more than democracy, underscores America's structural power even as it temporarily damages the country's soft power, catalyzes a more formidable balancing coalition against China, and leads to a more realistic form of globalization as well as renewed cooperation between the world's democratic states. In this essay, we lay out both scenarios and make a cautiously optimistic case that the brighter one could still materialize.

So much depends, however, on what choices America makes in a post-COVID world—on the way that the United States responds to the great structural questions that crisis has raised. The COVID pandemic reminds us that "American leadership" is not a cliché or a euphemism. It is arguably the single most important factor in determining whether the arc of history bends toward something better or something worse. For the more hopeful scenario we outline to materialize,

America must soon recover the tradition of enlightened global leadership it presently seems to have abandoned.

The World That Made the Pandemic

Whatever its long-term effects, COVID-19 already qualifies as the greatest shock to the international system since the 2007–9 financial crisis, and perhaps since September 11, 2001. Yet there is something puzzling about the way COVID has upended societies around the globe.

So far, the novel coronavirus that causes COVID appears to be significantly less lethal than the virus that caused the Spanish flu pandemic of 1918–19. Most of the world's population has access to vastly better medical care than it did one hundred years ago. But that pandemic did not shut down societies for months or threaten to destroy previously thriving national economies.[4] No one thinks of the 20th century as being broken into pre–Spanish flu and post–Spanish flu eras. This may be because the world had already been so profoundly disrupted by World War I. Or the fact that COVID has been both less lethal and more disruptive may reflect that many countries are now better able to survive national shutdowns, thanks to remote work and the availability of countercyclical fiscal policies. Perhaps we are worse off today because we are better off today. And this puzzle may simply show that societies place a higher value on saving human lives than they once did: they no longer view pandemics as tragic but essentially unavoidable phenomena.

The effect of COVID has been so outsized because it broke loose in a world where the stability, prosperity, and peace that so many people enjoyed after the Cold War was already being challenged by newer conflicts and cleavages. Five key trends—the pre-existing conditions—combined to increase the damage caused by the pandemic, while reducing the chances of a more effective response.

1. *The paradoxical state of globalization.* Pandemics have happened in eras of far less globalization than our own. Yet the intensely interconnected nature of the modern world is one reason this disease went in just weeks from being a "problem for China" to a global mega-crisis. The ease of global travel permitted the disease to hop from China to nearly every other continent before the nature or even the existence of the outbreak was widely understood. Extremely high levels of economic integration accelerated and magnified the economic pain. Just-in-time supply chains and integrated financial markets are boons to efficiency and prosperity in good times; they become transmission belts for disruption when things go bad.

Yet the trajectory of COVID-19 was also accelerated by a countervailing factor—the high level of populism and anti-globalization sentiment among key policy elites. That sentiment is a reaction to the dislocation globalization brings. But it had the perverse effect of slowing and hampering the coordinated response that would have been necessary to impede an aggressive disease from spreading in a highly globalized world. Leaders in the United States initially relied on border closures and travel restrictions as substitutes for, rather than elements of, a comprehensive national and international response; some officials welcomed COVID-19 as a spur to economic decoupling between America and China.[5] In a number of countries, populist sentiment—stoked by anti-globalization leaders—downplayed or even disparaged warnings from public health experts. Finally, anti-globalization sentiment in high-places undermined efforts to mount an early, multilateral economic or fiscal response.[6] In early 2020, the world had the *reality* of interdependence but lacked the *mindset* of interdependence necessary to manage it wisely.

2. *A combination of Chinese hyper-assertiveness and Chinese hyper-insecurity.* The best chance to prevent a pandemic would have been to limit the initial outbreak at its source. Yet doing so requires high levels of trust, transparency, and accountability within a political system. Most authoritarian polities would fall short in these areas; a Chinese system that has become increasingly personalized and neo-totalitarian failed miserably. Local officials squelched whistleblowers and suppressed news of the disease for crucial weeks in December and early January. Central officials and Xi Jinping himself then did likewise. Much of the pandemic's virulence and spread can be traced to this Chinese information blackout, which reflected the deep insecurity of a regime obsessed with threats to its rule.[7]

To prevent international embarrassment and isolation, China then blustered in ways that worsened the underlying global public health problem. Beijing employed economic and diplomatic pressure—whether explicitly or implicitly—to prevent countries such as Cambodia from shutting their borders to Chinese travelers or otherwise limiting their exposure.[8] Xi coerced the World Health Organization to delay reporting human-to-human transmission and otherwise to refrain from sounding the alarm while there was still time for stronger preventive action.[9] China then responded to the inevitable international criticism with a diplomatic offensive meant to obscure its early mistakes. All of these actions flowed from the growth of Chinese assertiveness dating back to 2008–9, and all hurt the chances of containing the outbreak.

3. *Surging great-power competition.* All things equal, we would expect a better global response to transnational threats in periods of low international tensions—when patterns of cooperation between leading powers are well established, positive-sum dynamics are prominent, and policy makers do not hope that a common danger will inflict asymmetric harm on a rival. When power and influence are more contested, however, mistrust impedes cooperation and zero-sum concerns come to the fore.[10]

By early 2020, this statement described US-China relations well. Despite a temporary truce in the post-2017 trade war, each side was deeply suspicious of the other's motives and actions; each viewed the other as an increasingly dangerous rival. That the COVID-19 crisis erupted amid widespread speculation about a "new Cold War" ensured that it was viewed through the lens of the competition.

This trend compounded Beijing's unwillingness to share information about the virus and its origins. Doing so would have seemed particularly dangerous for a regime locked in a spiraling competition with the United States. It meant that the early weeks of the crisis were characterized by escalating propaganda warfare and a dearth of meaningful high-level coordination. Most broadly, it ensured that the international dimensions of the US and Chinese responses to the crisis took on a mutually antagonistic rather than a mutually supportive quality, in opposition to the concerted stimulus that the two countries took in 2008–9.

4. *Deep strains in the liberal order.* A liberal international order is characterized by a dense web of international institutions and deep cooperation among like-minded states. One of the primary reasons for such an order is to respond collectively to common challenges that emerge from interdependence. If any crisis would be tailor-made for an interdependent, cooperative response, it would be a viral pandemic that does not respect borders, reaches every continent, and inflicts massive costs to economies and human lives. But such a response did not happen. The liberal international order did not produce a collective response because that order was beset by internal divisions, suspicions, and distractions.[11]

The cohesion of the order's core—the developed, democratic world—had been weakened by resurgent illiberalism. The European Union was plagued by persistent internal tensions, strong populist movements, and the distraction caused by Brexit. Political relationships between the United States and other key democracies were more strained than at any time since the 1970s; commercial and diplomatic disputes had depleted mutual trust and sympathy. Finally, the crisis revealed alarmingly high levels of institutional rot within key bodies such as the WHO, thanks to pressure exerted by authoritarian powers—namely, China—that had infiltrated the order without accepting its underlying values.[12]

In fairness, aspects of international cooperation—within Europe, for instance—did improve as the crisis progressed. The Federal Reserve kept the global economy afloat by stabilizing a wobbling financial system.[13] But if crises expose the underlying strength or weakness of everything they touch, COVID-19 showed that the liberal order was struggling.

5. *A leadership vacuum.* The liberal order does not function on its own; it requires a hegemonic power to catalyze collective action. Yet the United States refused to play that role. Extreme political polarization, heightened by the presidential impeachment saga and election-year gamesmanship, rendered Americans unable to reach even a common understanding of the threat.[14] Key aspects of contemporary American governance—denigration of expertise, a penchant for trafficking in untrue or misleading information, a resistance to systematic planning or preparation, a hyper-transactionalist foreign policy—left the United States particularly ill-placed to exercise global leadership and lent a lurching, unilateral quality to its response.[15] Other democratic countries were not capable of filling the resulting vacuum.

These five trends interacted in potent ways. Rising great-power competition fueled Chinese hyper-insecurity and hyper-assertiveness. Weak leadership and high levels of anti-globalization sentiment exacerbated strains within the liberal order. Deep interdependence and the rot within international institutions served as a recipe for trouble. Pandemics do not arise in a vacuum, nor is their trajectory determined entirely by the laws of science. Rather, intertwined geopolitical and geo-economic factors did much to shape the course of the disease.

The World after COVID, Take 1

What sort of world will COVID create? The negative scenario is not hard to envision; it seems that almost every analyst of global politics has described some variation of this outcome. Even assuming that the pandemic does go away—that we are in a world *after* COVID-19 rather than a world *of* COVID-19—this scenario involves dramatic regression along four key axes.

1. *The rollback of globalization.* If a world crisis were to be designed with deliberate intent to undermine globalization, it would look much like the global response to COVID-19. Nations closed their borders, curtailed information flows, decoupled from global supply chains, and mistrusted other nations. These actions, moreover, seemed to vindicate pre-existing discontent. While the young had

grown disenchanted with globalization's market dislocations, many older citizens in the United States and Europe had become disillusioned with globalization's permeable borders and high levels of immigration. As Francis Fukuyama observed shortly before the pandemic, "every generation's mental framework is shaped by the collective experiences that mark its members' formative years. . . . For people born after 1990, it is neoliberalism and its associated policies of fiscal austerity, privatization, and free trade that have taken on a negative valence."[16]

So far, there is little grounds for optimism that globalization will quickly reassert itself. Much international travel remains suspended; many firms assume that pre-existing supply chains, particularly those involving China, will not be quickly reconstituted. The increasingly zero-sum climate of US-China relations will not abate anytime soon, and will further accelerate the unwinding of globalization as it existed in December 2019.

2. *Decisive and adverse shifts in the balance of power.* Analysts have long been predicting the decline of the United States and the rise or resurgence of its challengers. Some of this has been driven by structural and secular trends, some of it by policy choices in numerous capitals. At first glance, COVID-19 appears to have hastened these shifts.

The stumbling response to the pandemic in Europe and especially the United States seems to have crippled the coalition that dominated global affairs since World War II. The damaged economies and diminished assets of the transatlantic powers have reduced their financial resources, while the global perception of America in particular has diminished. Nothing exemplified this more than the pathetic spectacle of the aircraft carrier USS *Theodore Roosevelt*. The world watched as this former avatar of American power projection limped into port at Guam, its crew waylaid by widespread infections, and its captain humiliatingly relieved from command because of a dysfunctional political dispute in Washington, DC.

Meanwhile the putative success of China in containing the pandemic, coupled with Beijing's aggressive diplomatic offensive combining economic aid and political warfare, seemed to lift China's global standing even higher. Typical is the argument of the Singaporean scholar Kishore Mahbubani that the geopolitical effects of the pandemic have "created a massive opening that China has taken full advantage of, on its way to victory over the post COVID-19 world."[17] Perhaps this time the prophets of American demise will finally be vindicated.

3. *The erosion and perhaps collapse of the liberal order.* The key institutions and relationships on which the world has traditionally depended in prior crises have

been absent or deficient in this one. The United Nations Security Council and United Nations itself have been nonentities; the World Trade Organization and International Monetary Fund have foundered in halting the spiral of protectionism and economic decline; the G7 cannot even agree to meet; the European Union initially did little to assist hard-hit member states; and the WHO was discredited as a mouthpiece for China and then abandoned by the United States. Much of this dysfunction stems from the US-China competition and its spillover into international institutions.[18] Yet frictions between the leading countries of the order—the United States and its democratic allies—have also increased rather than decreased; America, under the Trump administration, initially reacted to the crisis by increasing its estrangement from the relationships and institutions that make the order function. If American policy in particular continues in this direction for much longer, the strains on the liberal order could well become unbearable.

4. *The decline of democracy and the ascent of illiberalism and populism.* Democracy has suffered twin blows to its global standing. First, the public health response of many democracies to the pandemic has been weak. Democracies such as Italy, Spain, France, the United Kingdom, Brazil, India, and—most obviously—the United States have endured some of COVID-19's worst effects, and these harms have been compounded by governance failures. The slow and vacillating responses by many of these nations' leaders; the deficiencies in testing, in tracing, and in providing medical supplies; and the overwhelmed hospital systems have all displayed democratic shortcomings to the world.

The second blow has come from authoritarians and their aspiring imitators. Many autocrats have used the crisis to consolidate power and squelch dissent. From Belarus to Beijing to Brazil (the latter still a democracy but increasingly fragile), journalists have been jailed in growing numbers, and other dissidents have been targeted for state repression.[19] Other leaders such as Hungary's Viktor Orbán have imposed emergency laws and suspended civil liberties.[20] Dictators and would-be dictators are not letting this crisis go to waste, and their opportunism recalls the way in which other global crises, such as the Great Depression, led to global recessions of democracy.

If the Cold War ended with the triumph of democracies over authoritarian systems, perhaps the pandemic marks the end of the post–Cold War era, and the surprising reversal—the triumph of the authoritarian/populist model over democracy. And if the world order we have come to know features American dominance, deep globalization, an expanding liberal order, and the ascent of liberal political values, then perhaps COVID is pushing us into an entirely new era.

The World after COVID, Take 2

This pessimistic scenario is plausible, especially if one simply extrapolates from early responses to and effects of the crisis. But it is not foreordained. That American dominance, the liberal order, and other aspects of the pre-COVID status quo have continued for decades suggests that they possess a higher degree of resilience than many observers appreciate. Just as important, a closer look at some of the dynamics unleashed or highlighted by the crisis points to a more optimistic scenario that includes several opportunities for Washington and its allies. That scenario is, in many ways, the mirror image of the one previously described. We outline it here not because we believe it is certain to materialize but because we believe its plausibility indicates that the outlines of the post-COVID world are still very much up for grabs. In this scenario:

1. *The pandemic leads not to de-globalization but to re-globalization along geopolitical lines.* While trade, finance, and people flows all dropped markedly at the height of the pandemic, the fundamental drivers of long-term globalization—technology that shrinks distances, the quest for economic growth that spurs trade, and the recognition that global problems do not recognize borders—have not been undone. If anything, they are underscored. For example, the need for growth to reduce the crushing debt burden created by the pandemic-generated depression will, we believe, eventually produce a resurgence in global trade.

In some ways, the crisis may create opportunities for deeper globalization. As individual nations and leaders wrestle with the next phases of the COVID response, particularly antiviral therapies, vaccine development, contact tracing, and mass immunity, it will become clear that no one nation-state will be able to develop those alone. The resulting networks, some that evolve organically and others reinforced by institutional mandates and incentives, will create connective tissue binding nation-states together rather than furthering their distance. Similarly, the continuing decline in birth rates among industrialized nations, coupled with aging populations and increasing entitlement payments, will confront governments with unpalatable choices, the least unattractive of which will likely be increasing immigration to replenish the workforce.

The medium-term outlook could well be managed globalization, along two discernible directions. First, supply chains will likely diversify, with the risk premium justifying the inefficiencies of redundancy. In most cases, even with the advances of additive manufacturing, the costs of entirely onshoring production back to the United States will be prohibitive. But savvy firms should be able to generate more resilient production chains without complete onshoring, and those firms will have a competitive edge over others chasing the unicorn of autarky.

Second, globalization will increasingly occur within rather than across geopolitical lines. The quest for diversification and modest US-China decoupling will likely result in a diversion of trade and investment flows to other countries, particularly historic allies like Europe and Japan and other regions, such as South America and Southeast Asia, where the states have their own incentives to minimize their vulnerabilities to Chinese coercion. Geopolitical logic will reinforce and accelerate this trend since such deeper trade and economic integration could strengthen the "free world" economy for a competition with Beijing.[21] And globalization driven by the fourth industrial revolution plays against China's advantage in low-cost labor and in favor of the advantages enjoyed by the United States and its geopolitical allies—relatively highly educated work force and wealthy consumers.

2. *The pandemic does not result in dramatic, adverse shifts in the balance of power.* Even optimists would concede that America's geopolitical position has worsened somewhat as a result of the crisis. That China seemed to gain the upper hand in its fight against the spread of COVID-19 just as the United States and its major allies were slogging through the toughest phase of the lockdown reinforced the impression of waning Western, and especially American, power and created a perception that Beijing now enjoyed a window of opportunity to pursue its aims while Washington and its democratic allies were laid low.

If the psychological balance shifted rapidly, however, the material balance did not shift in a decisive or enduring way. The pandemic adversely affected *every* major economy and market: almost every geopolitical unit that has been touted at one time or another as a possible emerging disrupter of US primacy—the European Union, Russia, India, or Brazil—suffered a grievous economic wound. If anything, the flight of international investors *toward* the United States in the middle of the crisis underscored the fundamental sources of US structural strength.

The pandemic also underscores some fundamental Chinese problems. In contrast to the Great Recession of 2008–9, which largely exposed American financial weakness while foregrounding Chinese rising economic power, COVID has drawn attention to Chinese economic and political fragility.[22] "Wolf warriors" have not been able to obscure the reality that China botched its initial response to the spread of the virus and then botched its attempt to cover up this fact with crude propaganda and gifts of defective PPE.[23]

From the Chinese Communist Party's point of view, the most promising indicator is the fact that the pandemic shook global and American domestic confidence in the United States. Over the medium and long term, however, it is not clear that even this issue will redound to China's advantage. While American soft power and diplomatic prestige often attach in the short term to the successes and failures of a particular leader, they tend to reset quickly after the next electoral cycle. Previous declines in American soft power—under George W. Bush, for instance—were followed by sharp bounce backs, in some cases caused by nothing more than a change in the White House. If, a year from now, the United States is seen to be acting more competently at home and abroad, the deeper sources of American soft power and prestige may reassert themselves. And if the United States leads in developing and distributing a working vaccine—a big "if," but an area in which it is well positioned for success—then the soft-power bounce back could be substantial.

For China, by contrast, the long-term diplomatic trends seem more troubling. The fact that dozens of countries called for an international inquiry into the pandemic's origins, that international anger at China rose considerably on multiple continents, and that a number of countries that had previously accommodated China swung toward a harder line all indicated that Beijing may confront a more formidable balancing coalition in the years to come. Admittedly, forging an effective balancing coalition will require more skillful US diplomacy than of late. But it is quite possible that this pandemic will scathe China more than the United States.

3. *The liberal order holds and is revitalized.* As poorly as the institutions of the liberal order performed during the initial stages of the pandemic, they still command more legitimacy in the rest of the world than any plausible alternative. And unless the United States reacts to the crisis by simply abandoning the institutions and relationships it created—a prospect that does not seem as outlandish as it once might have—the more likely scenario could be reform and innovative new institutions rather than collapse.

Lamentations over the weaknesses of international institutions often go in tandem with expressions of nostalgia for a past golden era of multilateral cooperation. But such an era never existed. International institutions have always faced geopolitical challenges and criticism for their failings. Yet they adapted and endured, and that could happen again. What may emerge is a shift to a two-tiered order: one level involves the world's democracies and has a higher level of cohesion and ambition, and the second level is a broader order that involves a larger number of countries and a lower level of cohesion and ambition, reserved only for transnational issues such as pandemics and climate change.[24]

For example, the G7 could evolve into a D10 that includes the leading democracies committed to developing alternatives to technological dependence on China; the United Kingdom has already proposed such a reform. The EU is considering plans to deepen fiscal integration by making additional funds available to COVID-stricken economies. US military alliances are likely to prove even more relevant in the more competitive world that is now emerging; the imperative of decreasing economic dependence on autocracies could lead, over time, to trade and investment agreements that focus on deepening ties between America and like-minded democracies. And if the United States commits to fighting harder for influence in obscure but important institutions that China has sought to corrupt, the result could be (over time) to increase the effectiveness of those institutions.

Admittedly, the US suspension of participation in the WHO does not fit well with this assessment. Neither does the Trump administration's withdrawal from the Trans-Pacific Partnership, nor its penchant for trade wars with democratic allies. So, the crucial caveat here, and across all dimensions of the more optimistic scenario, is that this depends on whether the United States plays the role of leader or spoiler in the years ahead.

4. *The pandemic proves deadlier for autocrats and populists than for democrats.* Authoritarians and populists have short-term advantages in confronting a pandemic—for example, in implementing draconian public health measures and exploiting the demagoguery that accompanies suffering. But several months into the pandemic, there does not seem to be a lasting dictator's dividend. The nations that displayed the most effective responses are liberal democracies, including South Korea, Japan, Taiwan, Denmark, New Zealand, and Germany. Singapore, a soft-authoritarian city-state, is the main example of a non-democracy that marshaled an effective response and is almost the exception that proves the rule.

The performance of the world's foremost authoritarian regimes was somewhere between mediocre and catastrophic. China's delayed response to the coronavirus outbreak, once galvanized, drew on the advantages that authoritarianism offers, including mass lockdowns and mass surveillance.[25] Yet that response was necessary because the authoritarian system had prevented a more effective earlier response, and the pandemic almost certainly caused much higher numbers of infections and deaths than its government has admitted.[26] Iran, Russia, Turkmenistan, and North Korea also seem to have been hit very hard, with the damage obscured only by their lack of transparency. As mentioned earlier, many democratic nations have also underperformed. But the point is that neither type of political system has a monopoly on ineptitude of initial response, and democracies are still well positioned to win the governance challenge over the long term.

From a free press, to an independent judiciary, to opposition parties, to decentralized governance, to elections, democracies possess an ecosystem of self-correction that provide warnings when policies are not working, information channels for suggesting new approaches, policy laboratories for experimenting with different responses, and accountability channels for citizens to either reward or punish their elected leaders and the administrators who serve under them. Authoritarian systems, in contrast, eschew these mechanisms, any of which could threaten the autocrat's monopoly on power. In the near term, admittedly, such crises can provide political cover for leaders to consolidate control; they can also create the anger and resentment on which populist leaders thrive.[27] But authoritarians cannot indefinitely hide from the convergent pressures of disaffected citizens, dysfunctional health systems, eroding control, and economic stresses accentuated by the crisis, and their political systems tend to be more brittle than democracies when confronted by such challenges.

The greater challenge for democracies may be in shaping the global narrative about which system is performing better. That authoritarian information campaigns are often unconstrained by truth also creates propaganda advantages for autocratic regimes, at least in the short term. But one of the lessons of the Cold War is that authoritarian information campaigns trade short-run effectiveness for long-run persuasiveness, because they rely on a gap between truth and propaganda that becomes hard to sustain over time.[28] Shaping the global narrative will require better policy efforts than the democracies have shown thus far, but there is no reason they cannot compete.

Conclusion: From Crisis to Opportunity

The future is not binary; the world may well end up somewhere between these two scenarios. Or these two futures could unfold sequentially: in the near term, when the disruptions are greatest, the darker trends are most pronounced, but in the longer term, as the crisis eases, more favorable forces reassert themselves. Still, it is useful to frame the future against these two scenarios because they illustrate the range of likely outcomes. It is also possible that the alternatives for the future could be somewhat starker than we think. If the same factors that lead to a good (or bad) outcome on one dimension lead to a similar outcome on other dimensions, then the likelihood of the overall outcome leaning sharply one way or the other becomes higher. This raises what may be the most important factor in determining which way the future breaks: American policy.

If both the pessimistic and the optimistic scenarios are realistic enough to be plausible, only one is attractive from the vantage of a US policy maker. Most of the national interest goals that have driven American foreign policy since World War II would be harder to secure if the pessimistic vision proves true. Even critics from the so-called "restraint" school who criticize those goals as overly ambitious would likely prefer retrenchment from within the optimistic world rather than have such changes imposed by the harsh realities of the pessimistic world. The real debate among analysts is not whether the optimistic scenario is desirable but whether it is achievable.

If the pessimistic scenario is inevitable, US grand strategy must change profoundly. If globalization, the liberal order, and democracy itself are in inexorable decline, the United States must retreat. If the balance of power has shifted permanently, concessions to allies and rivals alike are unavoidable. If pandemics are the greatest threats facing the United States, "hard security" issues must be downgraded.[29]

No doubt global public health will receive more attention as a geopolitical security problem going forward than it did in the past several decades. For the foreseeable future, warnings about the next pandemic will have greater traction, and policy measures designed to better prepare for and head off the next pandemic will be taken more seriously—and funded more generously—than they were over the last decade. America will presumably invest more in stockpiling essential medical equipment and pharmaceuticals, constructing early warning mechanisms, strengthening bureaucratic response capabilities, and creating an infrastructure for the rapid development of vaccines. It *should* invest more in fortifying the international mechanisms needed for a global response to the next pandemic. If more Americans have already died from COVID-19 than all of America's wars since World War II, then national security priorities should be adjusted accordingly.

It does not follow, however, that there should be a fundamental reorienting of national security away from traditional state-based issues and toward the human security concerns of development and public health. When 9/11 vaulted terrorism to the top of America's national security agenda it did not, in fact, make the other concerns—what might be called the September 10 agenda—moot. The most trenchant critique of America's response to 9/11 is that it focused excessively on the novel threat, to the point that the country eventually lost ground in dealing with other threats. In the same way, the pandemic, and the social disruption it threatens, will interact with pre-existing national security concerns in ways that make them even more pressing, not less. Put simply, there are few if any significant national security challenges that have abated as a result of COVID. Rather than tempering existing patterns of conflict, or making irrelevant the clashes of interest and ideology that provoke them, in many cases the pandemic seems to be making these issues—from US-Russia tensions to the threat of an ISIS resurgence in the Middle East—worse.[30]

Most notably, if the Sino-American rivalry helped make the pandemic, then the pandemic is making a sharper Sino-American rivalry. As one of us has written elsewhere, COVID-19 appears to have convinced a large number of Americans what a long series of Chinese provocations in the South China Sea and other areas could not—that the regime in Beijing represents a significant threat to their physical well-being and livelihood. The crisis has also produced greater support in the United States for deepened ties with Taiwan, while tempting China to exploit the world's distraction by expanding its control in Hong Kong and its territorial claims from South Asia to the South China Sea.[31] Not least, the pandemic has revealed the stakes in the Sino-American competition for influence in international organizations and countries around the world.[32]

In short, the pandemic has made great-power competition more important, not less. COVID has surely proved that Americans are as likely to die as a result of the "soft" threats of the human security agenda as they are from the "hard" threats of the traditional security agenda. Yet it has also created near-term windows of opportunity for actors posing hard threats that will require the traditional tool kit and deep engagement to suppress.

The case for adapting US grand strategy on the margins, rather than radically restructuring it, is even more compelling if the optimistic scenario is within reach. And here the role for US policy is even more critical. COVID is interacting powerfully with pre-existing structural forces. But if structural trends constrain policy choices, then policy choices can also shape structural trends—particularly when the policies in question are those of the world's mightiest state. And on every dimension, the question of whether the pessimistic or the optimistic scenario materializes hinges to a great extent on US choices.

If the United States commits its vast power and prestige to deepening cooperation and economic integration with the democracies, to promoting a geopolitically informed globalization rather than a wholesale retreat from globalization, to reforming and competing for influence within the institutions of the liberal order that underperformed or were corrupted by authoritarian influence, and to developing the policies—not simply the rhetoric—of responsible competition with China, then the fluidity that the crisis has created may well redound to the advantage of America and the "free world." If the United States returns to a pattern of greater competency and responsibility in its statecraft, its soft power and prestige will probably once again prove resilient. Yet if the United States chooses a course of narrow economic nationalism, gratuitous provocation of its closest allies, retreat from institutions in which it does not get its way, and continued downgrading of efforts to promote democracy and human rights, and indefinite floundering in discharging its responsibilities at home and abroad, then the balance of possibilities may well tip in favor of the darker scenario.

The quality of US global leadership is inextricably a function of the quality of US political leaders—above all, the caliber of the president. And here the United States has been hamstrung. At almost every turn in the COVID crisis, the Trump administration has stumbled after choices that would make the pessimistic scenario more likely.

When China was hiding the true nature of the pandemic, the Trump administration was praising Beijing. By the time the pandemic was an undeniable global crisis demanding a coordinated response, the Trump administration acted alone through contradictory edicts rather than in close coordination with others. When the inherent unknowns of the science and public health response demanded caution, President Donald Trump offered reckless nostrums and inane conspiracies. When a more aggressive response might have better prepared us, the Trump administration did less; when a more cautious response might have eased the pain, the Trump administration did more. Throughout, the common thread was not what would best enable the country to overcome the crisis but what would best position the president to overcome a negative headline. And when trouble did materialize, the president's instinct in this crisis and throughout his presidency was to lash out—sometimes against allies, sometimes against rivals, but in ways more often destructive than helpful.

Bringing about the better scenario will require better American leadership in myriad ways. These include using the power to convene other nations for common goals; setting the agenda for what issues to focus on and how; providing economic, personnel, and technological resources toward international challenges; leading the gathering, analysis, and sharing of information on global problems; pioneering innovation and creative solutions; deploying leverage to induce or persuade those otherwise reluctant to make responsible choices; serving as a moral exemplar; demonstrating competence in policy design and implementation; and being willing to sacrifice narrow self-interest in favor of the enlightened self-interest that comes from pursuing a larger global good. This list is an implicit indictment of all that was lacking in American statecraft as the pandemic spread and a reminder of just how dramatically US performance will have to change to tip the balance from a dark future to a brighter one.

NOTES

1. G. John Ikenberry, "The Next Liberal Order," *Foreign Affairs*, July/August 2020; Robert Blackwill and Thomas Wright, *The Coronavirus, World Order, and the Future of American Foreign Policy*, CFR Special Report No. 86 (New York: Council on Foreign Relations, June 2020).

2. Anne Applebaum, "The People in Charge See an Opportunity," *The Atlantic*, March 23, 2020; Kurt M. Campbell and Rush Doshi, "The Coronavirus Could Reshape Global Order," *Foreign Affairs*, March 18, 2020; Kevin Rudd, "The Coming Post-COVID Anarchy," *Foreign Affairs*, May 6, 2020; Richard Haass, "A Cold War with China Would Be a Mistake," *Wall Street Journal*, May 7, 2020.

3. Lawrence Summers, "COVID-19 Looks Like a Hinge in History," *Financial Times*, May 14, 2020; Colin H. Kahl and Ariana Berengaut, "Aftershocks: The Coronavirus Pandemic and the New World Order," *War on the Rocks*, April 10, 2020.

4. Walter Scheidel, "The Spanish Flu Didn't Wreck the Global Economy," *Foreign Affairs*, May 28, 2020.

5. See "Wilbur Ross Says Coronavirus Could Boost U.S. Jobs," BBC.com, January 31, 2020.

6. Stewart Patrick, "The Multilateral System Still Cannot Get Its Act Together on COVID-19," CFR.org, March 26, 2020.

7. See "China Didn't Warn Public of Likely Pandemic for 6 Key Days," Associated Press, April 15, 2020; Shawn Yuan, "Inside the Early Days of China's Coronavirus Cover-up," *Wired*, May 1, 2020.

8. For example, Shannon Tiezzi, "China and Cambodia: Love in the Time of Coronavirus," *The Diplomat*, February 6, 2020.

9. Dave Makichuk, "German Intelligence Says Xi 'Pressured' WHO," *Asia Times*, May 20, 2020.

10. Hal Brands, "The Environment and Economy Have Become Great-Power Pawns," *Bloomberg Opinion*, November 18, 2018.

11. See Edward Fishman, "The World Order is Dead. Here's How to Build a New One for a Post-Coronavirus Era," *Politico*, May 3, 2020.

12. Hal Brands, "China's Global Influence Operation Goes Way beyond the WHO," *Bloomberg Opinion*, March 31, 2020.

13. For example, Justin Baer, "The Day Coronavirus Nearly Broke the Financial Markets," *Wall Street Journal*, May 20, 2020.

14. Frank Newport, "The Partisan Gap in Views of the Coronavirus," Gallup, May 15, 2020.

15. Karen Donfried and Wolfgang Ischinger, "The Pandemic and the Toll of Transatlantic Discord," *Foreign Affairs*, April 18, 2020; Katrin Bennhold, "'Sadness' and Disbelief from a World Missing American Leadership," *New York Times*, April 23, 2020.

16. Francis Fukuyama, "30 Years of World Politics: What Has Changed?," *Journal of Democracy* 31, no. 1 (January 2020).

17. Kishore Mahbubani, "How China Could Win Over the Post-Coronavirus World and Leave the U.S. Behind," *Marketwatch*, April 18, 2020.

18. Thomas Pickering and Atman Trivedi, "The International Order Didn't Fail the Pandemic Alone," *Foreign Affairs*, May 14, 2020.

19. Judith Miller, "The Virus, the Riots, and the Press," *City Journal*, June 10, 2020.

20. Michael Abramowitz and Arch Puddington, "Poland and Hungary Must Not Be Ignored," Perspectives, Freedom House, May 26, 2020, https://freedomhouse.org/article /poland-and-hungary-must-not-be-ignored.

21. Hal Brands, "Grand Strategy for a New Twilight Struggle," Center for a New American Security, April 11, 2019.

22. Jonathan Holslag, "The Rise of the Beijing Consensus," *The Guardian*, April 19, 2009; John Williamson, "Is the 'Beijing Consensus' Now Dominant?," *Asia Policy*, no. 13 (2012): 1–16, www.jstor.org/stable/24905162.

23. See "China Didn't Warn Public of Likely Pandemic for 6 Key Days," Associated Press, April 15, 2020; Yuan, "Inside the Early Days"; Makichuk, "German Intelligence Says Xi 'Pressured' WHO"; Laura Rosenberger, "China's Coronavirus Information Offensive," *Foreign Affairs*, April 22, 2020; David Gitter, Sandy Lu, and Brock Erdahl, "China Will Do Anything to Deflect Coronavirus Blame," *Foreign Policy*, March 30, 2020; "Coronavirus: Countries Reject Chinese-Made Equipment," *BBC News*, March 30, 2020; Gerry Shih, "China's Bid to Repair Its Coronavirus-Hit Image Is Backfiring in the West," *Washington Post*, April 14, 2020.

24. Fishman, "The World Order Is Dead."

25. Jessica Wang, Ellie Zhu, and Taylor Umlauf, "How China Built Two Coronavirus Hospitals in Just over a Week," *Wall Street Journal*, February 6, 2020.

26. Derek Scissors, "China's COVID Story: The Nonsense Continues," AEI.org, May 13, 2020.

27. Selam Gebrekidan, "For Autocrats, and Others, Coronavirus Is a Chance to Grab Even More Power," *New York Times*, March 30, 2020.

28. See, for instance, Alina Polyakova and Daniel Fried, "How Democracies Can Defend against Disinformation," *War on the Rocks*, May 30, 2018.

29. Ilan Goldenberg, "9–11 Swallowed U.S. Foreign Policy. Don't Let the Coronavirus Do the Same Thing," *Washington Post*, March 19, 2020.

30. "NATO Is Facing Up to Russia in the Arctic Circle," *The Economist*, May 14, 2020; Lara Seligman, "U.S. Military Fears Pandemic Could Lead to ISIS Resurgence in Syria," *Politico*, April 2, 2020.

31. Joshua Kurlantzick, "COVID-19 and the South China Sea," *Asia Unbound* (blog), Council on Foreign Relations, April 22, 2020.

32. See, for example, David Ignatius, "Trump's Pushback on China Results in an Important Win," *Washington Post*, March 10, 2020. Here the Trump administration

does deserve some credit for opening an intensified campaign to combat Chinese influence in obscure but important international institutions. Alas, the administration's penchant for withdrawing from institutions that it believes are functioning badly often has the effect of ceding the field to Beijing. See Brands, "China's Global Influence Operation."

Chapter Seventeen

COVID-19's Impact on Great-Power Competition

Thomas Wright

A fter the terrorist attacks on 9/11, the United States reoriented itself to focus on terrorist networks and rogue states. Congress created a new institution, the Department of Homeland Security. President George W. Bush made terrorism and counterproliferation the organizing principle of US national security policy. The administration adopted the 1% rule—if there was a 1% chance of something happening, it would be treated as an imminent danger. This doctrine would lead to the invasion of Iraq. Almost two decades later, the United States still wages a low-intensity, high-technology war against terrorist networks all over the world.

The coronavirus has surpassed 9/11 and the global financial crisis as the defining international event for the majority of Americans. Over 130,000 Americans have died to date, and over forty million have lost their jobs. More people are dying from COVID-19 globally than almost anything else.[1] The virus placed immense strain on globalization, brought travel to a virtual halt, exposed strains within the European Union, and poses the greatest challenge to the Chinese Communist Party since 1989. And that is as of this writing in June 2020. The crisis may be a long one that extends well into 2021.

Some experts believe that the COVID-19 crisis must lead to a radical transformation of US strategy. Alexandra Stark, a scholar at New America, wrote that

Thomas Wright is the director of the Center on the United States and Europe and a senior fellow in the Project on International Order and Strategy at the Brookings Institution.

"COVID-19 is likely to become another 9/11 moment, one that again reshapes Americans' conceptions of what security means. . . . Rather than taking a securitized approach to COVID-19, a new grand strategy must be fundamentally oriented around human well-being."[2] Joseph Cirincione, formerly head of Ploughshares, wrote in *The National Interest* that America "does not need all the weapons the majority once considered vital, nor are needed as many soldiers, airmen, or Marines at a time when America's best defense is global cooperation, not military confrontation."[3] Writing in *The Atlantic*, Peter Beinart called for Joe Biden to pursue a "radically different foreign policy" that recognized "the desperate need to improve international cooperation before the next pandemic hits."[4]

This approach would be in keeping with the 9/11 precedent and, indeed, with earlier examples of the United States' responses to strategic shocks. In addition, it would reorganize US foreign policy around the new danger and mobilize the resources of the nation to tackle it. In practical terms, this would mean elevating pandemics and the climate as the top national priorities, while seeking cooperation from other nations on these matters even at the expense of other interests.

However, this approach also runs the risk of making similar mistakes to the post-9/11 moment by misdiagnosing the nature of the challenge and focusing on one dimension of a strategy to the neglect of other important elements. Before the terrorist attacks, the Bush administration expected to focus on China. A year later, the administration called great-power competition obsolete because primacy made balancing irrational. The Bush administration would continue to play an important role in providing regional order, but it did not do as much as it should have to build new alliances and partnerships, particularly in Southeast Asia, where relationships were defined through the prism of counterterrorism. But the China challenge did not go away. Indeed, a few months after the attacks, a Goldman Sachs economist named Jim O'Neill coined the term "BRIC" (Brazil, Russia, India, and China) and predicted that their rise, in particular China's rise, would be the defining event of the decade.

Pandemic disease and climate change will remain significant dangers to societies around the world for some time to come. COVID-19 badly exposed America's lack of preparedness. The United States must genuinely expand its definition of national security to include pandemics, and it must invest much more in preventing a recurrence in the future. The United States is even further behind in tackling climate change and must do much more to prepare for the climate crises of the future.

But these are not the only challenges or crises. China has become more totalitarian, aggressive, and assertive; this arguably exacerbated the COVID-19 pandemic.

There is unfinished business from the financial crisis, and the broader crisis of globalization has been simmering for some time. Political interference by authoritarian states has worsened since the Russian attack on the 2016 election that went largely unanswered. US strategy needs to change, but it must respond to all of these challenges, not just the most recent.

The common thread of most of these challenges is that societies are interdependent and therefore vulnerable to one another at a time of increasing geopolitical and ideological competition between democracies and authoritarian regimes. Concentrating on one side of this equation while ignoring the other side is a strategic mistake. Focusing on transnational challenges and making international cooperation the primary goal of US grand strategy will not actually produce cooperation at the desired levels. Focusing only on great-power competition while ignoring the need for cooperation actually will not give the United States an enduring strategic advantage over China.

We have to move beyond the false dichotomy of transnational challenges versus hard security and better understand the strategic moment we are in, with all of its nuances. This essay looks at the implications of COVID-19 for great-power competition. What lessons can we learn? First, I look at the evolution of US grand strategy between 2016 and COVID-19. Second, I examine the impact of COVID-19 on the strategic debate and identify the strategic lessons we should learn from the crisis. Finally, I outline a "free world strategy" that deals with both transnational challenges and great-power competition by deepening cooperation with free societies on three areas—resilience, solidarity, and shaping the international environment.

The US Grand Strategy Debate from 2016 to COVID-19

The past four years in grand strategy have been dominated by a debate on the merits and demerits of the concept of great-power competition, which was the focal point of the Trump administration's 2017 National Security Strategy.[5] Upon taking office, the Trump team was able to take advantage of a broader bipartisan shift in the foreign policy community away from the notion that the major powers would converge on one model of liberal international order and toward a more geopolitically competitive concept of the world.[6] If Hillary Clinton had been elected, she was likely to have moved in this direction too. But the Trump administration put its own sheen on the concept. It was heavy on sovereignty and national interest, light on values and transnational challenges, and silent on the origins of the competition or America's end goal. Nevertheless, it was a significant shift and was backed up by the National Defense Strategy, which set the priorities for the Pentagon. It put the shift in even starker terms that the National Security Strategy stated that "inter-state strategic competition, not terrorism, is now the primary concern in U.S. national security."[7]

President Donald J. Trump was not fully on board. There is no record of him ever having spoken about the core tenet of the strategy—that of great-power competition. Even in his speech introducing the strategy, there was one line about Russia and China being great-power rivals, which he ad-libbed to convert it into a plea for cooperation with Russia on counterterrorism.[8] Trump had his own set of national security priorities, and geopolitical competition was not on it. In his speeches and remarks, he consistently highlighted four threats: (1) immigrants, (2) trade deals, (3) nuclear weapons (particularly in North Korea and Iran), and (4) allies taking advantage of the United States. His ferocious rhetoric on China, mainly motivated by trade, gave top cover for his administration's great-power rivalry.

The arrangement between Trump and his national security teams was an open marriage of sorts. They publicly committed to one another but did their own thing. For the officials, great-power competition was the substantive reason that justified staying and working for the president. It gave them a sense of purpose, and they made progress, beginning the process of reorienting the Department of Defense around a new mission. But substantive problems remained. Secretary of State Mike Pompeo and then National Security Advisor John Bolton were much more focused on Iran than on China. Bolton also had his own pet projects, such as Venezuela. Secretary of the Treasury Steve Mnuchin was skeptical of decoupling and tended to be more dovish on China. It was unclear what would happen if Trump actually struck a trade deal with Beijing. The Trump administration repeatedly rebuffed efforts by European leaders to work together on China. Although there was a dialogue with Asian allies, the president was unhappy with most of America's trade and basing agreements and sought to renegotiate on much more favorable terms.

The Trump administration was also never quite able to nail the values dimension of the competition with China, which most observers believed was a crucial distinction between the two sides. Trump was deeply suspicious of the notion that US strategy should be guided by a set of values, such as democracy, liberty, human rights, and a belief in the sovereign equality of nations. He was naturally drawn to strongmen, had a record of admiring the use of force against domestic opposition, felt that foreign policy should be purely transactional, and maintained that alliances were a mechanism through which smaller countries manipulated and took advantage of the United States. According to Bolton, Trump even told Xi Jinping that building concentration camps in Xinjiang was the right thing to do.[9] He also seemed to give Xi a green light for repression in Hong Kong. The rest of the administration would push the values dimension when they could, but they were heavily constrained by Trump.

Meanwhile, Americans began to change their strategic view, moving toward the great-power competition concept. Russia's interference in the 2016 election raised the specter of authoritarian interference in American elections and turned many Democrats into cold warriors. Xi's abolition of term limits signaled that he intended to remain in power for the rest of his life, turning China into a personality-centered dictatorship. Meanwhile, China's rapid advances in technologies, particularly artificial intelligence, facial recognition, and social credit scores, provided it with the means for a high-tech totalitarian society. China's behavior helped smooth the way for a tougher, more competitive approach in both parties, causing some to speak of a new consensus. The US-China competition is increasingly seen as a contest of systems—free societies and authoritarianism—that will directly shape the choices we make on technology, individual rights, the economy, and foreign policy.

It was not just the United States. European countries began to shift their approach toward China, away from one of economic engagement and toward one of limiting Chinese influence in Europe. This was summed up in the EU's 2019 document *EU-China: A Strategy Outlook*, which stated: "China is, simultaneously, in different policy areas, a cooperation partner with whom the EU has closely aligned objectives, a negotiating partner with whom the EU needs to find a balance of interests, an economic competitor in the pursuit of technological leadership, and a systemic rival promoting alternative models of governance."[10] On the eve of COVID-19, Europe remained committed to a policy of engagement with China, but it was also taking steps to protect itself against China's economic practices and to speak with one voice.

By the end of 2019, the Trump administration was communicating two dramatically different strategic messages to the world. For the senior officials, it was all about competition with China, including strengthening America's alliances and partnerships. For the president and a handful of his loyalist aides, it was America First, meaning a skepticism of alliances, a mercantilist foreign policy, and a dismissal of values that underpinned the post–World War II order.

Democrats embraced elements of the great-power competition concept, but they worried that the administration's version left no room for a substantive strategic dialogue with Beijing, making any cooperation on shared challenges all but impossible. It also effectively ruled out a strategic effort to forge a common front with America's allies in Europe. Nevertheless, there was some bipartisan support for a competitive approach toward China. Many Europeans who attended the 2020 Munich Security Conference in mid-February, weeks before COVID-19 ravaged Europe and the United States, commented that they were particularly struck by the tough line both parties took on China and the question of whether Huawei should be allowed to build Europe's 5G infrastructure.

Understanding the COVID-19 Moment

The COVID-19 pandemic was a stark reminder of the dangers that transnational threats pose to our societies and way of life. More people died in the United States than in all of the post–World War II conflicts combined. Over ten million people have been infected globally, which may be a considerable underestimate. The International Monetary Fund biannual report, *World Economic Outlook*, labeled the crisis "The Great Lockdown" and now estimates a reduction in global growth of 4.9% in 2020, making it the most severe recession since the Great Depression and far worse than the 2007–9 global financial crisis.[11] Even the countries that managed well—South Korea and Germany—paid a heavy economic price. Each nation's impulses were to respond nationally; there was little coordination with their neighbors. In the European Union, the most sophisticated and developed experiment in shared sovereignty short of formal nationhood, borders closed, and it was every country for itself, at least in the first month.

In the early days of the COVID-19 crisis, it appeared as though the deterioration in the West's relations with China might be slowed down or even reversed. Trump signed a trade deal with China, paving the way for a reelection campaign that emphasized his ability as a negotiator. He praised China's response to COVID-19 and expressed confidence in Xi. China, for its part, was consumed by the crisis and inwardly focused. The EU sent over fifty tons of protective equipment to China to assist their efforts. European officials said little about it, largely out of respect to Chinese authorities. French president Emmanuel Macron reportedly told a colleague that Chinese officials would remember Europe's support in the future.[12] Theoretically, COVID-19 opened a pathway for greater cooperation among the major powers on transnational challenges. Between the outbreak of SARS in southern China in 2002 and 2016, US personnel worked closely with China on pandemics. This fell apart during the Trump administration. The Centers for Disease Control and Prevention and the National Institutes of Health both reduced their presence inside China. Some observers suggested that, perhaps if the United States prioritized cooperation over competition, it may be possible to nurture a US-China partnership on this and other issues such as climate change.[13]

However, there are reasons to be skeptical. China has become much more repressive and secretive since Xi came to power, and this accelerated over the past four years. It is quite possible that cooperation on pandemics would have ended even without Trump, although he surely contributed to it. Xi's China sees transparency as a threat. It covered up the virus early on, failed to share crucial information with the World Health Organization and neighboring countries in a timely fashion, silenced the doctors who dissented, and refused to grant the international community access to China to investigate the origins of the virus.[14]

Moreover, if one sets aside the United States, China's relations with the rest of the world reveal some worrying patterns. It has become more aggressive, assertive, and bullying. In February 2020, it put considerable pressure on countries not to restrict travel with China, even as it prohibited domestic travel to and from Wuhan domestically. It asked donor countries to keep a low profile to save face. Later, it would freely impose its own travel restrictions on other countries, and it would demand that all those that received aid from China issue public declarations of support. China would threaten trade tariffs on Australia for daring to suggest an international investigation into the origins of the virus, and it would also launch a massive cyberattack on that country in June. Chinese forces engaged in a deadly clash with Indian troops along the border—the first time lives were lost in such a clash in forty-five years. It introduced a harsh new security law in Hong Kong, effectively ending one country, two systems.

Perhaps most instructive is China's diplomacy in Europe. The EU is eager to pursue a constructive and cooperative agenda with China. This year was supposed to see the first ever summit in Leipzig between Xi and all twenty-seven EU leaders, with a focus on an investment treaty, climate change, and Africa. Although the EU had turned more wary of China since 2015—largely for economic reasons—it is also wary of being drawn into the US competition with Beijing. COVID-19 presented China with the perfect opportunity to work with the EU and to attempt to drive a wedge into the heart of the transatlantic alliance. It did not turn out that way.

China behaved very assertively in Europe, seeking praise for foreign assistance, pressuring countries that criticized China's record, and trying to take advantage of the economic downturn to snap up crucial assets at knockdown prices and to push its 5G agenda. Its ambassadors were quickly labeled "wolf warriors" after the jingoistic Chinese action movie. The EU recoiled at its assertiveness and pushed back, tightening investment regulations and directly criticizing China for spreading disinformation.

We may need cooperation with China to tackle pandemic disease properly, but China's national and global response to COVID-19 should remind us that we should be realistic about how much cooperation we can get from China's Communist Party regime. It will be limited, imperfect, and hard to trust. As the rest of the world's experience shows, even if the United States were to approach China in a less hostile way, Xi's China is likely to remain secretive and assertive. It may also become increasingly aggressive in its actions.

What we learned from COVID-19 was that we are simultaneously facing near worst-case scenarios for transnational threats and great-power competition, with each exacerbating the other. And then there is a third problem—COVID-19 reveals an enormous governance gap between the United States and other democracies, such as South Korea, Germany, and Taiwan. The United States had shortages of key medical supplies. There was extremely weak leadership from the federal government. Some states performed well, but others did not. The result was an uneven patchwork of efforts that served, ultimately, to undermine rather than to strengthen one another. The results were clear. By midsummer, the United States had over three million cases, vastly more than any other nation, and over 130,000 fatalities. It was arguably the biggest failure of government since the Great Depression. Not all democracies performed well (Britain and Sweden, for instance, also did poorly), but those that did were able to take mass coordinated actions to limit social interaction early, kept to it in a disciplined way, and employed technology as part of a contact and tracing system. Experts have long argued that to be strong overseas, the United States must be strong at home and that it has a lot of work to do to prepare for 21st-century challenges. COVID-19 proves the point, if it were ever in dispute.

Toward a Free World Strategy

If a post-9/11-style revolution in American strategy—to focus on transnational threats at the expense of other problems—is undesirable, then how should we think about change? Should the United States simply try to do better at what it was already doing before Trump—invest more into tackling transnational challenges, seek reform and improvements to multilateralism and international institutions, narrow the counterterrorism fight, and gradually pivot to the Asia-Pacific? Should it try to do less internationally, passing the baton on to others and concentrating on the monumental task of domestic renovation and reform to recover not just from the COVID-19 crisis but also from decades of government dysfunction and underinvestment. Or, should the United States undertake more radical reforms and seek an organizing principle to guide its strategy?

A technocratic approach may sound attractive, but it offers little guidance on how to determine priorities or update US strategy for a changed world. What should our expectations be of a bilateral dialogue with China? What should the balance be between seeking cooperation on shared problems and competing with China? Should the United States aim for an inclusive form of multilateralism or work with like-minded democracies? Without a theory of the case, the United States is prone to strategic drift and will be forced to make decisions by the course of events rather than of its own volition.

Doing less internationally to focus on nation building at home misunderstands the nature of the domestic challenges we face. Pandemics, climate change, external interference in democratic processes, illiberal elements in domestic politics, and questions about the balance between technological advancement and individual rights are not unique to America. They are shared by free societies to some extent. And they must be dealt with collectively. The real challenges from other great powers will not go away or slow down just because Americans want to focus on the home front. In fact, they may accelerate—the pandemic, the recession, and doubts about America's commitment to its alliances sap the capacity of other democracies and makes the world more crisis prone.

So what should the United States actually do? As in any discussion of grand strategy, the answer in part depends on one's definition of the national interest. For all of its flaws as a strategic document, this may have been most clearly articulated in NSC-68, the highly classified assessment of the Soviet Union just before the outbreak of the Korean War. It stated that the fundamental purpose of the United States is to "assure the integrity and vitality of our free society, which is founded on the dignity and worth of the individual." To achieve this, NSC-68 called on the United States "to build a healthy international community" and a "world environment in which the American system can survive and flourish." This, the document said, "we would probably do even if there were no international threat."[15]

NSC-68 advocated for a highly active and ambitious US foreign policy. We can debate its relevance, but its definition of the national purpose captured the linkage between domestic welfare and the international in a way that many alternatives did not. Today, the United States finds its democracy and status as a free society challenged. The pandemic is an important piece of this. It revealed real shortcomings in the capacity of government to deal with an existential challenge to Americans' way of life. But it is far from the only piece.

Free societies are in trouble. As Freedom House has documented, the world has become less free over the past four years, due in large part to illiberal forces within democracies.[16] Many democracies also struggle to cope with fundamental challenges, including inequality, climate change, and the automation of work. Externally, free societies have the real threat of political interference from authoritarian states and networks of corruption. Other challenges, such as those arising out of artificial intelligence, loom large.

Placing the health, security, integrity, and prosperity of the free world as the centerpiece of US strategy is a way of integrating domestic, transnational, and great-power challenges in a way that actually sets priorities and helps to guide policy. The concept of the free world is one with a lineage dating back to just before World War II. According to the Swarthmore political scientist Dominic Tierney, internationalist Americans began to use the term "free world" in 1941 to press for entry into the war against the Nazis.[17] It took off in the early Cold War period but fell into disuse during the Vietnam War and was discarded after the fall of the Soviet Union. Its weakness was always that the world was more of a shaded gray than black and white.

Presidents would continue to pay it rhetorical homage. They would mention "leader of the free world," but no one took it seriously as a strategic concept. Recent developments give the term new meaning. The nature of freedom has been cast in doubt by new technologies, demagogues inside democracies, dictators in China and Russia, income inequality, climate change, and COVID-19. There is a question about what the United States stands for and why it competes with others. The free world is ripe for revival and redefinition.

In this new context, a free world strategy would have three core elements to it: (1) resilience, (2) solidarity, and (3) shaping the international system.

RESILIENCE

Resilience means ensuring that free societies are strong enough to withstand threats from within and from without. At a most basic level, it means investing in critical infrastructure, including public health, education, and research and development. However, it also means tackling corruption and oligarchy, protecting democratic institutions and the rule of law against erosion at the hands of populist nationalists, and reforming international tax and financial regulations. It means doing this with like-minded free societies and putting pressure on backward-sliding democracies, including Poland, or those that are on the verge of full-blown authoritarianism, such as Hungary.

Resilience also includes a strategic review about the extent and nature of our engagement with authoritarian countries—economically, culturally, politically, and technologically—to ensure that we are inoculated from any negative externalities of the authoritarian system. Vanderbilt professor Ganesh Sitaraman, who has written extensively about resilience, has outlined three strategic steps that should be taken: (1) selective disentanglement to uncouple "the American economy from Chinese corporations, investments, and the Chinese economy in sectors that are of critical importance to national security"; (2) diversification of economic partners; and (3) "a coherent development policy—an internal policy to support and strengthen innovation and industry."[18]

Solidarity

Authoritarian countries have become bolder in seeking to intimidate democratic countries, particularly small and middle powers. China uses its asymmetric economic power to make political demands on smaller countries and the private sector. It is not just China. Saudi Arabia cut off economic ties to Canada and reduced its investment in Germany after their foreign ministers criticized Riyadh for arresting women's rights activists and for Saudi policy in Yemen, respectively.

Authoritarian states can do this because the free world does not stand as one. Each nation must fend for itself. In a free world framework, the United States would begin to put together a political equivalent of Article 5 of the North Atlantic Treaty—when an authoritarian power seeks to illegitimately coerce a free society, there will be a collective response. Free societies would also work proactively to counter disinformation, corruption, and intelligence operations and to protect our technological infrastructure.

Shaping the International Order

China and other authoritarian states have made great inroads into the international order, shaping organizations like the World Health Organization and diluting international norms. Under the Trump administration, the United States has largely disengaged from these institutions. In a free world strategy, the United States would work with other free societies to strengthen liberal norms and to set up new structures where existing ones fall short. This coalition should also cooperate to reform and shape the global economic order—reducing corporate tax loopholes, tackling inequality, and regulating international finance. This is a form of competitive multilateralism whereby democracies actively contest illiberal values rather than cede the field to countries such as China.

There are challenges with a free world framework. It would be hard to institutionalize. After all, where would the line be drawn? Hungary certainly could not join but what about India, Brazil, or Poland? Some, including many Europeans, might see it as an anti-China alliance and would be reluctant to take part? This is why it should be informal—a goal of US strategy that should be practically pursued but not institutionalized. An expanded G7 with Australia, South Korea, and India could serve as a proxy of sorts, but its power would be as an organizing principle of US strategy.

The line-drawing issue has been problematic in the past. During the Cold War, countries could be part of the free world even if they were not free as long as they were committed to a balance of power that favored the democracies. One problem with that approach is that some countries may try to play both sides—leading to competitive outbidding by the superpowers to get autocracies in their column—and that authoritarianism at home can have negative spillover effects (e.g., on corruption). It is more important that the core of the free world maintain high standards rather than be as broad as possible. The free world could still ally with non-democracies on a transactional basis where there is a pressing strategic reason to do so, but they could not be part of that inner core unless they are making real progress on improving their domestic system of government. It would be acknowledged that there is something special and enduring about cooperation between democracies.

The pandemic shows why rivals must cooperate on shared challenges even as they compete ferociously in other spheres. The United States and the Soviet Union worked together on the nonproliferation treaty, arms control, and public health. Working with like-minded free societies must not preclude a dialogue and cooperation with China on shared challenges. In fact, it could facilitate it. If the United States and its allies and partners work together to agree on a common position, they can negotiate collectively from a position of strength with China and help to shape its choices. Cooperation between democracies and authoritarian powers will be difficult and limited in scope, but it is achievable if it is transactional and based on mutual interest. Democracies will have to think anew, though, about what cooperation with China would entail.

During the Cold War, arms control was only possible because strategists developed the counterintuitive concept of second-strike survivability whereby each superpower would be more secure if the other could absorb a first strike and retaliate, thus laying the foundation for mutually assured destruction. We need similar concepts to generate cooperation on transnational challenges. Perhaps such cooperation should be compartmentalized and sealed off from other parts of the relationship. Maybe the United States and China should try to cooperate on a partial decoupling to make each less vulnerable to the other. These are questions that US and Chinese officials must discuss in a renewed strategic dialogue.

The Post-COVID Moment

The COVID-19 crisis and its aftermath may be a rare reordering moment in the international order. US grand strategy is prone to massive oscillations after major crises. Americans would do well to avoid that this time. The strategy needs to change, but it must accommodate all of the developments underway, not just one. A focus on transnational challenges to the exclusion of great-power competition and hard security would only mean that a health and economic crisis would be accompanied by major geopolitical crises, compounding America's already mounting problems. The United States' top foreign policy priority for the next year must be defeating the virus and shaping the post-virus world. The strategic question is what follows that? What should guide US strategy for the next decade or two?

Deepening cooperation with other free and democratic societies, not just on geopolitical issues but also on shared domestic challenges, offers the most promising path forward. Americans want a strategy that is directly connected to their daily lives and the challenges they face. A free world strategy includes geopolitical interests in faraway places, but the core of it is about protecting liberty, prosperity, and democracy at home. It is less about the past—the liberal international order, alliances, and institutions—and more about providing solutions to modern problems, threats, and challenges, whether they are from new technologies, a virus, the environment, or a hostile foreign power. Great-power competition will continue in a free world strategy, but it will be shaped and limited by this doctrine in positive ways. It will reduce the risk that great-power competition will undermine American democracy and liberty at home by keeping to the forefront of our minds what the United States is competing for. If policy makers are serious about refining and improving the free society as a goal for a core group of like-minded states, it also allows them to avoid the excesses of the Cold War, including how the competition with the Soviet Union turned into a global contest spanning every region. A free world strategy also offers a framework to connect the foreign and domestic in a way that helps Americans realize the purpose set out in the Declaration of Independence. It is the right strategy for a nation and a world troubled on all fronts.

NOTES

1. "Covid-19 Has Become One of the Biggest Killers of 2020," *The Economist*, May 1, 2020, https://www.economist.com/graphic-detail/2020/05/01/covid-19-has-become-one-of -the-biggest-killers-of-2020.

2. Alexandra Stark, "Covid-19 Is This Generation's 9/11: Let's Make Sure We Apply the Right Lessons," New America, April 23, 2020, https://www.newamerica.org/weekly/covid -generations-911-lets-make-sure-we-apply-right-lessons/.

3. Joseph Cirincione, "Why America Needs to Rethink Its National Security Priorities," *The National Interest*, April 6, 2020, https://nationalinterest.org/feature/why-america -needs-rethink-its-national-security-priorities-141542.

4. Peter Beinart, "Even a Bolder Biden Will Only Go So Far," *The Atlantic*, May 20, 2020, https://www.theatlantic.com/ideas/archive/2020/05/bidens-grand-ambitions-dont-extend -foreign-policy/611863/.

5. The White House, *National Security Strategy of the United States of America*, December 2017, https://www.whitehouse.gov/wp-content/uploads/2017/12/NSS-Final-12-18-2017 -0905.pdf.

6. See, for example, Derek Chollet et al., *Building Situations of Strength: A National Security Strategy for the United States* (Washington, DC: Brookings Institution, February 2017), https://www.brookings.edu/wp-content/uploads/2017/02/fp_201702_ofc_re port_web.pdf.

7. Department of Defense, *Summary of the 2018 National Defense Strategy of the United States of America* (Washington, DC: Department of Defense, 2018), https://dod.defense .gov/Portals/1/Documents/pubs/2018-National-Defense-Strategy-Summary.pdf.

8. President Donald Trump, "Remarks by President Trump on the Administration's National Security Strategy" (The White House, December 18, 2017), https://www.white house.gov/briefings-statements/remarks-president-trump-administrations-national-secu rity-strategy/.

9. John Bolton, "The Scandal of Trump's China Policy," *Wall Street Journal*, June 17, 2020, https://www.wsj.com/articles/john-bolton-the-scandal-of-trumps-china-policy-11 592419564.

10. *EU-China: A Strategic Outlook* (Strasbourg: European Commission, March 2019), https://ec.europa.eu/commission/sites/beta-political/files/communication-eu-china-a -strategic-outlook.pdf.

11. *World Economic Outlook, April 2020: The Great Lockdown* (Washington, DC: International Monetary Fund, April 2020), http://imf.org/en/Publications/WEO/Issues/2020 /04/14/weo-april-2020; *World Economic Outlook Update: A Crisis Like No Other, An Uncertain Recovery* (Washington, DC: International Monetary Fund, June 2020), https://www .imf.org/en/Publications/WEO/Issues/2020/06/24/WEOUpdateJune2020.

12. Rym Momtaz, "Inside Macron's Coronavirus War," *Politico*, April 12, 2020, https://www.politico.eu/interactive/inside-emmanuel-macron-coronavirus-war/.

13. Peter Beinart, "Trump's Break with China Has Deadly Consequences," *The Atlantic*, March 28, 2020, https://www.theatlantic.com/ideas/archive/2020/03/breaking-china-exactly-wrong-answer/608911/.

14. For instance, see Bethany Allen-Ebrahimian, "Timeline: The Early Days of China's Coronavirus Outbreak and Cover-up," *Axios*, March 18, 2020, https://www.axios.com/timeline-the-early-days-of-chinas-coronavirus-outbreak-and-cover-up-ee65211a-afb6-4641-97b8-353718a5faab.html; "China Delayed Releasing Coronavirus Info, Frustrating WHO," Associated Press, June 3, 2020, https://apnews.com/3c061794970661042b18d5ae aaed9fae.

15. NSC-68 as published in Ernest May, ed., *American Cold War Strategy: Interpreting NSC-68* (New York: St. Martin's Press, 1993), 40.

16. *Freedom in the World 2020: A Leaderless Struggle for Democracy* (Washington, DC: Freedom House, March 4, 2020), https://freedomhouse.org/sites/default/files/2020-02/FIW_2020_REPORT_BOOKLET_Final.pdf.

17. Dominic Tierney, "What Does It Mean That Donald Trump Is Leader of the Free World," *The Atlantic*, January 24, 2017, https://www.theatlantic.com/international/archive/2017/01/trump-free-world-leader/514232/.

18. Ganesh Sitaraman, "Countering Nationalist Oligarchy," *Democracy: A Journal of Ideas* 51 (Winter 2019), https://democracyjournal.org/magazine/51/countering-nationalist-oligarchy/.

Chapter Eighteen

Building a More Globalized Order

Kori Schake

While the pandemic facilitated nationalist backlash against global supply chains and international organizations, it has actually revealed we need more globalization, not less. Our problem is overreliance on single-sourcing supplies rather than on a multiplicity of suppliers. Another issue is overreliance on a single international health organization malleable by the country in possession of its presidency rather than a web of many formal and informal groupings whose interests compete to produce Madisonian checks on power and provide a maximum of information as a basis for national and international action. Our vision for a better world should be an international order of greater connectedness and greater accountability. The method and means for attaining such an order should be to use the tools of free societies to protect and advance free societies.

What has made the American-dominated order cost-effective enough to be sustained by a reluctant hegemon is that the rules were beneficial enough to cajole voluntary compliance. Rather than construct an international order that maximized its dominance, the United States limited its direct power normatively, legally, and institutionally. It gave other states leadership roles and the ability to influence terms and institutions, which spread the burden of common problems more widely and made US dominance less objectionable than has been the case

Kori Schake is the director of foreign and defense policy studies at the American Enterprise Institute.

for previous hegemons. Leading with a light hand has served the United States well. Since the end of the Cold War, Republicans especially have clamored for changing the terms to US advantage and withdrawn from treaties and institutions they considered unduly constraining, believing the magnitude of American power alone is sufficient to safeguard the nation's interests.

The pandemic and associated policy failures in the United States have created an opening for renewed appreciation of international cooperation to create strategic depth and to identify and begin solving problems before they reach American shores. In the globalized order of our American creation, we are not strong enough to protect our interests alone. We should return to the aggravating work of coalition building, compromise, and institutional leadership so that we have the ability to see problems as they are developing and to address them before they affect American lives and grow to costlier dimensions. The only alternatives are leaving us poorer and more vulnerable to others creating an order hostile to our interests.

G. John Ikenberry's end-of-history vision of a self-sustaining liberal international order, operable even without American leadership, is not manifesting in the fifteen years of American retrenchment.[1] Middle powers have made some important contributions, but major initiatives elude without a hegemonic prime mover. It is also not clear that free world institutions are any more effective than those with universal membership; like-minded groups are more durable in agreement once compromise has been reached but are often much slower to reach it. Without the United States to drive ambitious multilateralism, middle powers are unlikely to become an effective counter-China coalition. But China's "wolf warrior" aggressiveness during the pandemic has given free societies the excuse to reevaluate policies and cooperate on both institutional and policy means for reining in China's ability to partake of the benefits of a rules-based order without shouldering its burdens, which is a good start.

The United States should not settle for a policy that is solely coercive of China, however. We are over-militarizing China policy, which plays to China's advantage since they have the easier military task, and it leaves on the sidelines the vitality and creativity of free societies. We should instead underwrite allied initiative, expand power-sharing institutions, and invest in a diplomatic and economic corps able to work bilateral relationships and drive policy agendas in overlapping multinational institutions—the G7 and an incipient D10 as well as the G20.

Pandemic recovery in the United States is certain to broaden the aperture of national security, incorporating health and preparedness and perhaps education. We should welcome those changes, as they will rebuild sources of domestic strength in the United States, which are essential to public support for an activist foreign policy that constraining China and expanding rules-based globalization will require.

The major consequences of the pandemic for the international order may be thus: renaissance in America of the value of international engagement, protection by free societies against China, and strengthening of the domestic foundations of American power.

The End of Globalization?

The COVID-19 pandemic has brought some elements of globalization to a screeching halt: movement of people across national boundaries has been completely stopped, shipping goods contracted to a tenth of their volume, and global supply chains have been revealed and questioned as countries limit export of medications, holding onto them instead for national consumption. Governments seeking to prevent crushing economic pain to their citizens are restricting assistance to foreign firms as they dispense stimulus to their own. Yet governments are not evil for preferential treatment of their own citizens, especially in a national emergency.

The United States closed its borders to immigration and barred any entry to travelers from China and other pandemic hot spots on the advice of the Centers for Disease Control and Prevention.[2] The enormous Keynesian splashing out of $2 trillion in economic stimulus was restricted to national recipients. Funding for vaccine development has likewise been national or geopolitical.

Some states, including the United States, go further, seeing economic opportunity in the pandemic to renationalize business lost to lower-cost international producers. America's trade representative accused China of profiteering off the pandemic. He said, "Onshoring America's public health industrial base is both a national imperative and the logical conclusion to draw from a pandemic that has exposed the weak underbelly of globalized supply chains and the risks of not domestically producing your essential medicines and medical countermeasures."[3]

But many of the constrictions on globalization are temporary. Businesses preceded government instruction, curtailing transport and closing shops for reputational or profitability reasons; as the pandemic recedes, those reasons will reverse direction. Draconian immigration restrictions are unsustainable and will quickly run up against the business case for both high-skilled and low-skilled labor. Green card applications are sure to rebound considerably, as will both legal and illegal immigration, once policy impediments become costly.

The activities currently impeded are also not the totality of globalization. Food has remained available and transportable through national screens on other goods. Skilled labor mobility in some fields like health care has been incentivized by relaxing credentialing.[4] Financial markets remain alarmingly volatile but robustly fluid across national borders.

Restrictions creeping into the globalized order and likely to be of long duration are not the result of the pandemic. Cross-border investment has never fully recovered from the 2008 global financial crisis. To the extent cross-border financial transactions are curbed, it is by government monetary policy that preceded the pandemic, as in China preventing convertibility of the renminbi, or using the pandemic as a geopolitical opportunity, as in the case of the United States proscribing pension funds from buying Chinese shares. The same dynamic affects cross-border data transmissions: enormous volumes yet also restricted by authoritarian government efforts to renationalize control or retain advantage in big data research for artificial intelligence.[5]

The *Economist* predicts "the pandemic will politicize travel and migration and entrench a bias towards self-reliance. This inward-looking lurch will enfeeble the recovery, leave the economy vulnerable and spread geopolitical instability."[6] Frictions will surely occur as national economies recover at different speeds. But the *Economist* is generalizing to the entirety of the world what is likelier to be a phenomenon specific to a regime type or even a specific country.

The increase of global connectedness has lurched forward and backward for centuries; it has never been a linear process, and we should not be overconcerned to see it reined back in some in ways that will diminish domestic opposition to the globalization that continues and that protects free societies from surreptitious foreign influence or overt aggression. The pandemic could just as well accelerate globalization into greater diversity of suppliers and markets, reducing single point reliance on China, in particular, to the advantage of other developing countries. That would be a net expansion of globalization, even if restricting it in one instance.

The greatest economic consequence of the pandemic probably will not be wholesale renationalization. Once economies begin to recover and dramatic stimulus measures end, businesses will return to seeking markets, investors, inexpensive supplies, and production centers. Governments worried about economic recovery are unlikely to override the business case for trade and foreign investment, with one exception.

China Rising?

The greatest economic consequence of the pandemic is likely instead to be geopolitical: free societies using policies occasioned by the pandemic to bifurcate technology, investment, education, and supply chains to exclude China. Hostility toward authoritarian regimes generally has been increasing as their incursions into free societies are exposed. But it had not been sufficient before the pandemic to exclude Russian money from the United States and the United Kingdom or to exclude Chinese government–affiliated companies from European and even rural American communications infrastructure.

China's policy decisions during the pandemic are fueling specifically Sinophobic attitudes. The rejection was already picking up speed before, but the pandemic has revealed China to be an unreliable partner—covering up existence of COVID-19, producing false data that misdirected other states' responses and inhibited protection of their populaces, grandstanding humanitarian contributions that turned out to be unhelpful, aggressively pursuing military advantage in contested territorial claims while other governments focus on public health, threatening states seeking international inquiry into origins of the pandemic, attempting to mobilize diaspora populations in free societies, and unleashing "wolf warrior" diplomacy to intimidate critics. China has managed to grab international opprobrium from the jaws of early advantage despite the mistakes of free societies.

No country has leaped economically so far and so fast as China since its 1979 jettisoning of Maoist economics, doubling the size of its economy every eight years until 2008.[7] Since 2008, however, gross domestic product growth has been trending downward to around 5.5% and has not yet settled into even a soft seabed.[8] The capital investments and productivity growth that drove China's rapid economic rise are producing diminishing returns, reforms necessary to stoke continued GDP growth have stagnated, and the middle-income trap that captures so many developing economies looms. A country that has so much to gain from Western tolerance of its continued partial participation in the rules of international order has nonetheless made sustainment of that position much more difficult by overtly rejecting the "responsible stakeholder" partnership on offer.

Whether the scattershot of aggressive policies is the result of disciplined government action, policy entrepreneurialism seeking to align with leadership preferences, or the irrepressible arrogance of a rising power shedding a policy of hiding its strength and biding its time, China has succeeded in turning both the national security and business communities against it. A general conclusion is forming, and not just among Western countries (in fact, they are some of the slowest to join), that China is seeking "to alter the norms that underpin existing institutions and put in place the building blocks of a new international system coveted by the Chinese Communist Party."[9]

The United States was not even the first mover; Australia was. Australia was the country that first excluded Huawei from its communications infrastructure in 2011 out of concern China might use access to sabotage power networks and other critical infrastructure.[10] Since then, the base of support has broadened. The Australian Parliamentary Joint Committee on Intelligence and Security concluded "that the Chinese Communist Party is working to covertly interfere with our media, our universities and also influence our political processes and public debates."[11] That is, preying on the openness of free societies to corrupt and corrode them.

And what has been surprising is how little effort China's government makes to disguise "the CCP's repurposing of globalization as an engine meant to power—and win global consent for—the party's progress toward 'the center of the global stage.'"[12] Britain's "golden era" of ties to China that Tory governments were banking on to buffer any economic damage from leaving the European Union has come to a screeching halt. The EU's lead diplomat Josep Borrell may make soothing noises, but the EU Commission's 2019 strategy considered China a "systemic rival" and the EU Parliament passed legislation condemning China's policy on Hong Kong.[13] Japan is reshaping its relations with countries on China's periphery by strengthening their coast guards to protect fisheries against Chinese intrusion and has teamed up with India to provide infrastructure financing to compete with China's Belt and Road Initiative.[14] Australia, India, Japan, and the United States have formed a "security conference of democratic states that seeks to strengthen democracy."[15] Gears are meshing in many countries to shield themselves from exposure to China.

What might have been handled as the economic jostling to create space and stature for a rising China has, in response to the belligerence of China's own actions, become a full-spectrum ideological struggle. Countries such as Germany that resent President Donald Trump's trade wars and distrust his aggressive ignorance are nonetheless being pulled into alignment with his policy direction by the activism of their own values-laden civil society. Countries such as Singapore that desperately do not want to have to choose between economic cooperation with China and hedging their bets by security cooperation with the United States see that space narrowing.

All this China might have avoided had it not burst from the penumbra of a more accommodating policy that professed to become a responsible stakeholder while continuing to flout decisions of the arbitration tribunal against it, trespass on territorial waters of its neighbors, have support for leadership roles in standard-setting international organizations, contest dominance of the next generation technologies while remaining intertwined with the universities and companies of the West, build military bases on artificial islands while the United States bleated ineffectually, lock poor countries into debt spirals while exporting its labor and capital excesses, and watch retrenchment destroy US alliances. China's policy choices may result in its worst outcome: the United States reorienting its national security strategy to focus on China and gaining allied support just as China's prospects of becoming a great-power challenger succumb to the limits of China's approach.[16]

The optimal policy for China was the strategy they adopted for the Paris Climate Agreement negotiations: demanding bilateral prior agreement with the hegemon as acknowledgment of stature while pleading the poverty of a developing country to claim the benefits others would receive, validating its partial compliance and creating the precedent of international agreement with special rules that apply only to it. The challenge for those who claim China's government consists of disciplined mandarins with a hundred-year strategic horizon is to explain why China has activated the antibodies against its continued rise now.[17] Its current policy choices seem more like trying to act to advantage to reshape the order before their window of opportunity closes.

America Sinking?

China is, of course, not the only country having a bad pandemic, politically and economically. Despite having months of warning plus a well-developed and funded public health infrastructure, the United States leads the world in COVID-19 infections and deaths, with the highest deaths per million population of any country in the world.[18] The president extols "cures" with no medical foundation and advocates dangerous social practices; enacts policies like visa cancellations that hurt education, innovation, and business creation; evidently has no national or international plan for managing either the pandemic or economic recovery; and retains the ardent support of Republicans in Congress and the party rank and file. American soft power has seldom looked less magnetic, its ability to shape the international order less persuasive.[19]

Yet, as Joseph Nye has argued, the United States has strong structural advantages: good neighbors, strong demographic trends that will keep the workforce expanding, an ecosystem for technology generation.[20] It has deep and fluid capital markets and corporate reporting requirements that make equities attractive. In addition to those advantages, it has dollar hegemony. What other country already running trillion-dollar-a-year deficits for consumption (rather than long-term investment) could get away with spending a tenth of its whole GDP in stimulus with no effect on interest rates? Exorbitant privilege indeed.

The United States also has an independent Federal Reserve that despite Trump's proclivity for narrow, nationalistic "America first" policies, has chosen to become central banker to the world: cutting interest rates, providing dollar swap lines, buying corporate bonds, dampening volatility, and reinforcing Treasury bonds as a safe haven for investors.[21] The pandemic has been an eye-popping example of the law of gross tonnage applied to economics: ships of large displacement set course and smaller craft navigate around them. In this case, the larger ship plotted a riskier course so that smaller craft would be in less danger. Where its political leadership has faltered, the dollar, capital markets, and government agencies—shielded by design from political influence—have succeeded.

The pandemic has been an elaborate morality play about the American political system, showcasing distributed power as governors, mayors, businesses, and civic groups set policy independent of or in contravention to federal demand. When the Trump administration cut funding to the World Health Organization, the Bill & Melinda Gates Foundation replaced it. Regional collectives of governors cooperated in absence of federal leadership. Converging in time with protests about police brutality and unequal justice, the military denuded its commander in chief of a praetorian guard by affirming its fealty to the Constitution, a ringing reminder of how little can be done with power unless a leader wins the political argument. American politics are messy, and they have always been messy. They are messy by design, restricting the concentration of power, tying elected officials tightly to public concern, and enabling porousness for influence by civil society.

The risk tolerance of the American public, even when obviously incurring danger, has been breathtaking, even terrifying, to behold. Americans are rebelling against the boredom of pandemic lockdowns, refusing scientific expertise about protection, treating public safety restrictions as unbearable tyranny, and tolerating thousands of new infections and hundreds of deaths each day. Former poet laureate Robert Pinsky has written, "American culture as I have experienced it seems so much in process, so brilliantly and sometimes brutally in motion, that standard models for it fail to apply."[22] We are the country whose Founding Fathers (bar one) published scurrilous diatribes under pseudonyms about one another; the country where a president (Andrew Jackson) challenged the Supreme Court to enforce its unwelcome verdicts, refusing to do so himself; the country that has impeached three presidents. It is an important cultural attribute, with a continuity from our immigrant composition through 19th-century settlers voluntarily moving into Comanche territory to policies like Chapter 11 bankruptcy's forgiveness of debt, and what Walter Russell Mead describes in *Special Providence* as "financial esprit."[23] A tolerance for volatility in public safety and prosperity marks out the country from other societies. The United States created the global financial crisis and was among the first economies to recover from it. With forty million Americans out of work and the economy contracting by 30% in the second quarter, American stock markets had both their lowest and highest bounds stretched during the pandemic.[24]

And while America's adversaries may crow about its objective failures, subjects in authoritarian regimes may also notice the limits of power forced on the president: governors and doctors unhesitatingly contradicting the president to reliably inform the public, and police and soldiers kneeling before protesters to acknowledge their demands. These subjects also see the accountability to policy decisions being forced by journalistic exposure or legal action against the government by appeal to the constitutional authority higher than law.

Even in failure, advantage in some ways still accrues to the United States, as Pulitzer Prize–winning journalist Dele Ologode points out: "The reason it has suffered this terrible blow to its reputation is because it holds itself to a higher standard and the world holds it to a higher standard. . . . The world is not protesting that Xi Jinping is locking up 1m Uighurs. . . . Nobody holds China to that kind of standard."[25]

What we have right in the US model is actually extraordinarily difficult for other countries to get right. Social cohesion may be more difficult amid diversity, but the challenge is not unique. China's looming demographic impoverishment could easily be overcome by immigration, but it lacks the cultural acceptance that makes the magnetism of America's appeal. How do you create an ecosystem accepting of change? Numerous countries want their own Silicon Valley but will not tolerate the boom-and-bust economies, build the wealthy and unfettered research universities, accept social and political upheaval of disruptive technologies at scale, or endure the cultural sanctimoniousness of tech culture. As General Ulysses S. Grant complained about his boss, Secretary of War Edward Staunton, "He could see our weakness, but he could not see that the enemy was in danger."[26] The same holds true for the United States and the West. We are excellent at diagnosing our own weaknesses and often give our adversaries and competitors unacknowledged benefit of our advantages in our assessments.

The pandemic and protests against police brutality are not the first blows to the attractiveness of America's image in the world. Those blows are legion. What makes them bruises but not mortal wounds has been two factors: (1) that many Americans shared in the condemnation, and (2) that our struggles are universal. We are not the only country in which citizens are not equal before the law, where police can be brutal, where grifters are elected to high office, or where politicians bungle disaster response. But we have the means to correct those problems, instead of suffering what Nigerian writer Chimamanda Ngozi Adichie terms "the oppressive lethargy of choicelessness."[27] And it is in the correcting that the dynamism of American society restores the country's stature. We are always one medical breakthrough, legislative compromise, or election away from deserving the power our society wields.

Durability of the Existing Order

If China ceases to rise and/or the US fails to recover, the international order could still be reshaped by states other than the great powers. There are at least four options: (1) the "rise of the rest," (2) cresting the BRIC (Brazil, Russia, India, and China) wave, (3) middle-power "coalitions of the competent," and (4) corrosion of the state system.[28] None appear imminent.

Fareed Zakaria's 2009 prediction of an emerging post-American world anticipated a fundamental redistribution of economic and political power to what had been considered the margins of the international order. "It is the birth of a truly global order."[29] That has not materialized, and the pandemic is likely to be much more devastating to developing economies since they rely on raw material demand and export-driven growth more than do the developed economies. The pandemic is also likely to put lesser-developed public health systems under crushing strain. Some marginal powers have dramatically advanced their visibility and potentially power through excellence in preparing for and handling the pandemic, but Taiwan's success is unlikely to translate into supplanting China's weight in the international order.

Excitement over the BRIC countries (South Africa was added in 2010) dimmed on the basis of their economic underperformance long before the pandemic hit and well before achieving the aspiration that "the dollar will be abandoned by most of the significant global economies and it will be kicked out of the global trade finance."[30] Collapse of commodity prices, corruption, and divergence of their economies make the grouping less meaningful than anticipated, while political frictions among members inhibit cooperative action (Brazilian president Jair Bolsonaro accused China of "buying Brazil"; India and China violently dispute their borders).[31] None of the five countries are weathering the pandemic particularly well. Brazil is second only to the United States in deaths. Russia's health system is buckling under cases. Vladimir Putin is forced to accept a fourfold decrease in oil production after six weeks of damaging dispute with Saudi Arabia and is pushed to delay the referendum on extending his presidency and further denting its legitimacy with the statistically improbable outcome.[32] So the BRICs are not replacing the existing order anytime soon.

In the absence of great-power success, or emergence of new power centers from the margins, an opportunity yawns open for middle-power cooperation to define the international order. John Ikenberry argued this would be the ultimate fulfillment of the liberal international order, when it did not require American power to sustain it.[33] That Elysian Field has not yet been attained. Ten signatories of the Trans-Pacific Partnership brought it into being even with the withdrawal of the United States, but, as Gideon Rachman has pointed out, it would not have coalesced without the American effort to get the deal in the first place. France's president Emmanuel Macron corralled fourteen European countries into an Intervention Initiative to claim strategic autonomy from the United States, but it has not actually done anything. The problem with "coalitions of the competent" is that they need a prime mover for their initiatives to reach escape velocity.[34] They can help sustain the order but are unlikely to redefine or expand it.

A final challenger to the existing order is entropy: rules corrode, institutions embrittle, great powers become unwilling or incapable of asserting order. American retrenchment and the lack of alternatives could simply produce the "emergence of a less cooperative and more fragile international system."[35] Beyond the *Economist*'s pandemic prediction, the international order could even return to the medieval model where states recede in importance and other groupings—businesses, religious organizations, cities—become the unit of action in the international order. Philip Bobbitt argues the end of international ideological competition casts into doubt the legitimacy of law, strategy, and the monopoly of violence on behalf of the state, meaning its purposes no longer suit the environment.[36]

Bobbitt's prediction may be borne out, but not for the reasons he anticipates. International coalitions of shared values transcending the geographic boundaries of states and creating competing loyalties, pervasive personal communications tools that challenge the state's control of information, and global transmissibility of money and people have created circumstances in which, for example, the US government can formally withdraw from the Paris Climate Agreement, roll back regulation of carbon emissions, and even sue the State of California for establishing standards higher than those required by the federal government. Still the actions of states, cities, businesses, philanthropists, and informed citizens making purchasing choices propel the United States into being the first country to meet its Paris Climate Agreement goals.[37] Distributed powers and mobilized publics may not destroy the state but can combine to act in its absence. Such a system would play to the civic strengths of free societies that enable such activity and benefit from diversity of activity.

The American experience of the COVID-19 pandemic suggests they cannot yet substitute for action of the federal state, however. Surely most citizens would have preferred a federal government using its international relationships and institutions as strategic depth: identifying burgeoning problems, utilizing international organizations like the World Health Organization and international relationships cultivated by the Centers for Disease Control and Prevention and federal intelligence services to get a robust understanding of pending dangers early, organizing the agencies for developing plans for assistance to affected populations that would tamp down spread, alerting governors to impending dangers so they can prepare in advance of infections, and coordinating international cooperation to create a common understanding and flow resources. These are things only the federal government has the breadth to do, and for sub-federal actors to figure out how to replace federal action takes costly time during a pandemic.

Because there continue to be constraints on acceptance of alternatives, it will be difficult to move from the equilibrium of this international order. So, advocates of the order have few practical alternatives to try to cajole the United States back into a more constructive posture. They may be aided in that task by Americans themselves. The US government's manifold failures during the pandemic may actually strengthen the current international order by demonstrating to Americans the value of their country constructively engaged in the international order we created to reduce the plagues, wars, and impoverishment that shaped the lives of World War II's survivors.

Connectedness and Accountability

American administrations of both stripes have missed important opportunities for multilateral advances; for example, no US president has expended the political capital to ratify the United Nations Convention on the Law of the Sea, even though we were a major force in its creation. We not only comply with its terms but also enforce them on other countries. But it must be acknowledged that in the past twenty-five years, Republicans have mostly lacked the creativity to pursue multilateral negotiations beyond trade. Instead, they have preferred to withdraw from treaties rather than renegotiate and to withhold funding from institutions not wholly in line with our policy preference. The Trump administration's bacchanalia of repudiation includes withdrawing from the Trans-Pacific Partnership; the Paris Climate Agreement; the Iran nuclear agreement; the UN Human Rights Council; the Intermediate-Range Nuclear Forces Treaty; the Open Skies Treaty; the UN Educational, Scientific, and Cultural Organization; and potentially the New Strategic Arms Reduction Treaty.

While Trump administration actions are damaging to structures of international cooperation and to American reliability as an international partner, they have occasioned a pendular swing toward greater support for alliances, immigration, and international trade among the public. This has resulted in a rare bipartisan congressional action to refuse funds for withdrawal of troops stationed in allied countries or repudiation of alliance commitments.[38]

Although Americans want a more internationally engaged America, they do not necessarily want the international order to remain exactly as it has been.[39] Concerns about allied free riding are not unique to the Trump administration—novel and self-defeating as their approach to achieving it may be. In fact, they parallel concerns about globalization: Americans favor them but are concerned political leaders are not preserving enough of their benefits for Americans. The experience of the pandemic should occasion reconsideration of what Nick Eberstadt terms "global integration without solidarity."[40]

China was admitted into economies, partnerships, standard-setting bodies, and institutional leadership roles without following the rules that constrained behavior of other states. And China has persisted in projecting its domestic practices onto international fora, kidnapping booksellers in Hong Kong, disappearing its own head of Interpol, manipulating the World Health Organization, violating the terms of its agreement with Britain about Hong Kong, reweighting the International Monetary Fund basket of currencies without making the renminbi convertible.

Forcing China to play by the rules will only be possible if the United States forms a united front with other countries also experiencing Chinese "exceptionalism." That means we need to prioritize our grievances and not pick fights—on trade or burden sharing or denigrating leaders—on all fronts. We need to create incentives and alternatives to China's monopoly positions, and that means further diversifying supply chains, not renationalizing them across the board.

The devastation wreaked by the pandemic on American lives and the economy is sure to engender recovery programs that expand the definition of national security beyond its current pinched and militaristic confines. These programs, too, could strengthen the existing international order by strengthening the domestic foundations of American power. For example, use economic recovery programs to repair and update infrastructure, make health care portable rather than reliant on employment to improve both health and labor mobility, generate broader-based prosperity, and expand access to quality education. These are not only social goods in themselves; they are necessary precursors for Americans to care about the shape of the international order.

The cost of rejuvenating the economy and smoothing over the disruptions caused by the pandemic is likely to create sustained downward pressure on defense spending. If indulged, this will incur increased risk of the United States losing its wars and will encourage challengers to test that proposition. But it will also likely create sustained downward pressure on spending for nonmilitary elements of American power. We already have a foreign policy that lurches toward the military; unless we spend the money and attention to balance our portfolio by expanding the size and capability of our diplomatic and economic professionals, our policies will become even more militarized. As the architect of the National Defense Strategy points out, our strategy for managing China is not over-militarized, but its execution is because the Department of Defense is the only arm of government carrying out the strategy.[41]

US policy in the Trump era has become a jeremiad of demands rather than the practice of diplomacy, that we can wring maximal gains out of every negotiation without creating enduring resentment. It is not and we cannot. We need to work through institutions such as ASEAN or the UN that may not be valuable to us but are to others. We need at least to tolerate institutions we do not participate in such as the International Criminal Court that serve others well and expend the effort to bring our own practice in line with the rules, by, for example, ratifying the Convention on the Law of the Sea. We even need to make compromises that advantage others to gain their voluntary cooperation, because that is less expensive than coercing compliance.

That international institutions and cooperation are imperfect is, however exasperating, immaterial to the fact that they are the genius of the American-led world order and our greatest lever to bring others into line with our practices. In 1945, when America stood astride the world like a colossus, comprising half of the world's GDP and with a military that had won wars on both sides of the world, it voluntarily restrained its own power by creating rules and institutions that shared power. It is through those rules and institutions that the United States shares the costs and responsibilities of solving problems before they take on costlier and more dangerous dimensions for us to bear alone.

NOTES

1. G. John Ikenberry, "The Future of the Liberal World Order: Internationalism after America," *Foreign Affairs* 90, no. 3 (May/June 2011): 56–68.

2. Joel Rose, "Immigration to the U.S. Comes to a Standstill during the Pandemic," NPR, May 20, 2020.

3. Jeff Stein, Robert Costa, and Josh Dawsey, "White House Aides Torn over Trade Hawk's Proposal as President Trump Weighs Action on China," *Washington Post*, April 29, 2020.

4. Silva Mathema, "Removing Barriers for Immigrant Medical Professionals Is Critical to Help Fight Coronavirus," Center for American Progress, April 2, 2020.

5. Danny O'Brien, "China's Global Reach: Surveillance and Censorship beyond the Great Firewall," Electronic Frontier Foundation, October 10, 2019; and Eiichi Tomiura, Banri Ito, and Byeongwoo Kang, "Cross-Border Data Transfers under New Regulations: Findings from a Survey of Japanese Firms," Vox, CEPR Policy Portal, March 14, 2020.

6. "Has Covid-19 Killed Globalization?," *The Economist*, May 14, 2020.

7. Wayne M. Morrison, *China's Economic Rise: History, Trends, Challenges, and Implications for the United States*, RL33534 (Washington, DC: Library of Congress, Congressional Research Service, June 25, 2019).

8. "World Economic Outlook Database," International Monetary Fund, April 2019.

9. Nadège Rolland, *China's Vision for a New World Order*, NBR Special Report No. 83 (Seattle: National Bureau of Asian Research, January 2020), 2, https://www.nbr.org/wp-content/uploads/pdfs/publications/sr83_chinasvision_jan2020.pdf.

10. Australian Signals Directorate chief Michael Burgess, quoted in Jamie Smythe, "Australia Banned Huawei over Risks to Key Infrastructure," *Financial Times*, March 27, 2019; and Meaghan Tobin, "Huawei Ban: Australia Becomes Increasingly Isolated among

Five Eyes Partners If UK Includes Chinese Firm in 5G Network," *South China Morning Post*, April 26, 2019.

11. Committee chair Andrew Hastie, quoted in Emily Baumgaertner and Jacqueline Williams, "In Australia, Fears of Chinese Meddling Rise on U.N. Bribery Case Revelation," *New York Times*, May 22, 2018.

12. Matt Schrader, "China Is Weaponizing Globalization," *Foreign Policy*, June 5, 2020.

13. Annabelle Timsit, "Parliaments Are on the Frontlines of Europe's Face-Off with China," Quartz, June 19, 2020.

14. Jay Tristan Tarriela, "How Abe Remade the Japan Coast Guard," *The Diplomat*, January 24, 2020.

15. Alyssa Ayres, "The Quad and the Free and Open Indo-Pacific," Council on Foreign Relations, November 20, 2018.

16. Michael Beckley, "China's Economy Is Not Overtaking America's," *Journal of Applied Corporate Finance* 32, no. 2 (Spring 2020): 10.

17. For example, see Michael Pillsbury, *The Hundred-Year Marathon: China's Secret Strategy to Replace America as the Global Superpower* (New York: St. Martin's Press, 2015).

18. "COVID-19 Coronavirus Pandemic," Worldometer, https://www.worldometers .info/coronavirus/?utm_campaign=homeAdvegas1?.

19. Arvind Subramanian, "The Coronavirus Is Accelerating America's Decline," MarketWatch, May 11, 2020.

20. Joseph Nye, "No, the Coronavirus Will Not Change the Global Order," *Foreign Policy*, April 16, 2020.

21. T. Rowe Price, "The Federal Reserve: Central Banker to the World," April 28, 2020.

22. Robert Pinsky, *Democracy, Culture, and the Voice of Poetry* (Princeton, NJ: Princeton University Press, 2002), 76.

23. Walter Russell Mead, *Special Providence: American Foreign Policy and How It Changed the World* (New York: Routledge, 2002), 232.

24. Mohammed el-Erian, "Wall Street Is Flourishing While Main Street Is Suffering," *Foreign Policy*, May 29, 2020.

25. Dele Olojode, quoted in David Pilling, "'Everybody Has Their Eyes on America': Black Lives Matter Goes Global," *Financial Times*, June 20, 2020.

26. Ulysses S. Grant, *Personal Memoirs of Ulysses S. Grant*, ed. Mary McFeeley and William S. McFeeley (New York: Library of America, 1990), lxx.

27. Chimamanda Ngozi Adichie, *Americanah* (New York: Random House, 2013), 341.

28. The terms come from Fareed Zakaria, Goldman Sachs, and Michael Fullilove, respectively.

29. Fareed Zakaria, *The Post-American World* (New York: W. W. Norton, 2009), 1–3.

30. Governor of Russia's Central Bank, Elvira Nabiullina, quoted in, "BRICs Morphing into Anti-dollar Alliance," Voice of Russia, July 3, 2014.

31. Sandrine Amiel, "What's BRICS for and Does It Still Make Sense?," *Euronews*, November 11, 2019.

32. Patrick Reevell, "Putin Granted Right to Extend Rule Till 2036 in Overwhelming Referendum Result," *ABC News*, July 1, 2020; "EU Calls for Investigation into Irregularities in 'Triumphant' Vote for Putin," *Radio Free Europe*, July 2, 2020.

33. Ikenberry, "The Future of the Liberal World Order."

34. "Who Runs the World?," *The Economist,* June 18, 2020.

35. Alexander Cooley and Daniel H. Nexon, "How Hegemony Ends: The Unraveling of American Power," *Foreign Affairs* 99, no. 4 (July/August 2020): 143–156.

36. Philip Bobbitt, *The Shield of Achilles: War, Peace, and the Course of History* (New York: Anchor, 2003), 667.

37. Julia Rosen, "Cities, States and Companies Vow to Meet U.S. Climate Goals without Trump. Can They?," *Los Angeles Times,* November 4, 2019.

38. Joe Gould, "Congress Moves to Block Trump's Germany Troop Withdrawal Plans," *Defense News,* June 30, 2020.

39. Dina Smeltz et al., "Rejecting Retreat," Chicago Council on Global Affairs, September 6, 2019.

40. Nicholas Eberstadt, "Can Pax Americana Survive the Coronavirus?," *Wall Street Journal,* June 19, 2020.

41. Jim Mattis, personal interview, June 18, 2020.

Chapter Nineteen

Could the Pandemic Reshape World Order, American Security, and National Defense?

Kathleen H. Hicks

The COVID-19 pandemic seems at once to be top of mind for international relations scholars while low on their list of enduring drivers. As economists and public health experts tally the virus's accumulating effects, prominent international relations scholars have generally limited their analysis to the ways in which COVID-19 is accelerating trends already underway. Structural explanations prevail. The US national security community appears more concerned but conflicted. Will the pandemic convince Americans to draw inward, amplifying nationalist sentiments and reducing the appetite for multilateral approaches? Or will it give new impetus for global engagement?

Making predictions in the middle of the pandemic is fraught. Yet history and recent events provide guides, and they point toward this pandemic mattering and mattering big. It will not only accelerate changes underway, but if policy makers are up for the challenge, it presents an opportunity to reshape the future of world order and national security. For defense watchers, this prospect is both daunting and fortuitous. The US defense world could use some reshaping if it is to contribute effectively to the nation's future.

Kathleen Hicks is senior vice president, Henry A. Kissinger Chair, and director of the International Security Program at the Center for Strategic and International Studies and the Donald Marron Scholar at the Kissinger Center for Global Affairs.

COVID-19 and the International System

Some prominent analysts have spoken of COVID-19 as "an accelerant" to trends already underway in the international system. "The pandemic and the response to it," one writes, "have revealed and reinforced the fundamental characteristics of geopolitics today."[1] COVID-19 is undeniably serving this accelerating function in several ways. Yet there is also evidence the pandemic may help reshape the international system. If democratic-minded nations can seize on this potential, the straight-line projections of the accelerant narrative would be inadequate to capture the force of COVID-19's effects.

The frame of competition among great powers, so prominent in US national security circles, is clearly playing out during the pandemic. In addition to continued foreign policy adventurism by Russia, Iran, and North Korea, China has attempted a multipronged influence campaign around COVID-19, including covering up and misinforming on the scale of cases inside China; undertaking health diplomacy, such as providing personal protective equipment (PPE) to Italy and other hard-hit countries; issuing official statements blaming others; and manipulating social media to divide Western countries.[2] Russia and Iran have undertaken less ambitious but similar efforts.[3] Ever audacious, Russia pointedly donated medical equipment to the United States in April 2020. President Donald Trump, for his part, has attempted to focus attention on China's inaction and dissembling at the outset of the outbreak, but he has done so using racist language about COVID-19, referring to it as "kung flu" and the "Chinese virus." Secretary of State Mike Pompeo has repeatedly called it the "Wuhan virus."[4]

As the pandemic turns up the heat between the United States and China, it is illuminating two facts at once. First, it underscores that the most important bilateral power dynamic for the coming decades is between these two countries. Second, however, it provides further evidence that bipolarity will be an inadequate description for the evolving international system.[5] Competition between the United States and China is not on pace to define the system to the same degree US-Soviet relations defined the Cold War era, and COVID-19 has set them back even further. Neither nation has fared well in managing the pandemic, with trust and confidence declining for both. The world is not nonpolar, but these two powers, it seems, have failed to generate magnetism sufficient to induce the levels of bandwagoning and/or balancing behavior expected of bipolar systems.

Instead, countries such as Germany and South Korea, and, but for Sweden, the European Union, have proved more adept and resilient in managing the crisis.

This may only fuel the degree of independence some states and entities are exerting from the United States and China, including other great (although lesser) powers, from the European Union (or France and Germany, if the reader prefers), the United Kingdom, and Japan to India to Russia. Several of these great powers, as well as Pakistan, North Korea, and soon potentially Iran, are also declared nuclear weapons states, further complicating simplistic bipolarity narratives.[6]

Then there are the transnational and subnational issues affecting the nature and expression of power itself. Even before COVID-19, several such trends were demonstrating their importance to the international system. Climate change stands out, given its potential to affect states' sources of strength—especially economic, demographic, and geographic—as well as their inclinations toward cooperation and conflict as they seek to mitigate and adapt to changes underway.[7] Also notable is the revolution in advanced technologies, which is proliferating know-how and production in fields like biology, information and computing, and robotics, both across states and below the state level. Shifts in military and economic power differentials could come from any of these vectors, but they are most likely to come at the intersection of several. For example, global information consumption, advanced computing algorithms, the availability of vast amounts of social media data, and automation are combining to influence operations of unprecedented scale. In many cases, these campaigns aim at dividing societies and nations, amplifying ideational challenges between autocracies and democracies, feeding ethnic nationalism, and amplifying concerns around globalization and internationalism.

As a pandemic, COVID-19 manifests the potential of transnational challenges to interstate relations and the operations of the international system. It is also begetting or accelerating a range of other transnational and subnational trends. In addition to spurring new influence operations, tension between globalization and nationalism is playing out around travel bans, support for the World Health Organization, and the search for supply-chain independence. Two prominent political scientists recently warned that amid COVID, "the world seems to be headed toward growing division and national self-reliance."[8]

Where mere acceleration of trends ends and reshaping of the international system begins is open to some debate. Still, it appears that a collective focus on the former is obscuring evidence of the latter. Just as jarring global events, like wars, have done in the past, it is worth asking whether COVID-19 may shift the trajectory of the international system toward greater order. Several scholars are skeptical the pandemic will or can do so.[9] Yet there are some early signals in domestic and foreign affairs that should not be quickly dismissed. Three of the most notable signs are moves by some democratic regional powers to balance nationalism with greater international engagement, the growth of citizen movements, and expanding public awareness of and push back against influence campaigns.

First, the abject failures of the United States and China to lead international COVID efforts is spurring greater voter engagement on internationalism inside the United States and other democracies, providing some green shoots of hope for a shift toward greater cooperation. In the wake of Brexit, when a further unwinding of the European Union seemed possible, the EU instead demonstrated substantial appetite for integration with its creation of a COVID-19 stimulus fund. Similarly, South Korean president Moon Jae-in used the banner "Corona Diplomacy" to convince the G20 to hold a virtual emergency summit on COVID in March 2020.[10] These democracies, largely performing well in meeting the pandemic's challenges, are developing more agency and moving to act cooperatively in the absence of global leadership from elsewhere. Recent polling suggests most of the US public shares this interest in greater global engagement and multilateral approaches to tackle security problems.[11]

Second, autocracy may be winning, but democracy is poised for a resurgence. The downward slide in global freedom is well documented and has been ongoing for nearly fifteen years.[12] Existing restrictions on citizen liberties in North Korea, China, Russia, and Iran have been accompanied more recently by backsliding in places like the United States, Hungary, and Saudi Arabia as well as substantial new repression in India. Unsurprisingly, attacks from right-wing extremists grew more than 230% from 2013 to 2018 in the United States, Oceania, and Europe.[13] COVID-19 and the societal restrictions imposed to combat it have already been used to generate new conspiracy theories and further fuel such extremism, resulting in neo-Nazi attacks in the United States.[14]

The decline of freedom is not standing unchallenged. Over the past decade, protest movements have been on the rise, growing more than 11% globally between 2009 and 2019 and above that level in the advanced democracies of Europe and North America. In 2019 alone, anti-government protests occurred in 114 countries.[15] A 2016 labor rights protest in India drew the largest protest crowds in history, estimated at more than 180 million people.[16] The five largest protest gatherings in US history have all occurred since the 2017 inauguration of President Trump, each significantly larger than his inauguration crowd.[17]

Where it is not repressed, people in the streets can translate into people at the ballot box. In the 2018 US congressional midterm election, almost 50% of the eligible voting population voted, the highest percentage of midterm voters since 1914. In 2014, just one midterm cycle earlier, turnout had been the lowest in seventy-two years, at 36.7%. This is not solely a US phenomenon; voting has surged in Europe as well. The December 2019 European Union parliament elections saw the highest EU turnout percentage since 1994.[18] The outcomes of these elections in the United States and Europe did not all point in one political direction. In several European countries, nationalist parties performed very well. Nevertheless, the degree of recent voter engagement is striking, juxtaposed as it is against global threats to freedom. In the first half of 2020, Chinese repression in Hong Kong and police brutality and systemic racism in the United States seem to have only propelled global protests and citizen mobilization.

Finally, there are signs that the pandemic is spurring greater democratic resilience to influence operations. As noted previously, China has substantially ramped up its disinformation efforts in the United States and around the world in the wake of its early failure to stem the pandemic.[19] China is not alone. Russia and Iran are suspected of similar information campaigns aimed at deflecting from their own pandemic challenges and seeding doubts and divisions in the West.[20] Such disinformation efforts align fully with the kind of gray zone tactics that periods of intense interstate competition breed. Compared to prior years, however, democracies around the world have been especially quick to "name and shame" China and others engaged in disinformation, calling early attention to the problem and providing early and direct health information to publics in ways that build trust in these democratic governments.

Of course, some disinformation efforts are coming from inside Western societies themselves. In the United States, President Trump, other elected officials, and those close to them have also lied and misled on public health safety issues arising during the pandemic. These efforts, while still deadly in their effects, have been blunted by the competence and airtime afforded to epidemiologists and other health professionals. Moreover, the pandemic's propensity to deliver outcomes that align to expert advice has helped push back against conspiracy theories and lies. Whereas the public had grown cynical about expertise prior to COVID-19, by April 2020, more than two in three Americans expressed trust in the Centers for Disease Control and Prevention and their doctors for accurate information. Fewer than one in four put great faith in President Trump's public health information.[21] This figure fell well below Trump's electoral polling, which suggests that even some of his supporters are distinguishing between his attractiveness as a political figure and his reliability as a public health leader. It is more difficult for disinformation to thrive in an environment where expertise is valued, and small gains may be built upon in other areas. The Black Lives Matter movement appears to be further spurring counters to disinformation. The capture of Ahmaud Arbery's and George Floyd's killings on video and the subsequent crowdsource debunking of antifa attacks are empowering citizens to use technology to reset popular paradigms of fact and fiction.

The pandemic thus may not only be shaping the international order, it may be shaping it in positive directions that previously seemed unlikely. Whether positive change now follows depends largely on the direction taken by great powers. Democracies have an opportunity for collective action. If they can capture it, the nature of their security and the order itself may improve. Nowhere is this possibility more tantalizing than in the United States.

National Security Anew

COVID's potential to reshape our world extends from the international sphere to the making of US national security. As of this writing, more than 130,000 Americans have died from COVID-19, with well over 2.3 million cases of the virus reported in the United States.[22] The economic impacts of the pandemic are historic in scale, generating sizable business closures and unemployment while prompting massive government stimulus spending. A pair of McKinsey analysts likens the moment to America's mobilizations for two world wars. Rather than ask residents to join a war effort beyond their homes, government incentives during COVID-19 are designed in part to help people socially distance and reduce non-essential activity.[23]

How could this seismic dislocation fail to affect how Americans pursue national security? History suggests Americans typically adjust policy agendas at home and abroad as world events emerge. The Soviet space program led to the National Defense Education Act, failures in Vietnam led President Richard Nixon to China, the dissolution of the Soviet Union begot new attention to small wars and ethnic conflicts, 9/11 shifted US focus to countering terrorists around the world and fighting regime-changing wars in the Middle East, and, most recently, Russian and Chinese coercion has led to renewed priority on "great-power competition." Yet these examples also demonstrate that Americans often react late, tend to "fight the last war," tune out foresight analysis, and at times reach for cures that are worse than the disease. The most important question for national security, then, is not *whether* COVID-19 will affect our conception of global challenges and US strategy but *how well* we meet the challenge.

The most immediate implication of COVID-19 for US national security will be to strengthen long-standing efforts to broaden the conception of security to encompass health, climate, and domestic economic and societal competitiveness. The stimulus packages already passed into law begin the needed reboot of the global health policy agenda, which had been a priority for multiple congresses and administrations prior to the Trump administration's evisceration of these programs. The goal now will be to shift from the "cycle of crisis and complacency" on global health to building enduring pandemic preparedness.[24]

This pandemic's legacy will also be felt in a more rapid embrace of climate change as a priority issue in national security. Health and climate are linked, and approaches to addressing them also share similarities: they typically require action at the local, national, and international level; the private sector and regular citizens meaningfully contribute to solutions for both; they affect everyone, but they will hit the world's most vulnerable first and hardest; they are best met with long-term, preventative policies; and many of the means to effect change lie outside the traditional national security tool kit. It thus bears exploring the implications of climate change more closely, as COVID-19 is likely to help it resonate as a national security issue with average citizens and security experts.

Heretofore a deeply partisan issue, climate change is increasingly a bipartisan priority for millennials and Generation Z voters. In the 2020 presidential election cycle, this cohort will be equal in size to baby boomers and their predecessors (aged 56 and older).[25] That climate change is a threat has long been accepted by the national security community. More than a decade ago, the US intelligence community concluded that "global climate change will have wide-ranging implications for US national security interests over the next 20 years."[26] With COVID, the politics, technology, and economics of climate change are finally catching up to analysts' concerns.

As a security issue, climate change multiplies security challenges in four major ways: (1) it threatens the existence of nations, (2) it makes weak states weaker, (3) it drives new contests among the strong, and (4) it imposes financial costs on security providers.

Eliminates territory: Sea level rise fueled by warming at the Earth's poles creates a near-term existential crisis for island nations, especially in the Pacific Ocean. For instance, the Marshall Islands, with its population of more than fifty-five thousand, expects to be underwater by 2030.[27] Nations in the Caribbean Sea, those at low altitude, and those with low-lying areas are also vulnerable to extinction or substantial dislocation.

Makes weak states weaker: Climate change accelerates instability by exacerbating underlying socioeconomic and political problems. It puts pressure on water resources, food production, and livelihoods and is affecting first many who are least able to cope. This includes nations that lack the governance practices and institutions to address the needs of their citizens. According to UN population projections, of the one hundred fastest-growing cities (by population), eighty-four are categorized as facing extreme risks of climate change and a further fourteen face high climate risks, mostly in Africa and Asia.[28] These results may be seen in the number and scale of humanitarian disasters, disease outbreaks, socioeconomic unrest, mass migration, crime, corruption, and intrastate violence, as well as interstate tensions. There is even a link to the flow of migrants from Central America across the US border, as climate change degrades farming conditions in places like Guatemala.[29]

Drives new geopolitical competition: Geopolitical competition is also playing out in climate change. Nowhere is this more evident than the Arctic. Since 2002, NASA estimates that the Arctic minimum sea ice has declined at a rate of 12.8% per decade.[30] The region is hotter today than it has been at any point over the last four thousand years. With sea lanes opening, transits of the Bering Strait have more than doubled in the past decade.[31] Russia, the United States, and other nations adjacent to the Arctic, and China, which is attempting to brand itself as a "near Arctic" nation, all have expressed interest in the Arctic's natural resources, including minerals and petrochemicals. These nations also find the promise of shorter shipping routes between East Asia and the Atlantic Ocean appealing. New coastlines are also generating new military facilities in strategic locations, especially by Russia.

Security provider costs: The Department of Defense's own capacity to respond to climate-related disasters is under strain. The US military operates in many areas of the world that face significant degradations from climate change, including within the United States. In 2018 and 2019, extreme weather at Tyndall Air Force Base (Florida), Marine Corps Base Camp Lejeune (North Carolina), and Offutt Air Force Base (Nebraska) inflicted more than $8 billion in damage.[32] Financial costs on the military are also borne when the US military deploys in support of civilian agencies at home, such as with forest fires and hurricanes, and overseas, such as with tsunami relief. The Pentagon must brace for budget and readiness impacts resulting from climate-related increases in the frequency and severity of natural disasters.

Health and climate are just two of the "nontraditional" issues propelled to the center of the national security agenda in 2020. The United States is stumbling in meeting the task of global economic competition and Russian and Chinese gray zone tactics like political, economic, and information coercion. These failures, taken together with COVID-19, the brutal killing of George Floyd, and the profoundly imprudent use of force against protesters in Washington, DC, have weakened US global standing. As I have argued elsewhere, healing America's domestic dysfunctions is a national security imperative.[33] The politicization and utter failure of US actions in response to COVID-19, and the spectacle of the Trump administration's strongman showmanship in the face of calls for racial justice, send signals of ineptness that play directly into competitors' narratives and plans. The United States cannot compete to secure its interests in the global arena when it is incapable of unifying and progressing its society at home.

With all that COVID-19 is revealing, US national security is primed for change. Advancing a more encompassing approach to security requires a new look at our national strategies, institutions, and investments. Disruptive collaboration that hones the nation's competitive edge will require trust and partnership between the government and the private sector. Competing effectively also requires pooled approaches with like-minded democracies. The US alliance system and international institutions need both repair and new vision. A next generation of diplomats must be grown. Information must be elevated as a significant element of foreign policy and economic statecraft expanded not only to coerce rivals' behavior but also to persuade friends and partners. In a world of growing multipolarity, the United States will need the collective strength of civil society, academia and businesses, and allies and partners to meet the challenge China and other authoritarian states present to its interests.

Implications for the Military

The United States will also still need its military. Acknowledging the many security needs that exist outside the military realm does not erase the reality that China, Russia, and other states are demonstrating the will and capability to use military forces to alter the character of the international system on terms that threaten American democracy and prosperity as well as the rule of law. Many Americans wrongly assume the nation retains a tolerable military edge to deter threats to its vital interests. The US advantage is eroding. Russia and China are aggressively pursuing advanced military capabilities, including in missiles, cyberspace, and space, and they are also using fait accompli tactics, disinformation, and proxy warfare to achieve relative gains.

The COVID-19 pandemic worsens many aspects of military competition for the United States. It is heightening the level of threat, requiring increased attention on the health and readiness of the armed forces, and expanding needs for defense support to civil authority at home and possibly abroad. These realities worsen the already troubled fiscal picture confronting the Department of Defense. Added to the sluggish pace of US adaptation to, or counterstrategy for, the high-low mix of capabilities and tactics potential adversaries are putting forth, prospects for defending against some classes of military threats are waning. As with national security more broadly, however, COVID-19 presents an opportunity to reshape rather than just accelerate current military trends seeming to favor Russia and China.

Military Threats in the Pandemic

Adventurism by China and Russia continues amid the COVID-19 outbreak. In the first half of 2020, China has renewed tensions with India over disputed border territory. It has also provoked skirmishes in the South China Sea with Vietnam and Malaysia, with the latter incident involving US and Australian vessels as well. It has stepped up its maritime activities near Taiwan, as has the United States, and near Japan. Perhaps most ominously, it has imposed a new national security law in Hong Kong that expands the Chinese Communist Party's digital and physical autocracy beyond its mainland.

Even as China agitates beyond its borders, the pandemic will almost certainly push back its military spending agenda. Using its own, usually rosy, assessments, the pandemic has damaged China's economy, with growth declining by 6.8% in the first quarter of 2020. Likely more telling of COVID's effects is China's announcement to forego any growth targets for this year.[34] Then, in May, China announced its smallest planned increase in defense spending in thirty years. The reported defense downshift is small, and future People's Liberation Army (PLA) budget trends bear monitoring. Beyond assessing shifts in its defense top line, understanding how China is spending its defense funds would shed light on COVID's impacts. China is not prone to provide such transparency, but it is reasonable to assume that it will divert military funds to cover costs related to the pandemic, including the PLA's role in domestic security, internal infrastructure projects, and force health and readiness expenses. Its industrial base is also likely suffering during COVID, due to worker absenteeism and possible work stoppages.

The Russian military, and likely its industrial base, are also suffering from mismanagement of the virus. First claiming no military personnel were infected,

Russia has been forced to announce some quarantines in its army.[35] The Russian defense budget was already projected to decline slightly in FY2021, and COVID's effects on the Russian economy, together with the collapse of oil prices, will pressurize it further. However, Russia has typically protected its highest-priority military projects during difficult times, and it is reasonable to assume President Vladimir Putin will attempt to do so again in the coming years.

To date, Russian aggression has continued during the pandemic. It undertook unsafe fighter maneuvers near US aircraft operating in the Mediterranean. It performed a direct-ascent antisatellite missile test, following on the heels of weapon-like satellite maneuvers near US space assets in February. Most notably, it stepped up the scale of its presence in Libya even as it remains engaged in Eastern Ukraine, Crimea, and Syria. As noted previously, its influence operations also continue apace, focused on influencing the forthcoming US presidential election, European democracies, and the transatlantic relationship.

The US Military and COVID-19

As China, Russia, and others grapple with the pandemic's effects on their economies and militaries, and continue to press against US interests, America's military is confronting its own challenges. Most immediately, it must attend to the health of service members and their families, as well as the broader defense workforce. Health and readiness are interdependent: health precautions impede some readiness measures, but a sick force cannot be a ready force. To date, the armed services have stayed relatively healthy and relatively ready. The most significant and public COVID-19 outbreak occurred on the USS *Theodore Roosevelt*, an incident that brought the resignation of an acting navy secretary and the firing of the vessel's captain. Overall, however, the number and severity of infections has been manageable. The Department of Defense cannot take for granted this will continue and thus must sustain focused attention—and investment—to ensure COVID-19 does not become a significant health and readiness challenge. This necessitates use of temporary quarantines, shifts in exercise plans, and other adaptations.

In addition to health and readiness concerns for its own, the Department of Defense also has a long history of providing defense support to civilian authorities in times of national emergency. President Trump declared COVID-19 to be just such a national emergency in March 2020, with a lackluster federal response following thereafter. After this very slow start, the Department of Defense has dedicated some attention and resources to its domestic support mission. It has not fully met the potential of its role in assisting contracting efforts through the Defense Production Act, and its early efforts to lend medical personnel and assets, such as hospital ships, were underwhelming. More recently, the president tasked the secretary of defense with co-leading Operation Warp Speed, which aims to rapidly produce and distribute a vaccine to Americans. It is too early to judge that effort.

The Pentagon's slow response in aiding civil authorities on COVID-19 stands in contrast to the speed with which it found itself embroiled in the White House's plans for countering Black Lives Matter protests. The ensuing civil-military crisis erupting in Lafayette Park and around Washington, DC, in June 2020 may generate further pressure to rebalance the national security enterprise away from military solutions. Trust between citizen and soldier is central to healthy civil-military relations in a democracy. Now more than at any other time in a generation, the military establishment may be called on to prove itself worthy of that trust, and of the investment American taxpayers make in it.

The pandemic is thus pressurizing defense spending by increasing demands on its resources at the same time economic and societal trends may be lowering the total funds available. Before COVID, the Trump administration was already signaling that the defense budget would likely be lower in a second term. At the beginning of 2020, the budget deficit was running at about $1 trillion, and deficit hawks were looking ahead to the potential for more constrained federal spending in a hoped-for second term. The pandemic has now eliminated the possibility of significant near-term deficit reduction. Stimulus funds to help the economy survive and recover from the coronavirus have ballooned the deficit to $4 trillion, with the potential for further spending to come. Together with the trust deficit the military now bears with some lawmakers and citizens, and the desire to invest in other areas of American competitiveness and national security, the new fiscal reality has only increased the pressure to constrain defense spending in the next presidential administration, no matter which candidate wins.

A squeeze on military spending will not be easily borne. The United States does not retain the advantages it once had, and the hurdles to cutting smartly are high. Despite the Winston Churchill adage, running out of money does not always generate more thoughtful approaches to strategy and, without strong leadership, can amplify rather than stamp out bureaucratic pathologies. Yet neither does having more defense dollars equate to better capabilities or likely victory. There are simply too many political and bureaucratic factors affecting how defense dollars are spent to make a direct correlation between inputs and outcomes one way or another. If US history provides any guide on these matters, it is that the nation at times reaches pivot points in which it acts to reshape its national security approach and America's military. COVID-19 cannot take full credit for bringing the United States to this point, but its role is larger than is currently acknowledged and certainly greater than a mere accelerant to the process.

It is not enough to reach a pivot point. One must also exploit it. Many changes are needed to compete effectively in the modern military realm, including limiting ongoing military operations and making greater use of collective approaches and nonmilitary foreign policy tools.[36] Three force development priorities particularly bear mention for reshaping America's defense in a post-pandemic world.

1. The United States must conceive, test, and constantly adapt its strategic and operational approaches in line with its goals. It must have theories of victory. The leadership of the Department of Defense spends most of its energy building budgets, monitoring current operations, and navigating acquisition issues. Its strategic and conceptual enterprises are too often backwaters. If the department is to change the way it fights, it must start with an enterprise-wide commitment to the operational art, tied to strategic purpose and experimented with routinely. Failure is an option, and the more it happens early and cheaply, the better for the evolution of thought and capability. If the US military is going to seize the advantage rather than react to advances made by others, its leaders must be selected, trained, and rewarded for these attributes.

2. In an era of competition and global threats, the United States would do well to ensure flexibility with a high-low mix of capabilities. Even as it takes a portfolio approach, the US military should prioritize in two crosscutting areas. First, it should capitalize on its own asymmetries, at the strategic (e.g., alliance), technological (e.g., undersea warfare), and operational (e.g., a ready and well-trained force) levels. If defense spending is cut substantially, many worthy investments may need to be slowed or shelved, so getting the asymmetries right will be vital. Second, it should ensure sufficient investment to close gaping weaknesses, especially in logistics, cyberspace, information operations, and space. Relative US advantages and weaknesses will shift over time, so this force development priority must interact with the prior one. The United States will need a systems approach in which it continuously assesses capability investments against current theories of victory while using its capability findings to inform the evolution of those theories.

3. The United States will need a global posture that acknowledges the pressure for speed of response with the need to provide sanctuary for follow-on forces. Allies and partners that are resident in Europe and Asia can and should provide significant elements of localized early response. Nevertheless, there are advantages for the United States in positioning certain types of capabilities close to potential adversaries. Ensuring strong relationships with allies and partners will be vital to ensuring needed access for American forces and for generating the capabilities and interoperability required during crises.

A shift in approach cannot come soon enough. The US rhetoric on competition is well outpacing the reality of its capabilities, both across society and within defense. Cultural change is not happening swiftly enough, hampered by a business-as-usual approach on personnel, conceptual art, experimentation, acquisition, and budget. The political will to take unpopular stances is low, including needed decisions to curtail some current production, to close underused installations, to redesign structures and operations, and to undertake substantial benefit reform. If the moment passes, COVID's legacy for the military may simply be to further expand the distance between the goals of American deterrence and its ability to credibly achieve them.

Conclusion

The ongoing COVID-19 pandemic is reshaping the world as we know it. The United States and China matter tremendously to the future order, but states are glimpsing a true world of anarchy facilitated by these two powers, and they are looking beyond their own borders for ways to manage it. The American public also sees disorder and the nation's contribution to it. Together with evidence of systemic dysfunction at home, the United States is beginning to grapple with the need for change and assessing the domestic and international elements that might strengthen Americans' safety, prosperity, and freedoms. Countervailing trends toward ethnic nationalism and government control coexist with these realities, as they have for at least the last decade. With all that the pandemic has exposed, however, the winds of change are blowing more clearly toward a chance for reform and renewal.

For defense watchers, these trends might be ominous. US defense spending is likely to decline in the coming years, under pressure from the reshaping of American national security and in the presence of fiscal challenges that the pandemic is substantially compounding. America's military is still needed, and it is in some trouble. Yet there is opportunity for the US military in the broader shifts under-way, from increased economic competitiveness to strengthened tools of statecraft to repaired relations with allies. The pandemic may just be the long-awaited gal-vanizing moment the United States needs to generate major improvements in its military and defense enterprise.

NOTES

1. See, for example, Richard Haass, "The Pandemic Will Accelerate History Rather Than Reshape It," *Foreign Affairs*, April 7, 2020, https://www.foreignaffairs.com/articles /united-states/2020-04-07/pandemic-will-accelerate-history-rather-reshape-it.

2. Edward Wong, Matthew Rosenberg, and Julian E. Barnes, "Chinese Agents Helped Spread Messages That Sowed Virus Panic in U.S., Officials Say," *New York Times*, April 22, 2020, updated April 23, 2020, https://www.nytimes.com/2020/04/22/us/politics/corona virus-china-disinformation.html; Michael Birnbaum, "E.U. Accuses China of Waging Pandemic Disinformation Campaign," *Washington Post*, June 10, 2020, https://www .washingtonpost.com/world/eu-accuses-china-of-waging-pandemic-disinformation-cam paign/2020/06/10/55af8a78-ab1f-11ea-a43b-be9f6494a87d_story.html.

3. Betsy Woodruff Swan, "State Report: Russian, Chinese and Iranian Disinformation Narratives Echo One Another," *Politico*, https://www.politico.com/news/2020/04/21/russia -china-iran-disinformation-coronavirus-state-department-193107.

4. On "kung flu," see, for example, Bruce Y. Lee, "Trump Once Again Calls Covid-19 Coronavirus the 'Kung Flu,'" *Forbes*, June 24, 2020, https://www.forbes.com/sites/brucelee /2020/06/24/trump-once-again-calls-covid-19-coronavirus-the-kung-flu/#6f5b50f61f59; On "Chinese virus" and "Wuhan virus," see, for example, Katie Rogers, Lara Jakes, and Ana Swanson, "Trump Defends Using 'Chinese Virus' Label, Ignoring Growing Criti-cism," *New York Times*, March 18, 2020, updated March 19, 2020, https://www.nytimes .com/2020/03/18/us/politics/china-virus.html.

5. See Michael J. Mazarr et al., *Understanding the Emerging Era of International Competi-tion: Theoretical and Historical Perspectives* (Santa Monica, CA: RAND Corporation, 2018).

6. See, for example, Jamie Smythe, "Australians Deliver Scathing Judgment of Trump's COVID-19 Response," *Financial Times*, May 13, 2020, https://www.ft.com/content /656cb0bb-0d4b-41eb-a601-2c74e00c802f; Lauren Vella, "Japan's Abe Calls for Support for World Health Organization after US Cuts," *The Hill*, April 17, 2020, https://thehill.com /policy/international/asia-pacific/493332-japans-abe-calls-for-support-for-world-health -organization; "France Expresses Doubt over China's Transparency as Covid-19 Toll Soars," *RFI*, April 17, 2020, http://www.rfi.fr/en/international/20200417-china-coronavirus-death -toll-increase-wuhan-france-emmanuel-macron-uk-usa-reactions; and Lowy Institute Poll, "Global Responses to COVID-19," accessed June 27, 2020, https://poll.lowyinstitute.org /charts/global-responses-to-covid-19.

7. Josh Busby, "Climate Change as Anarchy: The Need for a New Structural Theory of IR," *Duck of Minerva* (blog), April 1, 2019, https://duckofminerva.com/2019/04/climate -change-as-anarchy-the-need-for-a-new-structural-theory-of-ir.html.

8. G. John Ikenberry and Charles A. Kupchan, "Global Distancing," *Washington Post*, May 21, 2020, https://www.washingtonpost.com/outlook/2020/05/21/pandemic-international-cooperation-alliances/?arc404=true.

9. Haass writes, "The world today is simply not conducive to being shaped." Haass, "The Pandemic Will Accelerate History"; Ikenberry and Kupchan, "Global Distancing," strike a similar chord: "this moment does not lend itself to global realignment the way earlier crises did."

10. Minseon Ku, "The Limits of South Korea's 'Coronavirus Diplomacy,'" *The National Interest* (blog), March 30, 2020, https://nationalinterest.org/blog/korea-watch/limits-south-korea%E2%80%99s-%E2%80%9Ccoronavirus-diplomacy%E2%80%9D-138942.

11. "About six-in-ten (62%) think many of the problems facing the U.S. can be solved by working with other countries. Similarly, 61% think the U.S. should consider the interests of other countries rather than following its own interests alone." Mara Mordecai, "How Americans Envision a Post-Pandemic World Order," Pew Research Center, June 2, 2020, https://www.pewresearch.org/fact-tank/2020/06/02/how-americans-envision-a-post-pandemic-world-order/.

12. Sarah Repucci, "Freedom in the World 2020: A Leaderless Struggle for Democracy," Freedom House, accessed June 24, 2020, https://freedomhouse.org/report/freedom-world/2020/leaderless-struggle-democracy.

13. Seth G. Jones, Catrina Doxsee, and Nicholas Harrington, *The Right-Wing Terrorist Threat in Europe* (Washington, DC: Center for Strategic and International Studies, March 2020), 1.

14. See, for example, Katie Shepherd, "An Officer Was Gunned Down. The Killer Was a 'Boogaloo Boy' Using Nearby Peaceful Protests as Cover, Feds Say," *Washington Post*, June 17, 2020, https://www.washingtonpost.com/nation/2020/06/17/boogaloo-steven-carrillo/.

15. Samuel J. Brannen, Christian Haig, and Katherine S. Schmidt, *The Age of Mass Protests* (Washington, DC: Center for Strategic and International Studies, 2020), 1.

16. Brannen et al., *The Age of Mass Protests*, 7.

17. Brannen et al., *The Age of Mass Protest*, 1.

18. Daniel Clark, "EU Parliament: Voter Turnout in the European Elections 1979–2019," Statista, December 4, 2019, https://www.statista.com/statistics/300427/eu-parlament-turnout-for-the-european-elections/.

19. Wong et al., "Chinese Agents Helped Spread Messages."

20. See, for example, Swan et al., "State Report"; William J. Broad, "Putin's Long War against American Science," *New York Times*, April 13, 2020, updated April 14, 2020, https://www.nytimes.com/2020/04/13/science/putin-russia-disinformation-health-coronavirus.html.

21. Marley Coyne, "Americans Trust Doctors and the CDC—Not Trump—on COVID-19, Survey Reports," *Forbes*, April 30, 2020, https://www.forbes.com/sites/marleycoyne/2020/04/30/americans-trust-doctors-and-cdc-not-trump-on-covid-19-survey-reports/#3c33acf0cc6c.

22. "Coronavirus in the U.S.: Latest Map and Case Count," *New York Times*, accessed June 25, 2020, https://www.nytimes.com/interactive/2020/us/coronavirus-us-cases.html.

23. Gary Pinkus and Sree Ramaswamy, "What History Can Teach Us about the Economic Impact of the Coronavirus Pandemic," *Fortune*, June 1, 2020, https://fortune.com/2020/06/01/coronavirus-economic-impact-historical-analysis-covid-19/.

24. The CSIS Commission on Strengthening America's Health Security, *Ending the Cycle of Crisis and Complacency in U.S. Global Health Security* (Washington, DC: Center for Strategic and International Studies, November 18, 2019), 1.

25. On the generational composition of the electorate, see Anthony Cilluffo and Richard Fry, "An Early Look at the 2020 Electorate," Pew Research Center, January 30, 2019, https://www.pewsocialtrends.org/essay/an-early-look-at-the-2020-electorate/. On generational and partisan views of climate change, government policy, and alternative energy, see Cary Funk and Alec Tyson, "Millennial and Gen Z Republicans Stand Out from Their Elders on Climate and Energy Issues," Pew Research Center, June 24, 2020, https://www.pewresearch.org/fact-tank/2020/06/24/millennial-and-gen-z-republicans-stand-out-from-their-elders-on-climate-and-energy-issues/.

26. Quote from the National Intelligence Council, "National Intelligence Assessment on the National Security Implications of Global Climate Change to 2030, June 25, 2008," provided in *Findings from Select Federal Reports: The National Security Implications of a Changing Climate* (Washington, DC: White House, May 2015), 2, https://obamawhitehouse.archives.gov/sites/default/files/docs/National_Security_Implications_of_Changing_Climate_Final_051915.pdf.

27. Susanne Rust, "Marshall Islands, Low-Lying U.S. Ally and Nuclear Testing Site, Declares a Climate Crisis," *Los Angeles Times*, October 11, 2019, https://www.latimes.com/environment/story/2019-10-11/marshall-islands-national-climate-crisis.

28. Megan Rowling, "Fast-Growing African Cities at 'Extreme Risk' from Climate Change: Analysts," Reuters, November 13, 2018, https://www.reuters.com/article/us-africa-climatechange-cities/fast-growing-african-cities-at-extreme-risk-from-climate-change-analysts-idUSKCN1NJ00F.

29. Gena Steffens, "Changing Climate Forces Desperate Guatemalans to Migrate," *National Geographic*, October 23, 2018, https://www.nationalgeographic.com/environment/2018/10/drought-climate-change-force-guatemalans-migrate-to-us/.

30. National Aeronautics and Space Administration, "Arctic Sea Minimum," accessed June 27, 2020, https://climate.nasa.gov/vital-signs/arctic-sea-ice/.

31. Heather A. Conley and Matthew Melino, *The Implications of U.S. Policy Stagnation toward the Arctic Region* (Washington, DC: Center for Strategic and International Studies, May 2019), 3–4.

32. Congressional Research Service, "Military Installations and Sea-Level Rise," CRS: In Focus, July 26, 2019, https://fas.org/sgp/crs/natsec/IF11275.pdf; Steve Liewer, "Flood Recovery at Offutt Could Cost $1 Billion and Take Five Years," *Omaha World-Herald*, September 16, 2019, https://www.omaha.com/news/military/flood-recovery-at-offutt-could-cost-1-billion-and-take-five-years/article_8f4fff1a-ff4e-5265-bf73-3d6df6be94e8.html.

33. Kathleen Hicks, "Now What? The American Citizen, World Order, and Building a New Foreign Policy Consensus," *Texas National Security Review* 1, no. 1 (November 2017): 117–118, https://tnsr.org/2017/11/now-american-citizen-world-order-building-new-foreign-policy-consensus/.

34. Tang Ziyi, "Update: China Scraps GDP Growth Target, Boosts Budget Deficit amid Coronavirus Pandemic," May 22, 2020, Caixin Global, https://www.caixinglobal.com /2020-05-2/china-ditches-gdp-growth-target-for-2020-101557274.html.

35. For an overview of COVID's implications for the Russian armed forces, see Mathieu Boulegue, "How Is the Russian Military Responding to COVID-19?" *War on the Rocks*, May 4, 2020, https://warontherocks.com/2020/05/how-is-the-russian-military -responding-to-covid-19/.

36. For a fuller treatment of these issues, see Kathleen Hicks, "Getting to Less: The Truth about Defense Spending," *Foreign Affairs*, March/April 2020, 56–62.

PART VII / Sino-American Rivalry

Chapter Twenty

The United States, China, and the Great Values Game

Elizabeth Economy

G lobal crises inevitably raise questions of global leadership. As the world confronts a dramatically changing climate, a pandemic, a global economic recession, and an ongoing refugee crisis, it seeks competent leaders that both model best behavior and bear a greater share of the burden in responding to these challenges. But in the midst of the COVID-19 pandemic, when the world came calling, both superpowers, the United States and China, fell short. The United States flailed helplessly, unable to overcome a lack of presidential leadership, a partisan divide, and a broken health care system.[1] On the global stage, the United States abdicated leadership in spectacular fashion. Its moves to divert personal protective equipment (PPE) away from other countries,[2] as well as its suspension of funding and subsequent move to withdraw from the World Health Organization (WHO),[3] served as defining and devastating symbols of the Trump administration's "America First" mantra. China, in contrast, sought to grasp the mantle of global leadership. It provided material and technical support for much of the world and pledged significant assistance to meet the challenge of future pandemics. Its response was marred, however, by both a lack of transparency and accountability that enabled the virus to spread within China and abroad and its self-aggrandizing

Elizabeth Economy is the C. V. Starr Senior Fellow and director for Asia studies at the Council on Foreign Relations and Distinguished Visiting Fellow at the Hoover Institution at Stanford University.

and coercive diplomacy.[4] Moreover, any hope that the two powers would together step up to coordinate a global response was quickly quashed by the efforts of each to offload blame onto the other. The WHO also failed its mandate to array the world's resources to ensure the timely and transparent transmission of best policy options and practices in combating the pandemic.[5] The triumph belonged to the middle and large powers, such as Taiwan, South Korea, and Germany, who boasted competent leaders and resilient systems. They managed to arrest the spread of the virus at home and offer assistance to others in need. Nonetheless, they lacked the heft and reach to lead globally in a sustained manner.

The failure of global leadership in response to the COVID-19 pandemic illustrates the much larger challenges in global governance that the world confronts today. The institutions, norms, and values of the current international order are not adequate to meet the range of needs and demands of the world's peoples; some need to be bolstered, while others need to be reformed. At the same time, the pandemic also laid bare the scope and scale of China's ambition to reshape the geostrategic landscape and reform international institutions to reflect its preferred norms, values, and policies. For decades, China has maintained a low-profile foreign policy and selectively adapted to the current international order, contributing to a widespread belief that the country was on a path, however long and tortuous, to becoming a "responsible stakeholder" in the international system. Yet since coming to power in 2012, Chinese Communist Party (CCP) General Secretary and President Xi Jinping has advanced an alternative vision of the international order and China's place within it. As China's behavior over the course of the pandemic underscores, this vision poses a threat to a number of norms underpinning the current order, including freedom of navigation and overflight, free trade, open societies, and the rule of law, as well as to the international institutions embodying these norms. Xi seeks to create what he has characterized as "a community of shared destiny for mankind"—a rules-based order in which the norms and values of authoritarian countries and those of democratic systems coexist and are protected equally.

The United States, for its part, has signaled that, at least for the duration of the Trump administration, it can no longer be relied upon to serve as the standard-bearer for the current international order. President Donald Trump understands international institutions and multilateral arrangements more as constraints than enablers of US power and influence. He has devalued the role of alliances and withdrawn from some international institutions, while ignoring the norms inherent in others. Yet the United States does not want to cede global leadership to China. It has recognized China as a "strategic competitor" and "revisionist power" and adopted a strategy to compete with, counter, and contain China—erecting bulwarks against Chinese initiatives to reorder the global order, while aggressively encouraging its allies and partners to join in the effort.

For much of the rest of the world, Chinese behavior and the US posture have created an increasingly complicated and challenging situation. Neither superpower offers an attractive world vision, but countries are being asked—and sometimes coerced—to choose sides in ways suggestive of a cold war. In response, a number of officials and foreign policy experts have offered alternative frameworks, in which China and the United States compete but also seek out areas of cooperation. One such approach, "coopetition"—a concept borrowed from the business world—acknowledges competition as a defining feature of the bilateral relationship but also underscores the advantages to be realized from cooperation in certain well-defined areas to produce a greater good.[6] Others have drawn on an idea from the natural sciences, "coevolution," to suggest that the United States and China naturally share broad areas of common purpose and should identify opportunities to learn from the other, change, and adapt for mutual benefit.[7] Both coopetition and coevolution offer the two countries the opportunity to reset the relationship and embark on a new diplomatic endeavor that takes cooperation as a core strategic objective—a good in and of itself. And both approaches, if fully realized, would contribute to a world order led by the United States and China that was more stable and better able to respond to global challenges.

Yet the COVID-19 pandemic also raises the question of whether the future of the world should rely so completely on the intentions, capabilities, and actions of China and the United States. China's wide-ranging attacks on the basic norms and institutions underpinning the current rules-based order and the United States' determination to reduce its support for many of the international institutions that support this order make China in particular, but also the United States, destabilizing forces within the international system. In this current reality, it is worth exploring the opportunities for other countries, many of which displayed governance capabilities superior to those of China and the United States during the pandemic, to play a larger role in shaping the future international order, its institutions, values, and norms.

China Reaches for the Crown

In a short essay published in *Noema* in June 2020, "China: Threat or Opportunity?," former Singaporean diplomat Kishore Mahbubani argues that even as America's geopolitical influence has receded and China's has expanded, Beijing has no interest in providing global leadership. According to Mahbubani, China has "benefited from the rules-based global order" and has "no desire to overturn this order."[8] More than two hundred US scholars and analysts expressed a similar view in a letter published in the *Washington Post* in July 2019, in which they argued that it was "not clear" whether Beijing saw global leadership as "necessary or feasible," and in any case, while China might be "seeking to weaken the role of Western democratic norms within the global order," it was "not seeking to overturn vital economic and other components of that order" because China, itself, had benefited from that order.[9]

Despite their apparent confidence in the staying power of the current rules-based system, Xi's stated intentions and policies over the past almost decade suggest otherwise. Xi has called for China to "lead in the reform of the global governance system"[10] and to create a "community of shared destiny," in which universal values and the institutions and multilateral arrangements that support them, such as the US-led alliance system, no longer define the international order.[11] Xi has further advanced China as a model for other countries, claiming that "the China model for a better social governance system offers a new option for other countries and nations who want to speed up their development while preserving their independence."[12] (While there is no one clearly accepted definition of this model, at its heart it is a variant of authoritarian capitalism, characterized, as University of Michigan professor Yuen Yuen Ang has described, by extensive state control over political and social life, including the media, internet, and education, and an economy that reflects a mix of both market-based practices, as well as the strong hand of the state in core sectors of the economy.[13])

Xi's objectives in promoting a China model and calling for reform of global governance institutions are both defensive—to protect China from international criticism—and offensive—to ensure that international norms and values align with and serve Chinese values and political and economic priorities. States and international institutions that reflect China's values on human rights and cyber-governance, for example, are less likely to criticize Beijing's labor and reeducation camps in Xinjiang and more likely to support China's negotiating stance in international institutions on the primacy of cyber-sovereignty. And they may also embrace Chinese trade, investment, and security ties in support of these norms and values. To advance these objectives, Xi has moved both strategically and opportunistically, using China's sovereignty claims, its Belt and Road Initiative (BRI), its position within international institutions, and its economic prowess to incentivize and coerce actors to align their practices with Chinese preferences.

Chinese Ambitions Meet COVID-19

The story of COVID-19 is still evolving, but its implications for China's position on the global stage are already emerging. While the international community lauded China for its ability to mobilize its vast resources to combat the pandemic, Beijing's approach has also raised doubts about its model, the nature of its international influence, and the desirability of Chinese leadership on the global stage.

As China's leaders moved to control the spread of COVID-19, a high degree of political centralization and the deep penetration of the CCP into Chinese society enabled them to quarantine more than one hundred million people,[14] to deploy significant financial and human capital to construct hospitals and makeshift quarantine centers,[15] and to command enterprises across the country to manufacture the PPE necessary to meet the Chinese and later international demand.[16] In addition, the government's already operational surveillance technology and close ties with Chinese technology companies allowed it to track and contain the spread of the virus in much of the country. Yet this same authoritarian model also enabled the spread of the virus within China and beyond the country's borders. The tight control over information, as well as the lack of transparency, an open media, and the rule of law, delayed the transmission of critical information that could have contained the spread of the virus in its initial stages. Millions of Chinese left the city of Wuhan, the epicenter of the epidemic, to travel during the Lunar New Year, many unknowingly carrying the virus with them. The Chinese government manipulated and destroyed information regarding the true number of cases and deaths, further putting Chinese citizens and the rest of the world at risk.[17] (Still, today, there is no accurate accounting of the number of COVID-19-related cases and deaths in China, with some outside estimates placing the number of cases in China in January 2020 at thirty-seven times the official number.[18]) Chinese citizens rose up to challenge the official narrative, undertaking their own investigations into the number of cases and deaths, creating maps that tracked the virus's path, developing trusted platforms for citizens to access verified information, and even criticizing Xi and the CCP directly for their handling of the virus. The message to the rest of the world: if the Chinese people don't trust their government, why should it? By March 2020, the government had arrested over eight hundred Chinese citizens for pursuing independent inquiries and publicly questioning the government's actions.

At the same time, Xi took advantage of the pandemic to extend China's reach into the politically contested regions that it claims as its sovereign territory, including much of the South China Sea, Taiwan, and Hong Kong. In the South China Sea, China has consistently ignored the 2016 ruling by the Permanent Court of Arbitration that deemed its claims unlawful and has continued to take destabilizing actions to realize its claims. Beijing used the distraction of the pandemic to establish two districts to oversee the Paracels Islands and Macclesfield Bank, which are also claimed by Vietnam and Taiwan, and name eighty different features in the South China Sea, fifty-five of which were underwater. At the same time, Chinese vessels rammed and sunk a Vietnamese shipping boat and threatened Malaysian and Indonesian ships.[19] Beijing also took advantage of the pandemic to enforce its political norms within Hong Kong. China's National People's Congress passed a draft national security law that dramatically curtails Hong Kong citizens' political and civil rights.[20] According to many international experts, the law breaches the "one country, two system" principle and the city's de facto constitution, the Basic Law.[21] Finally, China used the pandemic to enforce its sovereignty claims over Taiwan. Unification with Taiwan is a top priority for Xi,[22] and as the pandemic spread, Beijing insisted on treating Taiwan as a province of China. The Chinese leadership initially refused to allow Taiwan the right it granted countries to charter planes to bring their citizens home from Wuhan, claiming that the Taiwanese had been "well cared for."[23] It also rejected entreaties by Taiwanese officials to grant them direct access to World Health Organization briefings on COVID-19 or to permit Taiwan to participate as an observer member of the World Health Assembly gathering, the annual meeting of the WHO's plenary body.[24]

Beyond its immediate neighborhood, China has also sought to extend its values and normative preferences to other countries through the BRI, its grand-scale global infrastructure plan. While many countries have courted BRI investment, the Chinese-led projects have also resulted in widespread popular protests in host countries around Chinese lending, environmental, and labor standards.[25] And some countries, which have incurred significant debt due to BRI projects, have sought to cancel or renegotiate additional Chinese investment.[26] Over time, the Chinese leadership has also opportunistically expanded the BRI to advance its security and political ambitions. For example, China established its first military base in Djibouti and has helped develop and manage more than seventy ports and terminals in thirty-four countries, several of which now provide People's Liberation Army (PLA) navy ships with convenient docking and refueling opportunities.[27] Equally significant, Beijing has used the BRI to export its values and norms around human rights and internet governance. As cyber legal experts Kadri Kaska and Maria Tolppa note, China treats the internet not as a technological environment but rather as an information space that needs to be "protected from subverting state power, undermining national unity [or] infringing upon national honour and interests."[28] To this end, Beijing hosts two- to three-week seminars for BRI countries on how to conduct online censorship and surveillance, providing both the policy framework and the surveillance technology.[29] Tanzania, Zimbabwe, and Vietnam have all modeled their cybersecurity laws after that of China.[30]

China's bold moves to transform the geostrategic landscape are further reinforced by a quieter but highly effective effort to transform values and norms within international institutions. China now holds the top position in four of the fifteen United Nations specialized agencies—more than any other country—and it uses its leadership to enforce its own normative preferences. For example, as head of the International Civil Aviation Organization (ICAO), it has blocked people who support Taiwan's membership in the ICAO from the organization's Twitter feed.[31] And, even as it has used the BRI to gain adherents for its norms around human rights and internet governance, it has pushed to have these same norms codified in UN agreements. In 2019, for example, China successfully advanced an anti-cybercrime pact that supports its preference for cyber-sovereignty and grants authoritarian governments much greater leeway to censor online political dissent.[32]

While human rights activists and scholars have long expressed alarm about China's norm and standard setting within the UN, the extent of China's influence became a matter of global concern during the pandemic. In particular, the WHO's calls for the international community to avoid imposing travel bans or otherwise isolating China, its reluctance to declare a Public Health Emergency of International Concern, and its praise for the Chinese government's handling of the crisis raised serious questions in the minds of many observers about undue Chinese influence.[33] This was not the first time that the relationship had come under scrutiny. Scientific experts had also criticized the WHO for its 2019 decision to include traditional Chinese medicine (TCM) in its International Classification of Diseases (a document that validates certain treatments and medicines for doctors to diagnose patients) without subjecting TCM practices to the same rigorous testing demanded of Western medicine and treatments included in the document.[34]

Underlying much of China's success in shaping global norms is its ability to deploy its economic power either to incentivize or to coerce other actors into accepting its preferences. In October 2019, the United States was rocked by the case of Houston Rockets General Manager Daryl Morey, who tweeted, "Fight for

Freedom, Stand with Hong Kong." In response to the tweet, Chinese companies cancelled all licensing deals for Rockets merchandise, and the Chinese government banned all CCTV broadcasts of NBA games and reportedly called on the NBA to fire Morey. State-owned CCTV went even further to state that "any remarks that challenge national sovereignty and social stability are not within the scope of freedom of speech,"[35] suggesting that the Chinese government had the right to apply the same standards of free speech it practices at home to actors abroad. Chinese diplomacy during the COVID-19 pandemic displayed this same coercive element. While Chinese diplomats provided PPE and medical support to tens of countries, they also demanded that the countries express public gratitude for the PPE and for China's "great effort and sacrifice" on behalf of the rest of the world.[36] If countries did not publicly thank China, Beijing threatened to withhold its medical supplies.[37] Australia's call for an international investigation into the origins of the coronavirus triggered an even more dramatic response. China's ambassador to Australia Cheng Jingye suggested that the Chinese people would stop sending their children to study in Australia, drinking Australian wine, and eating Australian beef. Within two weeks of the ambassador's remarks, Beijing banned more than one-third of Australia's beef exports and levied an 80% tariff on Australian barley.[38]

China is advancing an alternative world vision in which freedom of navigation, free trade, open societies, and the rule of law are no longer the normative backbone of the international system. Instead, the norms and values of authoritarian states would equally shape or perhaps even dominate the world's governance structures. While the Trump administration has displayed little interest in donning the mantle of global leadership traditionally worn by the United States, it has also refused to cede the mantle to China.

The United States Abdicates . . . but Not Entirely

China's effort to assume the mantle of leadership in global governance reflects one tectonic shift in the global order; the United States' abdication of leadership on the global stage is another. Waving a banner of "America First," President Trump has argued that the United States has sacrificed its own interests in support of other countries—that it has borne an unfair share of the burden of global security and fallen victim to unequal trade deals that have disadvantaged the American people. He devalues allies and multilateralism, viewing them as constraints on American interests and power, and he has reduced the United States' global commitments by withdrawing from some multilateral institutions and ignoring others. On just his third day in office, President Trump ended US participation in the final stage of negotiations around the Trans-Pacific Partnership, the twelve-nation trade deal that would have been the largest regional trade accord in history.[39] In short order, he also announced the withdrawal of the United States from the United Nations Human Rights Council, the UN Educational Scientific and Cultural Organization, the Paris Climate Agreement, the Iran nuclear deal, and the Intermediate-Range Nuclear Forces Treaty.[40] In the midst of the COVID-19 pandemic, President Trump also pledged to stop funding and then to withdraw entirely from the WHO. In addition, the president's transactional approach to diplomatic engagement—suggesting that history and historical obligation are fungible and everything is open to negotiation—has cost the United States credibility with its allies and partners.

US domestic politics have also harmed US standing on the global stage. In particular, according to a Pew Research Center poll, President Trump's inflammatory rhetoric around Muslims, efforts to restrict immigration from Muslim-majority countries, construction of the border wall, and perceived lack of care for ordinary people all contributed to a 50% drop in confidence in the president among the citizens of the United States' top allies within just his first six months in office.[41] The chaotic response of the Trump administration to the pandemic, failures of the US health care system, and evidence of pervasive racial injustice also have tarnished the United States' image and contributed to a sense of relative US decline.

The result of the United States' retreat from leadership, both intentional and not, is an international order that is headless and increasingly vulnerable to Chinese ambitions and influence. Yet despite its failure to project an affirmative policy in support of the current international order, the Trump administration has moved aggressively to prevent a Chinese-led order from emerging. The Trump administration has labeled China a "strategic competitor" and "revisionist power" that seeks to replace the United States as the dominant power in Asia and to refashion the international system to serve its own self-interest.[42]

This new assessment of Chinese intent has led the Trump administration to conclude that the traditional policy of "engage but hedge" is no longer adequate to the task of managing the bilateral relationship and to adopt a policy best understood as "compete, counter, and contain." The administration devotes significant effort to denying China its ambitions of realizing its sovereignty claims, spreading its influence through the BRI, and setting norms and standards in the United Nations and other international organizations. The United States has also hardened its defenses against efforts by China's state-led technology sector to enhance its competencies through the acquisition of US intellectual property and financial capital.[43] Far from going it alone, the Trump administration has alternately cajoled and bullied allies and partners to join in this effort.

With regard to the BRI, for example, the United States has loudly and publicly accused China of practicing predatory loan policies and weak governance standards.[44] The administration and Congress established a new institution, the US International Development Finance Corporation, and passed new legislation, the Asia Reassurance Initiative Act, to enable the United States and its partners to better compete with the BRI. The United States also joined with Australia and Japan to create the Blue Dot Network, a certification process for companies and countries seeking to ensure high-quality infrastructure projects.[45] As a result of US efforts, many countries have revisited the terms of their BRI deals, slowed down or cancelled projects, and reconsidered new Chinese investment.

The Trump administration has adopted a similar approach to addressing China's normative challenge to freedom of navigation in the South China Sea. The administration has publicized Chinese illegal activities in the region and has ramped up its freedom of navigation operations from three in 2016 to nine in 2019.[46] It also has persuaded Australia, Japan, Vietnam, the United Kingdom, France, and India, among others, to increase their multilateral maritime patrols.[47] And unlike previous US administrations, the Trump White House did not hesitate to cancel cooperative activities when China flouted international law. For example, when China continued to militarize contested features in the South China Sea's Spratly Islands, the United States Navy disinvited Beijing from its 2018 Rim of the Pacific Exercise.[48]

In the trade and investment realm, the United States has long criticized China's unfair practices, such as barriers to market access, intellectual property theft, and state subsidies, among others, and the Trump administration has also targeted the bilateral trade deficit as an issue of central concern, using tariffs to force a trade deal in which China has agreed to purchase an additional $200 billion in US products. At the same time, in ways that give credence to Cold War analogies, where trade and investment intersect with national security and human rights, the administration has embarked on an effort to decouple the US economy from that of China. In these areas, the Trump administration seeks to prevent China's economy from benefiting from US technological know-how or financial capital and to prevent Chinese and US companies from participating in activities that contribute to Chinese human rights abuses. While the Trump administration has conducted most of its trade policy through bilateral negotiations with China, it has encouraged other countries to adopt similar trade and investment policies around national security and human rights. Most notably, the United States has launched a global campaign to persuade countries to bar the deployment of Huawei's 5G technology in their telecommunications infrastructure on the grounds that the company poses a national security threat.[49]

Even in areas President Trump considers low priority, such as the United Nations, the administration has developed a robust effort to push back against Chinese initiatives. President Trump has long denigrated the United Nations, calling it an "underperformer" and "not a friend of democracy," and he has complained about the large share of the United Nations' budget paid by the United States.[50] Nonetheless, his foreign policy team has targeted the United Nations as an important arena in which to counter Chinese influence. In March 2019, and then again in September 2019, the Trump administration successfully prevented the inclusion of the BRI in the reauthorization resolution for the UN mission in Afghanistan, despite the fact that the reference had been included for the three years prior. Jonathan Cohen, acting US permanent representative to the United Nations, argued that China was "using Security Council resolutions as a platform for inappropriately promoting self-serving initiatives," further criticizing the BRI for its "known problems with corruption, debt distress, environmental damage, and lack of transparency."[51] And in March 2020, the Trump administration also helped prevent China from assuming leadership of the World Intellectual Property Organization by working with allies and lobbying other countries.

Cold War 2.0

In the face of this hardening competition, many officials and analysts believe the United States and China are edging toward, or are already in the midst of, a cold war.[52] Chinese State Councillor Wang Yi, for one, has asserted that the relationship is at risk of arriving at a "new Cold War,"[53] while Oxford historian Timothy Garten Ash has urged everyone to "call a spade a spade" and acknowledge that the two countries have already arrived at such a state.[54] Others, however, view US-China economic interdependence as a mitigating factor and argue that the two countries are far from "locked in an implacable ideological struggle that seeks to end in the demise of the other."[55]

Certainly, parallels can be drawn between the Cold War that characterized much of the US relationship with the former Soviet Union and the current conflict between the United States and China. Although China is not engaged in an effort to export communist ideology, it is exporting elements of authoritarianism. It has also established alliances (albeit not treaty alliances), such as the Shanghai Cooperation Organisation, with like-minded actors to support its controversial positions on anti-terrorism, internet governance, and human rights. The ideological divide between the United States and China is also reinforced by both countries' efforts to develop separate innovation and manufacturing supply chains for advanced technologies. And while military conflict between the United States and China remains hypothetical, the South China Sea, Taiwan, and the competing claims of China and Japan over the Diaoyu/Senkaku Islands all have the potential to draw the United States and China into a larger conflict. Any Chinese moves to develop additional military bases could also help create the conditions for the establishment of hardened military alliances or security blocs.

Even if the dimensions of the US-China conflict do not align precisely with those of the United States and former Soviet Union, there are few signs that either country is prepared to find a way out of the relationship's downward spiral. But there is also little appetite globally for the United States and China to allow tensions in the relationship to solidify into a new cold war. Few, if any, countries would welcome the demand to align with one or the other great power and sacrifice the economic and security benefits of a less polarized world. Moreover, the prospects for addressing global challenges—climate change, pandemics, refugees, and financial crises—are all diminished in a world characterized by sharp divides and a zero-sum mentality.

Coopetition and Coevolution

Concern over the prospect of a US-China cold war has contributed to growing support for a number of alternative conceptions for the US-China relationship, such as coopetition and coevolution, that recognize the inevitability of competition between the two countries but attempt to stabilize it by introducing a renewed focus on cooperation. In coopetition, for example, the overall relationship between the United States and China is defined by competition, but the two countries would work to identify particular policy challenges that could be better addressed through cooperation. For example, China and the United States might compete in a wide variety of areas in the biotech space but could establish a partnership to develop a vaccine for COVID-19 that they would deliver at no cost to the rest of the world.

Coevolution is even more ambitious in its belief that the United States and China can find a path forward together. As outlined by former Acting Assistant

Secretary of State for East Asia and Pacific Affairs Susan Thornton, there is virtually no area in which China and the United States cannot coevolve. In East Asian regional security, for example, China should "evolve to see the value of the constraining effects of the U.S. security presence in the region," and the US is "going to have to evolve in respecting legitimate Chinese security concerns." Even in the value-laden arena of global governance and international institutions, Thornton suggests that the United States should acknowledge China's complaints that it didn't have a say in establishing in the international system and that the United States should "work with China on reforming these institutions, since they need changing anyway."[56]

Both coopetition and coevolution are attractive in their confidence that areas of cooperation can be expanded and areas of competition can be bounded if both countries simply commit to the effort. Yet to be operationalized effectively, both frameworks, and in particular coevolution, must at least acknowledge, if not address, some of the underlying realities of Chinese behavior that complicate their chances of success. For example, coopetition assumes that both players will act in good faith, but Xi Jinping has left behind him a string of broken promises and agreements, including, for example, a promise not to militarize the seven artificial features in the South China Sea and the 2015 US-China Cyber Agreement on cyber economic espionage. Coevolution, for its part, assumes a greater commonality of values and interests between China and the United States than China's behavior around human rights and internet governance might suggest. Thornton, for one, does not believe China intends to "overturn the international system" because it has "served China well." In this context, her argument that the United States and China should reform international institutions together becomes a more realistic project. Finally, as more than three decades of US "engagement" with China demonstrate, there is a risk in establishing cooperation as an objective or a good in and of itself. It encourages the actor more committed to cooperation to excuse or even ignore the other's missteps or malign actions out of fear that cooperation otherwise will not ultimately be realized.

The Third Way

The COVID-19 pandemic revealed a number of important and unfortunate truths about the current international rules-based system. First, it lacks a worthy leader that is willing and able to place its narrow self-interests second to the greater global good. Second, its institutions cannot be relied on to organize an effective response to a significant global challenge. Third, and most important, in the near term, its norms and institutions face a serious and persistent threat from China. Taken together, these conclusions suggest a set of three priorities for ensuring that the current rules-based order is reinvigorated and reformed in ways that better enable it to meet ongoing global challenges and emergent crises.

First, the world's market democracies should take as their greatest strategic priority a recommitment to the norms and values, as well as the institutions, that underpin the current international order. In practical terms, this means pushing back consistently against Chinese efforts to undermine the rules-based system. Notwithstanding the claims of some observers and analysts to the contrary, China poses a direct and sustained threat to international norms and values, including freedom of navigation, free trade, and good governance and human rights. Moreover, as the pandemic underscored, if left untended, international institutions, such as the WHO, risk being captured by China in ways that are harmful to the interests of the larger international community.

Importantly, this effort to bolster the current rules-based order is most accurately and powerfully framed as a value and norm-based contest, not as a US-China competition. The ongoing conflicts in the South China Sea, for example, should be understood not as a battleground for regional security primacy between the United States and China but as what it is: a normative challenge by China to freedom of navigation that should engage not only the United States but also all parties to the United Nations Convention on the Law of the Sea. A bilateral US-China framework elevates every issue into a signal of relative power and influence and naturally advantages China. As the rising power, any relative Chinese gain becomes a win, even if the United States retains the dominant position. The US-China competition frame also enables Beijing to claim that US actions are motivated solely by its desire to avoid losing its primacy to China.[57] Moreover, as the pandemic demonstrated, the world cannot consistently rely on the United States to bolster international norms and institutions. All market democracies must be prepared to step up to assume a degree of leadership in defending the current international system.

The world's advanced market democracies should also reach out to a broader array of countries in their efforts to ensure a more robust and resilient international rules-based system. They should use pre-existing democratic alliance structures and organizations, such as NATO, the Organisation for Economic Cooperation and Development, and the G7, to develop partnerships with still-developing economies to reinforce the value of the international system's norms and institutions. For example, as the advanced market economies consider the creation of trusted supply chains for national security–related goods, they could structure opportunities for developing economies to participate.

Second, advancing the norms of the current international order and restraining the advance of the China model is only one element in ensuring the long-term resilience of the rules-based order. As Hans Kundnani has suggested, the international order must be not only defended but also reformed.[58] Already, for example, there have been calls for the WHO to be more transparent in its reporting on member state compliance with international health regulations.[59] In addition, there are important insights to be gained from the values, norms, and policies of the countries that most successfully combated the pandemic. What do they suggest, for example, for global governance debates around issues such as individual privacy and collective security or the importance of adhering to norms of transparency?

Finally, the United States should continue to call out China on its efforts to subvert the values and norms of the rules-based order and not shy away from a relationship characterized overwhelmingly by competition. Still, there is room for consideration of coopetition, if not coevolution, to help stabilize the bilateral relationship in ways that can also contribute to spur positive outcomes on the global stage. Even at the height of the Cold War, the United States and the Soviet Union cooperated on a series of arms control treaties that significantly advanced global security. The United States and China could similarly partner to address a current global challenge, such as climate change. Given that the two countries contribute 42% of the world's total emissions of the greenhouse gas, carbon dioxide,[60] there is perhaps no other issue on which the two countries could make as immediate and significant a contribution to global security and, in the process, perhaps stave off further deterioration in the bilateral relationship.

NOTES

1. Elizabeth Economy, "The Hydra vs. the Headless Horseman: China and the United States," *Asia Unbound* (blog), April 15, 2020, https://www.cfr.org/blog/hydra-vs-headless -horseman-china-and-united-states.

2. "Coronavirus: US Accused of 'Piracy' over Mask 'Confiscation,'" *BBC News*, April 4, 2020, https://www.bbc.com/news/world-52161995.

3. Harold Hongju Koh, "Trump's Empty 'Withdrawal' from the World Health Organization," Just Security, May 20, 2020, https://www.justsecurity.org/70493/trumps-empty -withdrawal-from-the-world-health-organization/.

4. Steven Erlanger, "Global Backlash Builds against China over Coronavirus," *New York Times*, June 17, 2020, https://www.nytimes.com/2020/05/03/world/europe/backlash -china-coronavirus.html.

5. "The Role of WHO in Public Health," World Health Organization, accessed June 24, 2020, https://www.who.int/about/role/en/.

6. Josh Keller, "Coopetition? American and Chinese Views on Competition and Co-operation," interview with US-China Business Council on April 9, 2019, YouTube video, 8:56, https://www.youtube.com/watch?v=04KZKAD0Gcs.

7. Susan Thornton, "Can We Live with China?" (lecture, 2019 Annual Charles Neu-hauser Memorial Lecture delivered at Harvard University, Cambridge, MA, March 4, 2019), https://fairbank.fas.harvard.edu/events/neuhauser-lecture-featuring-susan-thornton-can-we-live-with-china-a-roadmap-for-co-evolution/.

8. Kishore Mahbubani, "China: Threat or Opportunity?," *Noema*, June 15, 2020, https://www.noemamag.com/china-threat-or-opportunity/.

9. M. Taylor Fravel et al., "China Is Not an Enemy," *Washington Post*, July 3, 2019, https://www.washingtonpost.com/opinions/making-china-a-us-enemy-is-counterproduc tive/2019/07/02/647d49d0-9bfa-11e9-b27f-ed2942f73d70_story.html.

10. Kevin Rudd, "Xi Jinping, China and the Global Order: The Significance of China's 2018 Central Foreign Policy Work Conference," Asia Society, June 26, 2018, https://asiasociety.org/sites/default/files/2019-01/Xi%20Jinping_China%20and%20the%20Global%20Order.pdf.

11. Jacob Mardell, "The 'Community of a Common Destiny' in Xi Jinping's New Era," *The Diplomat*, October 25, 2017, https://thediplomat.com/2017/10/the-community-of -common-destiny-in-xi-jinpings-new-era/.

12. "Full Text of Xi Jinping's Report at the 19th CPC National Congress," *China Daily*, last updated November 4, 2017, https://www.chinadaily.com.cn/china/19thcpcnationalc ongress/2017-11/04/content_34115212.htm.

13. Yuen Yuen Ang, "Autocracy with Chinese Characteristics," *Foreign Affairs* 93, no. 3, (May/June 2018): 39–46, https://www.foreignaffairs.com/articles/asia/2018-04-16/auto cracy-chinese-characteristics.

14. "Over 100 Million in China's Northeast Face Renewed Lockdown," *Bloomberg News*, May 18, 2020, https://www.bloomberg.com/news/articles/2020-05-18/over-100 -million-in-china-s-northeast-thrown-back-under-lockdown.

15. Emily Feng, "China Has Built over 20 Mass Quarantine Centers for Coronavirus Patients In Wuhan," NPR, February 24, 2020, https://www.npr.org/2020/02/24/808995258 /china-has-built-over-20-mass-quarantine-centers-for-coronavirus-patients-in-wuha.

16. Kevin M. Sutter, Andreas B. Schwarzenberg, and Michael D. Sutherland, "COVID-19: China Medical Supply Chains and Broader Trade Issues," Congressional Research Service, April 6, 2020, https://crsreports.congress.gov/product/pdf/R/R46304.

17. Lu Haitao, "Wuhan, Endless Queues for Ashes of Coronavirus Dead Cast Doubts on Numbers," *AsiaNews.it*, March 27, 2020, http://www.asianews.it/news-en/Wuhan, -endless-queues-for-ashes-of-coronavirus-dead-cast-doubts-on-numbers-49673.html.

18. Christopher Moulton et al., *COVID-19 Air Traffic Visualization: COVID-19 Cases in China Were Likely 37 Times Higher Than Reported in January 2020* (Santa Monica, CA: RAND Corporation, 2020), https://www.rand.org/pubs/research_reports/RRA248-3.html.

19. Ben Westcott and Brad Lendon, "Pressures Increasing on Indonesia and Malaysia in the South China Sea," CNN, June 8, 2020, https://www.cnn.com/2020/06/07/asia/china -malaysia-indonesia-south-china-sea-intl-hnk/index.html.

20. "'中华人民共和国香港特别行政区维护国家安全法 (草案)' 对四类危害国家安全的犯罪行为和刑事责任作出明确规定," *Xinhua*, June 18, 2020, http://www.xinhuanet.com/2020-06/18/c_1126130350.htm.

21. Both of these documents were agreed to by China and Great Britain in advance of the 1997 handover.

22. Teddy Ng and Lawrence Chung, "Chinese President Xi Jinping Urges Taiwan to Follow Hong Kong Model for Unification," *South China Morning Post*, January 2, 2019, https://www.scmp.com/news/china/politics/article/2180391/chinese-president-xi-jinping-urges-taiwan-follow-hong-kong-model.

23. George Liao, "China Refuses Taiwan's Request to Evacuate Citizens from Wuhan," *Taiwan News*, January 28, 2020, https://www.taiwannews.com.tw/en/news/3865894.

24. Louise Watt, "Taiwan Says It Tried to Warn the World about Coronavirus. Here's What It Really Knew and When," *Time*, May 19, 2020, https://time.com/5826025/taiwan-who-trump-coronavirus-covid19/.

25. Oyuna Baldakova, "Protests along the BRI: China's Prestige Project Meets Growing Resistance," Mercator Institute for China Studies, December 10, 2019, https://merics.org/en/analysis/protests-along-bri-chinas-prestige-project-meets-growing-resistance.

26. Agatha Kratz, Allen Feng, and Logan Wright, "New Data on 'Debt Trap' Question," Rhodium Group, April 29, 2019, https://rhg.com/research/new-data-on-the-debt-trap-question/.

27. Glenn P. Hastedt and William F. Felice, *Introduction to International Politics: Global Challenges and Policy Responses* (Lanham, MD: Rowman & Littlefield, 2019).

28. Kadri Kasa and Maria Tolppa, "China's Sovereignty and Internet Governance," International Centre for Defence and Security, June 2020, https://icds.ee/wp-content/uploads/2020/06/ICDS_EFPI_Brief_Chinas_Sovereignty_and_Internet_Governance_Kadri_Kaska_Maria_Tolppa_June_2020.pdf.

29. Adrian Shahbaz, "Freedom of the Net 2018: The Rise of Digital Authoritarianism," Freedom House, 2018, https://freedomhouse.org/report/freedom-net/2018/rise-digital-authoritarianism.

30. Shahbaz, "Freedom of the Net."

31. Bethany Allen-Ebrahimian, "UN Aviation Agency Blocks Critics of Taiwan Policy on Twitter," *Axios*, January 27, 2020, https://www.axios.com/as-virus-spreads-un-agency-blocks-critics-taiwan-policy-on-twitter-e8a8bce6-f31a-4f41-89e0-77d919109887.html.

32. Kristine Lee, "It's Not Just the WHO: How China Is Moving on the Whole U.N.," *Politico*, April 15, 2020, https://www.politico.com/news/magazine/2020/04/15/its-not-just-the-who-how-china-is-moving-on-the-whole-un-189029.

33. Andrew Joseph and Megan Theilking, "WHO Praises China's Response to Coronavirus, Will Reconvene Expert Committee to Assess Global Threat," *Stat*, January 29, 2020, https://www.statnews.com/2020/01/29/who-reconvene-expert-committee-coronavirus/.

34. "The World Health Organization Decision about Traditional Chinese Medicine Could Backfire," *Nature*, June 5, 2019, https://www.nature.com/articles/d41586-019-01726-1.

35. Stephen Wade and Tim Reynold, "With China Rift Ongoing, NBA Says Free Speech Remains Vital," Associated Press, October 8, 2019, https://apnews.com/cacbc722f6834e64814f82b14752682c.

36. Sarah Zheng, "Wolf Warrior Diplomats," *South China Morning Post*, March 23, 2020, https://www.scmp.com/news/china/diplomacy/article/3076384/chinas-wolf-war riors-battle-twitter-control-coronavirus.

37. Bethany Allen-Ebrahimian, "Beijing Demanded Praise in Exchange for Medical Supplies," *Axios*, May 6, 2020, https://www.axios.com/beijing-demanded-praise-in-exc hange-for-medical-supplies-16f5183e-589a-42e5-bc25-414eb13841b0.html.

38. "China Punishes Australia for Promoting an Inquiry into Covid-19," *The Economist*, May 21, 2020, https://www.economist.com/asia/2020/05/21/china-punishes-australia -for-promoting-an-inquiry-into-covid-19.

39. "Trump Executive Order Pulls Out of TPP Trade Deal," *BBC News*, January 24, 2017, https://www.bbc.com/news/world-us-canada-38721056.

40. Zachary B. Wolf and JoElla Carman, "Here Are All the Treaties and Agreements Trump Has Abandoned," CNN Politics, February 1, 2019, https://www.cnn.com/2019/02/01 /politics/nuclear-treaty-trump/index.html.

41. Eric Levitz, "Poll: Trump Has Hurt America's Image in the Eyes of the World," *New York Magazine*, June 27, 2017, https://nymag.com/intelligencer/2017/06/trump-has-hurt -americas-image-in-the-eyes-of-the-world.html.

42. "Trump's National Security Strategy and China," ChinaFile, December 19, 2017, https://www.chinafile.com/conversation/trumps-national-security-strategy-and-china.

43. Takashi Kawakami and Taisei Hoyama, "Trump's Blacklist Squeezes 200 Chinese Companies as Net Widens," *Nikkei Asian Review*, November 19, 2019, https://asia.nikkei .com/Economy/Trade-war/Trump-s-blacklist-squeezes-200-Chinese-companies-as-ne t-widens.

44. Krishnadev Calamur, "China vs. America in a Financial Game of 'Risk,'" *The Atlantic*, October 18, 2017, https://www.theatlantic.com/international/archive/2017/10/china -investments/543321/.

45. "2019 Indo-Pacific Business Forum Showcases High-Standard U.S.-Investment" (fact sheet, US Department of State, November 3, 2019), https://www.state.gov/2019-indo -pacific-business-forum-showcases-high-standard-u-s-investment/.

46. John Power, "US Freedom of Navigation Patrols in South China Sea Hit Record High in 2019," *South China Morning Post*, February 5, 2020, https://www.scmp.com/week-asia /politics/article/3048967/us-freedom-navigation-patrols-south-china-sea-hit-record-high.

47. Scott Harold et al., *The Thickening Web of Asian Security Cooperation: Deepening Defense Times among U.S. Allies and Partners in the Indo-Pacific* (Santa Monica, CA: RAND Corporation, 2019), https://www.rand.org/content/dam/rand/pubs/research_reports/RR 3100/RR3125/RAND_RR3125.pdf.

48. Helene Cooper, "U.S. Disinvites China from Military Exercise amid Rising Tensions," *New York Times*, May 23, 2018, https://www.nytimes.com/2018/05/23/world/asia /us-china-rimpac-military-exercise-tensions.html.

49. Emily Stewart, "The US Government's Battle with Chinese Telecom Giant Huawei, Explained," *Vox*, August 19, 2019, https://www.vox.com/technology/2018/12/11/1813 4440/huawei-executive-order-entity-list-china-trump.

50. "Factbox: What Trump Has Said about the United Nations," Reuters, September 17, 2017, https://www.reuters.com/article/us-un-assembly-trump-comments-factbox/factbox-what -trump-has-said-about-the-united-nations-idUSKCN1BS0UO.

51. "US Says China's Belt and Road Project Has Problems with Corruption, Debt, Opacity and Environmental Damage," *Hong Kong Free Press*, March 17, 2019, https://hongkongfp.com/2019/03/17/us-says-chinas-belt-road-project-problems-corruption-debt-opacity-environmental-damage/.

52. Jeffrey Bader, *U.S.-China Relations: Is It Time to End the Engagement?* (Washington, DC: Brookings Institution, September 2018), https://www.brookings.edu/wp-content/uploads/2018/09/FP_20180925_us_china_relations.pdf.

53. "Beijing Says US Is Pushing China to 'Brink of a New Cold War,'" Deutsche Welle, May 24, 2020, https://www.dw.com/en/beijing-says-us-is-pushing-china-to-brink-of-a-new-cold-war/a-53550524.

Stephen Collinson, "What's Happening between the US and China Is No Cold War," CNN, May 8, 2020, https://www.cnn.com/2020/05/08/world/meanwhile-in-america-may-8-intl/index.html.

54. Timothy Garton Ash, "The US and China Are Entering a New Cold War: Where Does That Leave the Rest of Us?," *The Guardian*, June 20, 2020, https://www.theguardian.com/commentisfree/2020/jun/20/us-china-cold-war-liberal-de.

55. Iskander Rehman et al., "Policy Roundtable: Are the United States and China in a New Cold War?," *Texas Security National Review*, May 15, 2018, https://tnsr.org/roundtable/policy-roundtable-are-the-united-states-and-china-in-a-new-cold-war/.

56. Susan Thornton, "Prospects for Co-evolution in Sino-American Relations" (2019 Barnett-Oksenberg Lecture on Sino-American Relations, Shanghai, China, May 15, 2019), https://www.ncuscr.org/event/barnett-oksenberg-lecture-sino-american-relations/2019/transcript.

57. "How Should China Respond to a Changing US: Fu Ying," *People's Daily*, September 12, 2018, http://en.people.cn/n3/2018/0912/c90000-9499699.html.

58. Hans Kundnani, "What Is the Liberal International Order?," German Marshall Fund of the United States, May 3, 2017, https://www.gmfus.org/publications/what-liberal-international-order.

59. Julian Borger, "US Gives G7 a List of Reforms It Wants WHO to Undertake," *The Guardian*, April 30, 2020, https://www.theguardian.com/world/2020/apr/30/us-gives-g7-countries-a-list-of-reforms-it-wants-who-to-undertake.

60. Hannah Ritchie and Max Roser, "CO_2 and Greenhouse Gas Emissions," Our World in Data, last updated December 2019, https://ourworldindata.org/co2-and-other-greenhouse-gas-emissions.

The US-China Relationship after Coronavirus

Clues from History

Graham Allison

Coronavirus struck like a flash of lightning that illuminates for an instant distant horizons otherwise obscured. The impact of this pandemic highlights three central realities of world order—and disorder.

First and most fundamentally, coronavirus magnifies the underlying structural reality that will be the defining feature of world order and disorder for as far as any eye can see. In what we are coming to recognize as the Great Rivalry, a rising China is seriously threatening to displace a ruling United States from its accustomed position at the top of every pecking order. In twelve of sixteen cases over the last five hundred years, such Thucydidean rivalries ended in war.

Second, despite this inevitable and inescapable rivalry, coronavirus also provides a vivid reminder that each nation faces external threats it cannot defeat by itself acting alone. However unnatural, however uncomfortable, each must come to recognize the other as its insufferable but inseparable conjoined twin. As American and Russian Cold Warriors learned painfully as they acquired superpower nuclear arsenals capable of destroying their adversary, neither could survive a nuclear war. To coexist rather than co-destruct, both came to recognize the necessity to constrain their competition.

Graham Allison is the Douglas Dillon Professor of Government at Harvard University and author of *Destined for War: Can American and China Escape Thucydides's Trap?*

Third, this deadly pathogen has condemned the United States and China, despite their hostility, to work together, at least to the extent necessary to ensure their national survival and well-being. In their search for a new strategic rationale for their relationship, perhaps they can find a way forward by combining an ancient Chinese concept of "rivalry partners" and an insight President John F. Kennedy came to after having survived the Cuban Missile Crisis. He called for the United States and the Soviet Union to coexist in a "world safe for diversity."

Each of these central realities is best understood through the lens of Applied History: the explicit attempt to illuminate current challenges and choices by analyzing the historical record.[1] First, we need to assess how coronavirus will change the nature of world politics. In a tweet: much less than most of the commentariat is currently claiming.

"A Possession for All Time": Applying History to Clarify the Coronavirus

Imagine a conversation between two great Applied Historians: Thucydides and George Marshall. Thucydides asserted that "as long as humans are human, the future will resemble the past." In contrast to the celebrated playwrights of classical Greece who left Oedipus no choice about killing his father and marrying his mother, Thucydides analyzed the past in order to inform future statecraft. As he explained in the introduction to his *History of the Peloponnesian War*, his purpose was to help future political leaders, soldiers, and citizens understand war so that they could avoid mistakes made by their predecessors. As the founder of realpolitik, as well as history, his analysis of the great war that destroyed the two leading city-states of Greece begins with underlying structural realities and basic motives of human behavior. In his summary, these were "fear, honor, and interest." Thus, as he wrote, he hoped his history would be "a possession for all time."[2]

In their classic *Thinking in Time: The Uses of History for Decision Makers*, Ernest May and Richard Neustadt hold up Marshall as a model Applied Historian for his ability to think in "time-streams"—seeing connections between the past, present, and future. In their summary, "The essence of thinking in time-streams is imagining the future as it may be when it becomes the past—with some intelligible continuity but richly complex and able to surprise."[3] Both in directing America's war effort and in constructing the European Recovery Act, Marshall was sensitive to choices that could set the course of events on a different path. As May and Neustadt put it, he knew that "what matters for the future in the present is departures from the past, alterations, changes."[4]

If these two men lived today, what might they say about the impact of this novel virus and the pandemic it has caused? Marshall would likely ask, "What will change?" Thucydides might answer, "Not the fundamentals."

When facing immediate threats to survival, human beings respond: me and mine first. As long as states remain the primary units in international relations, and heads of state remain dependent on support from the citizens of their state for their jobs, President Donald Trump will not be the only leader who puts his own nation first.

Thucydides would thus be skeptical of the claims now being made by many in the American foreign policy establishment that coronavirus means the end of international relations as we have known it. He would likely remind us of the proclamations of an "end of history" at the end of the Cold War. He might contest Henry Kissinger's proposition that "the coronavirus pandemic will forever alter the world order" and require "the post-coronavirus order."[5] He would likely reject the president of the Council on Foreign Relations' claim that "today and for the century ahead, the most significant threats that we face are less other states than a range of transnational problems."[6] He would not agree with Larry Summers's assertion that post-coronavirus, we will live in a "world where security depends more on exceeding a threshold of co-operation with allies and adversaries alike than on maintaining a balance of power."[7] And he would find delusional the "great awakening" many international observers have hailed in which enlightened leaders embrace the solidarity of all 7.7 billion inhabitants of planet Earth, create a "one world" vaccine, and bury petty nationalisms in a new era of globalism.[8]

If one small nuclear bomb devastates the heart of a great city, or a state launches a bioterrorist attack a hundred times deadlier than COVID-19 against an adversary's major airport hubs, or China takes advantage of the world's preoccupation to forcefully reintegrate Taiwan with the mainland, Thucydides would expect that those who have been unhinged by this novel virus will return to Earth.

A shared interest in defeating coronavirus will not override the US-China competition and redefine the future of the relationship. Instead, coronavirus will become yet another element in the greatest geopolitical challenge of our lifetime.

A Great Thucydidean Rivalry

In speculating about the world after coronavirus, Thucydides would begin with structural realities. Just as he identified that the rise of Athens and the fear it inspired in Sparta made war nearly inevitable, he would note that the defining feature of international politics going forward will continue to be an analogous rivalry between a rising China and a ruling United States. Coronavirus has now become another dimension along which these rivals are waging their competition. How each nation addresses this challenge and how their response affects their nations' gross domestic products (GDPs), their citizens' confidence in their government, and their standing in the world will become another strand in this rivalry.

"THE BIGGEST PLAYER IN THE HISTORY OF THE WORLD"

What has happened to the relative power of the United States and China since the US victory in the Cold War introduced what most of the American national security establishment thought would be a unipolar era in which America would lead, other nations would take their assigned place in the new "liberal international rules-based order," and peace would be ensured by McDonald's Golden Arches?[9] In two words: tectonic shift. Never before in history has a rising power ascended so far, so fast, on so many different dimensions. Never before has a ruling power seen its relative position change so quickly.[10]

After nearly half a century of competition, when the Cold War ended and the Soviet Union disappeared, in 1991, the United States was left economically, militarily, and geopolitically dominant. But that was then. Although GDP is not everything, it does form the substructure of power in relations among nations. The US share of global GDP—nearly one-half in 1950—has gone from one-quarter in 1991 to one-seventh today.[11] China has been the chief beneficiary of this transformation. In the past generation, its GDP has soared: from 20% of the US level in 1991 to 120% today (measured by the metric that both the CIA and the International Monetary Fund judge the best yardstick for comparing national economies: purchasing power parity, or PPP).[12]

In Asia, the shift in the economic balance of power has been even more dramatic. Having emerged as the world's largest exporter and second-largest importer, China is the top trading partner of every other major East Asian country, including US allies.[13] As an aggressive practitioner of economic statecraft, Beijing does not hesitate to use the leverage this provides, squeezing countries such as the Philippines and South Korea when they resist Chinese demands. Globally, China is also rapidly becoming a peer competitor of the United States in advanced technologies. Today, of the twenty largest information technology companies, nine are Chinese.[14] Four years ago, when Google, the global leader in artificial intelligence (AI), the most significant advanced technology, assessed its competition, Chinese companies ranked alongside European companies. Now, that state of affairs is barely visible in the rearview mirror: Chinese companies lead in many areas of applied AI, including surveillance, facial and voice recognition, and financial technology.

China's military spending and capabilities have surged as well. A quarter century ago, its defense budget was one-sixteenth that of the United States; now, it is one-third and on a path to parity.[15] Moreover, this is the difference when measured in market exchange rate. If converted to PPP, China's defense budget is already as large as—and possibly larger than—the United States' defense budget.[16] Unlike the United States, China's priority military missions include "internal domestic security." But whereas the US defense budget is spread across global commitments, many of them in Europe and the Middle East, China's budget is focused on East Asia. Accordingly, in specific military scenarios involving a conflict over Taiwan or in the South China Sea, China may have already taken the lead.

Short of actual war, the best tests of relative military capabilities are war games. In 2019, Robert Work, a former US deputy secretary of defense, and David Ochmanek, one of the Department of Defense's key defense planners, offered a public summary of the results from a series of classified recent war games. Their bottom line, in Ochmanek's words: "When we fight Russia and China, 'blue' [the United States] gets its ass handed to it."[17] As the *New York Times* reported: "In 18 of the last 18 Pentagon war games involving China in the Taiwan Strait, the US lost."[18]

In short, as the Singaporean statesman and world's premier China watcher Lee Kuan Yew once told me: "The size of China's displacement of the world balance is such that the world must find a new balance. It is not possible to pretend that this is just another big player. This is the biggest player in the history of the world."[19]

When a rising power threatens to displace a ruling power, alarm bells should sound: extreme danger ahead. Thucydides explained this dangerous dynamic in the case of Athens's rise to rival Sparta in classical Greece. In the centuries since then, this story line has been repeated over and over. The last five hundred years saw sixteen cases in which a rising power threatened to displace a major ruling power. Twelve ended in war.[20]

No argument that fails to ask the "Marshall question" is complete. After listening to, or indeed making a compelling case for a proposition, Marshall would often say, "Just one more question: How could I be wrong?" I can identify a dozen ways and am sure participants in the forum can think of more. Many forecast a significant slowdown in China's extraordinary growth rate and, indeed, have been doing so annually for the past two decades. Of course, as Stein's Law says: a trend that cannot continue indefinitely won't. But predicting that something will happen is much easier than saying when it will. President Xi Jinping's attempt to revitalize the Chinese Communist Party as the Leninist Mandarin vanguard of 1.4 billion people may flounder. As Lee Kuan Yew told him directly, he's trying to put 21st-century apps on a 20th-century operating system.[21] China's military may behave recklessly and provoke a military confrontation that China loses—and that could lead to the overthrow of its new emperor. Xi could slip in his bathtub. And so forth. While US planners must consider all reasonable contingencies, basing our strategy to meet the China challenge on the expectation that the Chinese economy or political system fails would be a mistake.

Unless Xi is unsuccessful in his ambitions to "Make China Great Again," China will continue challenging America's accustomed position at the top of every pecking order. If Xi succeeds, China will displace the United States as the predominant power in East Asia in his lifetime. Unless the United States redefines itself to settle for something less than number one, Americans will increasingly find China's rise discombobulating.

As Thucydides explained, the objective reality of a rising power's impact on a ruling power is bad enough. But in the real world, these objective facts are perceived subjectively—magnifying misperceptions and multiplying miscalculations. When one competitor "knows" what the other's "real motive" is, every action is interpreted in ways that confirm that bias. Moreover, beyond reality and psychology, Thucydidean dynamics are derived by a third factor: domestic politics. As we are now seeing vividly in the current US presidential campaign, a fundamental axiom of electoral politics declares never let a serious competitor get to your right on a matter of national security. Thus, both campaigns seek to protect their candidate from claims that he is "soft" on China and to demonstrate that he will be tougher in combating this rival than his opponent.

Are confrontation and competition inevitable? Yes. But is war—real bloody war—inevitable? No. To repeat, no. Debate about whether this competition would become "Cold War II"—a rivalry waged along every azimuth excluding uniformed combatants attacking the adversary's soldiers or citizens—began with Vice President Mike Pence's de facto declaration of cold war against China in earnest in late 2018.[22] While the many differences between today's world and the world in which the "Wise Men" shaped America's Cold War strategy are at least as crucial as the similarities, one key likeness stands out. As in the Cold War, rivalry has begun to metastasize through every dimension of the US-China relationship, including the coronavirus. In turn, each nation's response to the coronavirus has magnified the sources of their Thucydidean rivalry.

One Coronavirus, Two Systems

In this competition to be number one, coronavirus presents a preview of "one crisis, two systems" performance—displaying vividly each government's weaknesses and strengths.[23] The imperative for the US and Chinese governments today is to act to defeat this scourge. But as each attempts to do so, it must recognize that its response to the coronavirus crisis will have profound consequences for the larger rivalry for leadership. From economic growth over the next twelve months, to its citizens' confidence in their government, and each nation's standing around the world, successes and failures in meeting a test that has captured the mind of the world will matter hugely.

Unfortunately, most of the US commentary about this aspect of the current crisis has focused on China's effort to manipulate the narrative. Where did the coronavirus first appear? In China. Who failed to nip the crisis in the bud? Chinese authoritarianism has displayed all its ugly features in suppressing initial reports, delaying transmission of bad news to superiors and dissembling. Of course, China is vigorously selling its story line and attempting to rearrange the facts to show itself in the best light. Despite the Chinese government's best efforts to rewrite history, it cannot disguise the fact that there is much in this case for which China deserves blame. But the effort by many in Washington as well as the Blob (the foreign policy establishment) to make this the primary story line is escapist— an attempt to duck responsibilities for their own failures. Focusing on the words in this case rather than the deeds misses the mountain behind the molehill.

Unlike the rhetorical debate about this issue, or governments' attempts to shape a narrative, coronavirus is providing a test in which citizens can see for themselves who delivers and who does not. Crises are, in effect, showtime, when the curtain is drawn and the lights are up. Whatever the words and promises that have gone before, the audience can judge for itself whether those on the stage can play their instruments or sing. Governments' claims about their capabilities and rhetoric about who or what is the greatest fade as the truth is revealed.

Markets are now betting that China has essentially succeeded in the first battle in this long war. After a bungling start that wasted weeks and imposed significant costs on itself and on the world, once China's President Xi and his team grasped the magnitude of the challenge, they acted boldly and decisively to contain its spread and then to defeat it. To do this, they drew a cordon sanitaire around not only the eleven-million-person city of Wuhan, but the entire province of Hubei with its sixty million people—in effect, quarantining a population the size of New

York and California combined. They then flooded this province with health workers supported by thousands of People's Liberation Army soldiers, imposed a lockdown in which citizens had to shelter in their apartments, and conducted massive testing. When individuals were found to be infected, or even thought to be likely to be contagious, they were separated strictly from the healthy population. Announcements from the Chinese government can never be taken at face value. Its government has manipulated data and even the criteria for what counts as a new case. But despite this noise, at this point, the evidence from all sources suggests that these efforts have actually succeeded in bending the curve of infections toward zero.

On the other hand, the United States remains mired in this mess. It has experienced more infections and more deaths than any other country on the planet; closed down its own economy and society, leading to an economic decline larger than any experienced since the Great Depression; added $3 trillion to its national balance sheet; and is still struggling to find its way. The current patchwork reopening of its economy and society has been followed by waves of new infections and poisonous political recriminations.

Lest the reader despair at this point, a reminder from history may be in order. Democracies are notoriously slow to awaken to change but when finally aroused and focused are ferocious in their response. American democracy's record provides the extreme case of this weakness. Had any of its wars been declared over at the end of the first quarter—from the Revolutionary War to the Civil War to World Wars I and II—we would have lost. Despite our miserable record in the first rounds of what promises to be an extended war against coronavirus, it is much too soon to count us out. Historically, when finely focused, Americans have proved indomitable.

Since the coronavirus crisis will be testing us for many months, if not years to come, no one can be sure today what these results will show six months from now or this time next year. But if an impartial Martian strategist were to judge America's and China's performance in this war today, the answer would be clear: the USA lost.

The geopolitical consequences of these responses for the United States and its rivalry with China must be assessed in four dimensions: (1) impact on each nation's GDP, (2) impact on citizens' confidence in their government, (3) impact on each nation's capacity and will to assist other nations as they attempt to ensure the lives and well-being of their citizens, and (4) impact of all of the above on the reputations of the United States and China and their standing in the eyes of governing classes in every other nation.

The Chinese government understood and accepted that its response would hit the economy hard. But after a single quarter in which its economy declined by almost 7%, China reopened for business and has now returned to positive growth in the second quarter and beyond.[24] The American response has caused its economy to suffer a sharper decline than in any equivalent period in the Great Depression and has put the United States on track to enter 2021 with a GDP smaller than it had last year.[25] If China now returns to robust economic growth, on the one hand, and the United States teeters on the brink between an extended recession and a genuine depression for months, the gap between the GDP of China and the United States will grow.

The initial missteps in responding to coronavirus raised serious questions about China's party-led government and especially about its president, who as "COE"— chief of everything—has projected a "cult of competence." But the rapid turnaround and the results that followed have renewed Chinese citizens' confidence in their leader and in their form of government—especially as they watch the United States continuing to stumble. Coronavirus has amplified America's dysfunctional democracy in an already vicious election year. Moreover, if an authoritarian government demonstrates competence in ensuring its citizens' most basic human right—the right to life—as a democratic, decentralized government flounders, propaganda about China's virtues or vices will be a sideshow.

Nations that have successfully managed challenges within their own borders have the resources to lend a helping hand to those desperately seeking assistance. After World War II, the United States accounted for half of the world's GDP. It therefore had the means to conceive and launch the Marshall Plan for Europe. That allowed a devastated Britain, France, Germany, and Italy to survive, recover, and become parts of the American NATO alliance against the Soviet Union. As Germany's great end-of–Cold War Chancellor Helmut Kohl never tired of saying, in the ruins of a defeated country, as a teenager who was cold and hungry, he received his first overcoat and food from American soldiers who had less than a year before been in deadly conflict with Nazi armies.

Which way is aid flowing in this crisis? With whom have both the United States and France placed orders for millions of face masks?[26] Who is the major supplier to the world of protective equipment, ingredients for tests, ventilators, and other medical supplies? As the United States has wrestled with its ally France over whose delivery of masks from China comes first, China has provided protective equipment and medicines to more than one hundred countries, focusing in particular on countries it sees as important in its campaign for global influence.[27] Italy is one of these, and Italians who were overwhelmed by endless videos of hospitals being overrun and lines of coffins will not soon forget who provided protective equipment, ventilators, and hundreds of doctors and who, including their EU partners and the United States, sent get-well cards. China's usurpation of the role the United States has played for the past seven decades as the benevolent provider of assistance to states in their most desperate moments may become the metaphor for historians writing the requiem for the American century.

In addition, the United States and China are each doing everything in their power to win the vaccine race. Anyone who has any doubts about which population the winner will vaccinate first is still in need of a dose of reality.

Moreover, we should never forget the larger canvas. There China's meta-narrative is a story of its inevitable rise and America's irreversible decline. A nation that began the century with a GDP less than a quarter of America's has now overtaken the United States to create an economy larger than ours. A military that was forced to back down in the Taiwan Strait Crisis of 1996 when the United States sent two carriers to the theater has over the past two decades built up an arsenal of "carrier-killer" missiles that would force the United States to make different choices today. In the aftermath of the 2008 financial crisis, China's leadership was emboldened by its success in returning to rapid growth as the United States was stuck in secular stagnation. Unless the United States can find a way to meet the current coronavirus challenge, China could be tempted to take greater risks, including forcibly bringing Taiwan under Beijing's rule.

In sum, as the United States and China navigate the coronavirus crisis, they are simultaneously facing off in the competition between their two fundamentally different conceptions of governance. Americans and Chinese will see how well—or poorly—their form of government ensures their safety. Others around the world will draw conclusions about the relative strengths and weaknesses of an American-style decentralized democracy with its core commitment to individual liberty, on the one hand, versus China's party-led autocracy in which order is the paramount political value, on the other.

Inseparable Conjoined Twins

Despite this rivalry, coronavirus also provides a vivid reminder that each nation faces external threats it cannot defeat on its own. Even if one nation succeeds in driving the rate of new domestic infections to zero, when its citizens return from abroad, they can bring it with them, creating further waves of infections. This dilemma illuminates a fundamental feature of the relationship first learned by American and Soviet cold warriors: the United States and China, like the United States and Soviet Union, are insufferable but inseparable conjoined twins.

COLD WAR WISDOM

After exploding its first bomb in 1949, the Soviet Union rapidly developed a nuclear arsenal so substantial and sophisticated that it created what nuclear strategists recognized as mutual assured destruction, or MAD.[28] This described a condition in which neither the United States nor the Soviet Union could be sure of destroying its opponent's arsenal with a nuclear first strike before the enemy could launch a fatal nuclear response. Under such conditions, one state's decision to kill another is simultaneously a choice to commit national suicide. President Ronald Reagan's one-liner captures the central truth: "A nuclear war cannot be won and must therefore never be fought."

If Reagan was right, then between nuclear superpowers, the menu of viable strategic options cannot include nuclear attack. In rivalries between nuclear superpowers in which neither has dominance on every rung up the escalation ladder from conventional war, the use of conventional military forces to attack the adversary also becomes almost unthinkable—for anything short of a threat to national survival. History saw these constraints emerge in the Cold War, beginning with the Berlin blockade of 1948, and the US government's refusal to come to the rescue of Hungarian freedom fighters when they rose up in 1956 or Czech freedom fighters trying to escape Soviet domination in 1968.

Cold War strategists learned that survival under these conditions necessitated shaping the competition around five Cs: caution, communication, constraints, compromise, and cooperation. To guard against the risk of their "cold" war turning "hot," the United States and the Soviet Union accepted—for the time being—many unacceptable facts on the ground. These included Soviet domination of the captive nations of Eastern Europe and the Communist regimes in China, Cuba, and North Korea. In addition, the rivals wove an intricate web of mutual constraints around the competition, constraints that President Kennedy called "the precarious rules of the status quo." To reduce the risk of surprise nuclear attacks, for instance, they negotiated arms control treaties that provided greater transparency and instilled greater confidence in each party that the other was not about to launch a first strike. To avoid accidental collisions of aircraft or ships, they negotiated precise rules of the road for air and sea. Over time, both competitors tacitly agreed to each other's three nos: (1) no use of nuclear weapons, (2) no direct overt killing of each other's armed forces, and (3) no overt military intervention in each other's recognized sphere of influence.

Nevertheless, while superpower arsenals create what students of security studies have called a "crystal ball effect" that reminds policy makers of the devastating consequences of war and thus engenders additional caution, in confronting the Soviet Union in the Cuban Missile Crisis, President Kennedy still took what he judged to be a one-in-three chance of nuclear war.[29]

Nuclear weapons, in effect, made the United States and the Soviet Union (and now Russia) inseparable conjoined twins. While each still had a head, a brain, and the will to act, their backbones had been fused to become one. In their united breast beat a single heart. On the day that one stopped the other's heart from beating, both would unquestionably die. As awkward and uncomfortable as this metaphor is, it captures the defining fact about the US relationship with the Soviet Union in the Cold War. And it remains the defining truth many 21st-century Americans imagine somehow vanished when the Cold War ended. While the Soviet Union disappeared, its superpower arsenal certainly did not.

Today, China has developed a nuclear arsenal so robust that it creates a 21st-century version of MAD with the United States. Thus, however evil, however demonic, however dangerous, however deserving to be strangled it is, the United States must struggle to find some way to live with it—or face dying together.

21st-Century Mini-MADs

The shared fate of the United States and China does not stop with mutual assured nuclear destruction. In our interconnected world, it instead goes beyond to a number of "mini-MADs," challenges that threaten mutual assured "defeat," if not "destruction," for both countries that neither can overcome alone.

Viruses carry no passports, have no ideology, and respect no borders. When droplets from an infected patient who sneezes are inhaled by a healthy individual, the biological impact is essentially identical whether the person is American, Italian, or Chinese. When an outbreak becomes a pandemic infecting citizens around the world, since no nation can hermetically seal its borders, every country is at risk. The inescapable fact is that all 7.7 billion people alive today inhabit one small planet Earth. As President Kennedy noted in explaining the necessity for coexistence with the Soviet Union in facing mutual, existential nuclear danger: "We all breathe the same air. We all cherish our children's future. And we are all mortal."[30]

Pandemics are one mini-MAD. Climate change is another. Given the fact that every citizen on planet Earth lives inside a single biosphere, unless the United

States and China—as the number one and number two emitters of greenhouse gases, respectively—can find ways to restrain emissions or limit their effects, by century's end, citizens could find the climates in both countries unlivable. The Paris Climate Agreement took a small step toward recognizing this fact and beginning to act to address the challenge. President Trump's withdrawal from the pact and denial of the problem is hard to understand.

Financial crises, like the events of 2008 that occurred after the collapse of Lehman Brothers, which produced a Great Recession and threatened a second Great Depression, can also only be managed if the two largest economies in the world work together. In 2008, they did. As former secretary of the treasury Hank Paulson—the key player for the United States in that event—has said, the Chinese cooperation in coordinating a Chinese fiscal stimulus was at least as important, and perhaps more important, than American action in what could have become a global depression.[31] (And those who have forgotten the political consequences of the Great Depression of the 1930s should google *fascism* and *Nazism*.)

Rivalry, indeed intense rivalry, between the United States and China is inevitable. But coronavirus is a reminder that in key arenas of international affairs, neither country can live without the other.

Condemned to Cooperate

As long as the United States and China depend on each other for their security in the face of mutual threats, cooperation will be as much a defining feature of world order as rivalry. This deadly pathogen has condemned the United States and China, despite their hostility, to work together, at least to the extent necessary, to ensure their national survival and well-being.

Victory for each will require an effective vaccine. In the current race for that vaccine, we see both the benefits of cooperation and the inevitability of rivalry. Even as both countries rush to create a vaccine that will almost certainly be used on the winners' own population first, important aspects of its development have been team efforts. By quickly sequencing the genome of the virus and posting it on the Web, China provided essential data for scientists around the world. Joint ventures between a German biotech firm and a Chinese partner, Harvard Medical School and Guangzhou Institute, and others underscore the fact that science advances fastest when scientists everywhere combine their strengths.

RIVALRY PARTNERS

The United States' core national interest is "to preserve the United States as a free nation with our fundamental institutions and values intact," as the defining statement of Cold War strategy put it.[32] But could that goal be achieved in a world that also included an Evil Empire, as Ronald Reagan rightly called the Soviet Union? Or, today, in a world with a rapidly rising authoritarian China?[33]

In the first chapter of the Cold War, leaders we now revere as the "Wise Men" answered "no." George Kennan's Long Telegram identified the Soviet Union as "a political force committed fanatically to the belief that with the United States there can be no permanent modus vivendi."[34] According to Kennan's diagnosis, the Soviets "believed it was necessary that our society be disrupted, our traditional way of life be destroyed, the international authority of our state be broken, if Soviet power was to be secured."[35] As America's first secretary of defense, James Forrestal, put it: Soviet Communism is "as incompatible with democracy as was Nazism or fascism."[36]

But after having survived the Cuban Missile Crisis in which he confronted the prospect of a nuclear war that could have killed hundreds of millions of people, President Kennedy had second thoughts. In the most significant foreign policy speech of his career, delivered just five months before he was assassinated, Kennedy signaled a major shift in American Cold War strategy. While never wavering in his conviction that the Soviet Union was evil and the US-led free world good, he nonetheless concluded that an unconstrained effort to bury Soviet-led totalitarianism had become unacceptably dangerous.

Going forward, the United States and Soviet Union would have to find ways to constrain their competition and even compromise: to live and let live in a world of diverse political systems with diametrically opposed values and ideologies. In a bit of rhetorical jiujitsu that stood President Woodrow Wilson's long-standing call for a "world safe for democracy" on its head, he insisted that hereafter, the priority in the Cold War would be to build a "world safe for diversity."[37]

What led President Kennedy to such a dramatic change of mind? The experience of existential nuclear danger. He really believed that the confrontation in which he had stood eyeball-to-eyeball with the Soviet leader Nikita Khrushchev could have ended in nuclear Armageddon. Having survived, as he gave thanks, he vowed that hereafter he would do everything in his power to ensure that neither he nor any of his successors would ever have to do that again.

Could Kennedy's insight offer clues for Americans and Chinese strategists today as they think about how to escape Thucydides's Trap? Could it be enlarged and enriched by a concept of "rivalry partnership" that emerged a thousand years ago in ancient China?

Rivalry partners sounds like a contradiction. But it describes the relationship the Song Emperor of China established with the Liao, a Manchurian kingdom on China's northern border, after concluding that his armies would not be able to defeat them. In the Chanyuan Treaty of 1005, Song China and Liao agreed to compete aggressively in some arenas and simultaneously to cooperate intensely in others. In a unique version of Chinese tributary relations, the Chanyuan Treaty required the Song to pay tribute to the Liao, who agreed to invest that payment in economic, scientific, and technical development in Song China.[38]

Sustaining this rivalry partnership required managing recurring crises and adapting to new conditions. Nonetheless, the era of peace between the two rivals that followed lasted 120 years. Moreover, the payments created an early form of a market, stimulating economic growth in China that supported the development of arts and learning in what Chinese historians now describe as a "golden era."

The question today is whether American and Chinese government leaders could find their way to a 21st-century analogue of the Song's invention—one that would allow them simultaneously to compete and cooperate.

The toxic cocktail of pride, arrogance, and paranoia engulfing both rivals is a serious challenge to cooperation. But what may be an alien concept to world leaders today is normal for the leaders of our most dynamic companies. Apple and Samsung, for example, are fierce competitors in selling smartphones. But Samsung is also Apple's essential supplier of components for smartphones.[39] Coronavirus makes incandescent the impossibility of identifying China clearly as either foe or friend. Rivalry partnership may sound complicated, but life is complicated.

Conclusion

What lasting impact will coronavirus have on relations between the United States and China? While the future is uncertain, I'll record my bet that Thucydides will be a better guide than those who are now proclaiming a transformation of international relations.

Could a rivalry partnership in a world safe for peaceful competition between diverse political systems serve as the starting point for a new strategic concept for managing the dangerous dynamic between China and the United States today? For political leaders unable to see shades between black and white, this may prove too demanding. If so, Thucydides would say they chose their fate. But since our survival is at stake, we must hope that political leaders learn from history to navigate a complicated, difficult, challenging rivalry—one in which the United States and China have both competing interests and shared interests they have to manage in order to survive.

NOTES

1. For more information, visit the Harvard Kennedy School Belfer Center's Applied History Project website, https://www.belfercenter.org/project/applied-history-project.

2. Thucydides, *The History of the Peloponnesian War*.

3. Richard E. Neustadt and Ernest R. May, *Thinking in Time: The Uses of History for Decision Makers* (New York: Free Press, 1986), 253–254.

4. Neustadt and May, *Thinking in Time*, 251.

5. Henry Kissinger, "The Coronavirus Pandemic Will Forever Alter the World Order," *Wall Street Journal*, April 3, 2020.

6. Richard Haass, "A Cold War with China Would Be a Mistake," *Wall Street Journal*, May 7, 2020.

7. Lawrence Summers, "Covid-19 Looks Like a Hinge in History," *Financial Times*, May 14, 2020.

8. Others include Stewart M. Patrick, "COVID-19 and Climate Change Will Change the Definition of National Security," *World Politics Review*, May 18, 2020; Samantha Power, "How the COVID-19 Era Will Change National Security Forever," *Time*, April 14, 2020; and Anne-Marie Slaughter, "Redefining National Security for the Post Pandemic World," *Project Syndicate*, June 3, 2020.

9. *New York Times* columnist Thomas Friedman proclaimed the "Golden Arches Theory of Conflict Prevention" in 1996: "When a country reaches a certain level of economic development, when it has a middle class big enough to support a McDonald's, it becomes a McDonald's country, and people in McDonald's countries don't like to fight wars; they like to wait in line for burgers." See Friedman, "Foreign Affairs Big Mac I," *New York Times*, December 8, 1996; and Graham Allison, "The Myth of the Liberal Order," *Foreign Affairs*, July/August 2018.

10. This section builds on and expands Graham Allison, "The New Spheres of Influence," *Foreign Affairs*, March/April 2020; and Allison, "The U.S.-China Strategic Competition: Clues from History" (discussion paper, Harvard Kennedy School Belfer Center for Science and International Affairs, February 2020).

11. "World Economic Outlook Data Mapper," International Monetary Fund, October 2019; "World Development Indicators Data Bank," World Bank, October 28, 2019, https://datacatalog.worldbank.org/dataset/world-development-indicators.

12. "References: Definition and Notes: GDP Methodology," CIA World Factbook, n.d., accessed July 15, 2019, https://www.cia.gov/library/publications/the-world-factbook/docs/notesanddefs.html; Tim Callen, "Purchasing Power Parity: Weights Matter," International Monetary Fund, December 18, 2018, https://www.imf.org/external/pubs/ft/fandd

/basics/ppp.htm. For the judgment of the world's leading central banker, Stanley Fischer, see Graham Allison, *Destined for War: Can American and China Escape Thucydides's Trap?* (New York: Houghton Mifflin Harcourt, 2017), 11–12.

13. "Direction of Trade Statistics," International Monetary Fund, accessed July 15, 2019, https://data.imf.org/?sk=9D6028D4-F14A-464C-A2F2-59B2CD424B85.

14. "Internet Trends Report 2018," Kleiner Perkins, May 30, 2018, https://www.klein erperkins.com/perspectives/internet-trends-report-2018/.

15. SIPRI Military Expenditure Database, accessed February 3, 2020, https://www.sipri .org/databases/milex.

16. Allison, "The U.S.-China Strategic Competition."

17. Center for a New American Security (CNAS), "How the U.S. Military Fights Wars Today and in the Future," March 7, 2019, YouTube video, 13:09, https://www.youtube.com /watch?v=m1DtXOuUoMo.

18. Nicholas Kristof, "This Is How War with China Could Begin," *New York Times*, September 4, 2019. Former defense official David Ochmanek also remarks that a key takeaway of fifteen years of wargaming is that "we're 0-for-18" in CNAS, "How the U.S. Military Fights Wars Today and in the Future," March 7, 2019, YouTube video, 31:21, https://www.youtube.com/watch?v=m1DtXOuUoMo.

19. Graham Allison, Robert D. Blackwill, and Ali Wyne, *Lee Kuan Yew: The Grand Master's Insights on China, the United States, and the World* (Cambridge, MA: MIT Press, 2013), 42.

20. For more information, visit the Harvard Kennedy School Belfer Center's Thucydides's Trap Case File website, https://www.belfercenter.org/thucydides-trap/case-file.

21. Allison et al., *Lee Kuan Yew.*

22. Graham Allison, "The US Is Hunkering Down for a New Cold War with China," *Financial Times*, October 12, 2018.

23. This section builds on and expands Graham Allison, "In War against Coronavirus: Is China Foe—or Friend?," *The National Interest*, March 27, 2020.

24. "Preliminary Accounting Results of GDP for the First Quarter of 2020," National Bureau of Statistics of China, April 20, 2020, http://www.stats.gov.cn/english/PressRelease /202004/t20200420_1739811.html; "Economists Are Increasingly Optimistic about China's Economic Recovery and GDP Growth," *Fortune*, June 23, 2020.

25. Nelson D. Schwartz, Ben Casselman, and Ella Koeze, "How Bad Is Unemployment? 'Literally Off the Charts,'" *New York Times*, May 8, 2020.

26. For French purchases, see "France Has Ordered over 1 Billion Face Masks, Most from China: Minister," Reuters, March 28, 2020. For US purchases, see Jonathan Swan and Joann Muller, "Inside the Start of the Great Virus Airlift," *Axios*, March 29, 2020.

27. "China Keeps Engine Roaring to Ensure Global Medical Supplies amid Pandemic," *Global Times*, March 29, 2020. See also Chad P. Bown, "COVID-19: China's Exports of Medical Supplies Provide a Ray of Hope," Peterson Institute for International Economics, March 26, 2020.

28. This section builds on and expands Allison, *Destined for War*; Allison, "The U.S.-China Strategic Competition."

29. Theodore Sorensen, *Kennedy* (New York: Harper & Row, 1965), 705.

30. John F. Kennedy, "American University Commencement Address," June 10, 1963.

31. Henry Paulson, "The U.S. and China at a Crossroads" (press release, Paulson Institute, Chicago, IL, November 7, 2018), https://www.paulsoninstitute.org/press_release/remarks-by-henry-m-paulson-jr-on-the-united-states-and-china-at-a-crossroads/.

32. US Department of State Policy Planning Staff, "NSC-68: United States Objectives and Programs for National Security," April 7, 1950.

33. This section builds on and expands Graham Allison, "Could the United States and China Be Rivalry Partners?," *The National Interest*, July 7, 2019.

34. George Kennan, "The Long Telegram," February 22, 1946.

35. Kennan, "The Long Telegram."

36. John Lewis Gaddis, *The United States and the Origins of the Cold War, 1941–1947* (New York: Columbia University Press, 2000), 298.

37. Kennedy, "American University Commencement Address."

38. Peter Lorge, *War, Politics and Society in Early Modern China, 900–1795* (London: Routledge, 2005).

39. "Rivalry between Apple and Samsung in Smartphones Will Grow Fiercer," *The Economist*, September 14, 2017.

Chapter Twenty-Two

Building a New Technological Relationship and Rivalry

US-China Relations in the Aftermath of COVID

Eric Schmidt

Containing COVID-19 requires opposite moves. Stopping the virus requires radical separation—of the sick and the healthy, of communities stricken and those spared, of nations whose borders are ordinarily open to people and goods. In a better world, this radical separation would be paired with intense cooperation—cooperation in finding and distributing a vaccine, restarting the world economy, and pooling resources to prevent future outbreaks. COVID-19 marks one of the first times that we as a species have faced a sudden global crisis with modern communications linking us seamlessly together. It could easily be a unifying moment.

Instead, in fewer than six months, the outbreak of COVID-19 has cracked the bridge that was thoughtfully constructed between the United States and a rising China in the years since Henry Kissinger's 1971 visit to Beijing. Rather than cooperating with each other and sharing the burden of global leadership at a moment of crisis, Washington and Beijing turned their animus on each other. The

Eric Schmidt is an accomplished technologist, entrepreneur, and philanthropist. He joined Google in 2001 and helped grow the company from a Silicon Valley start-up to a global leader in technology alongside founders Sergey Brin and Larry Page. Eric served as Google's chief executive officer and chairman from 2001 to 2011, as well as executive chairman and technical advisor. Under his leadership, Google dramatically scaled its infrastructure and diversified its product offerings while maintaining a strong culture of innovation. In 2017, he cofounded Schmidt Futures, a philanthropic initiative designed to help exceptional people do more for others by applying science and technology thoughtfully and working together across fields.

present friction, despite the two nations' economies sharing a deep structural interdependence, showcases how easily domestic policy and decision making in both countries can destabilize a relationship that had been growing more fragile for some time. Even as China surpassed Mexico and Canada to become the United States' largest trading partner in April 2020, informed commentators are now talking of a new cold war and wondering whether Taiwan will be the next domino to fall after Hong Kong's wholesale absorption into the mainland's system of governance and control.[1]

Prudent leadership is needed to transcend the present tensions and establish a new framework for how the United States and China will cooperate and compete in the years to come. The framework must place technology as its central axis. Advanced technology is at the core of US-China competition and cooperation in global markets today. While calls for "decoupling" are reaching a higher decibel than ever before, leaders of both countries must resist the temptation to isolate industries and talent. We cannot—and should not—attempt the kind of expansive decoupling being called for by some. Neither coexistence nor global progress is possible unless the leaders of both countries find ways to revive cooperation even as the two countries enter a new phase of economic competition intensified by deep ideological differences and geopolitical rivalry.[2]

Five elements will underlie a recalibration of the relationship in such a way that preserves sovereignty and security, enables US companies to win the great game of platform competition now under way in global markets, and lets the United States continue to reap the beneficial aspects of interchange. They are as follows: (1) some purposeful decoupling of specific linkages that introduce unacceptable vulnerabilities; (2) continuing cooperative research, which brings significant joint benefit; (3) a clear commitment to commercial interchange between tech sectors; (4) greater collaboration in shared challenge areas; and (5) gearing up to win the platform competition through greater federal investment in research and development (R&D).

Before exploring each element in turn, we must first understand why COVID has become an inflection point in the relationship between the two dominant actors in the global system and how the underlying intensification of technological competition brought us to this point.

What the Virus Wrought

While greater cooperation may emerge in time, the early months of the pandemic have been characterized by radical separation. There is a new fragility in the world, which we feel collectively. Leaders seem driven by rapid-fire response to events, neglecting reason or long-term perspective. This dynamic is especially evident between the United States and China. One of the first breaks in cooperation occurred when N95 respirator masks produced by foreign-owned factories in China were effectively nationalized by the Chinese Communist Party without sufficient consultation. When China's own demand for medical-grade masks stabilized as the Wuhan outbreak subsided, China then pursued a ruthless and ultimately counterproductive program of "mask diplomacy" that tied the export of scarce medical supplies to coercive ends.[3] Conditions for receiving lifesaving shipments included recipients making public statements of support for the Chinese Communist Party, heads of state giving thanks beside Chinese aircraft delivering supplies, or, most perniciously, recipients agreeing to a greater market share and dropping security concerns for telecommunications company Huawei. It was not Beijing's finest moment.

Nor was it Washington's best hour. As the outbreak grew in the United States, escalating accusations about the origin of the virus and questions about early transparency around the threat it posed produced a disastrous break in diplomacy for international health, with the United States ultimately defunding the World Health Organization and President Xi Jinping of China effectively pledging to replace the US contribution with Chinese funds. Coming after the US withdrawal from the Paris accord on climate, it was a second major retreat by the United States from an established framework for global cooperation.

With neither the United States nor China joining together in any of the global COVID vaccine coalitions striving to optimize R&D and production, analysts have raised the specter of a dangerous kind of "vaccine nationalism" playing out. These fears only grew when Gustave Perna, the four-star general appointed to run Operation Warp Speed, the US government's vaccine initiative, was asked whether the list of countries that the United States was prepared to cooperate with includes China: "It does not," he responded.[4] A successful vaccine candidate held by the United States or by China could swiftly become an instrument of geopolitical competition, slowing the global administration of inoculum that is the one assured way to end the pandemic and restart the global economy. The costs to the world of China and the United States failing to cooperate are high.

The Deeper Fissure

When we ask ourselves why the rivalry has intensified, technology explains it to a much more significant extent than do the recent breakdowns induced by

COVID. China's new technological prowess applied to an ambitious global agenda has destabilized the relationship. In emerging technology—in particular, artificial intelligence (AI) and 5G (fifth-generation mobile broadband)—Chinese and American companies are competing over platform dominance in global markets. Platform technologies are assemblages of hardware, software, and services that, by virtue of network effects, quickly become invincible in their sectors. Think Facebook and Weibo in social media, Google and Baidu in search, Amazon and Alibaba in online retail. Leveraging the positive feedback loop that results from rapid expansion, platform technologies often expand to other sectors and services. The future will increasingly become a battle over platform technologies dominated by a small number of companies from information-rich countries.

While both governments harbor ambitions of leading the world in research, applications, and market share, the Chinese government has acted most vigorously in support of its "national champion" companies. As recently as May 2020, President Xi announced that Beijing will invest $1.4 trillion over six years to accelerate the rollout of 5G wireless networks, improve technology infrastructure, and develop new AI systems. Huawei's runaway market dominance in 5G is in fact the first platform technology of the internet age in which a Chinese firm has a breakout lead over the United States and other Western competitors, which have fallen behind in the race to develop and deploy the next generation of telecommunications technology. China, like the United States, is building an innovation system in which networks of knowledge, talent, and entrepreneurism drive advances so rapidly that few others will ever catch up.

Part of the reason why our government is not yet matching Beijing's aggressive backing of science and technology is that many Americans still have an outdated vision of China, viewing it, in essence, as a still-developing nation rather than a peer with aspirations for global influence on par with the United States. In three generations, China transformed from having a per capita income of about $90 in 1960 to about $10,000 today. China has already passed the United States in gross domestic product based on purchasing power parity. China poses a larger economic challenge to the United States than the Soviet Union did. As a leading historian recently noted, "the Soviet Union could never draw on the resources of a dynamic private sector. China can."[5] Now, the Chinese government has ambitions—and specific plans, with promises of billions of dollars in funding— to surpass the United States in areas such as quantum communications, supercomputing, aerospace, 5G, mobile payment, new energy vehicles, high-speed railway, financial technology, and AI.

Already today, China has almost twice as many supercomputers as the United States. It has approximately fifteen times the number of deployed 5G base stations as the United States.[6] By 2025, Chinese researchers are expected to overtake American researchers in the 1% of most-cited scientific papers in AI.[7] By 2030, China is expected to spend more than the United States on overall R&D, in absolute terms.[8] Sometime after 2030, the Chinese economy likely will become larger than ours.[9]

China's rapid technological progress unsettles Americans for many legitimate reasons. China is challenging the most important engine of American economic power—its innovation system. Americans believe that China's ambition to dominate the world's digital infrastructure will, whether through design or impact, create a new geopolitical reality. Americans see China's technological ambition through the lens of its authoritarian system and its use of technology at home to maintain control. Americans also resent that China's growth has been delivered in part by restricting the access of US firms to its domestic market, by theft of intellectual property, by forced technology transfer, and by other odious coercive economic tools. The United States welcomed China into the global trading system and welcomed Chinese students into American universities; and from the American perspective, that move has cost Americans jobs, hurt the American middle class, and is now threatening US leadership abroad. Chinese leaders, meanwhile, see US actions meant to hinder the growth of China's technology companies as the overreaction of a declining power unwilling to allow China to exercise influence commensurate with its stature.

While the race for global market share in platform technologies may at first glance appear zero-sum for the firms involved, a web of underlying connections makes it anything but. Technical collaboration among US and Chinese researchers and the interlocking set of commercial activities between each country's technology economy are a major driver of wealth and progress for both countries and for the world. Preserving the beneficial aspects of this research, talent, and market ecosystem is essential for economic reasons. The question, given present tensions, is how.

A New Technological Relationship

To move beyond the current dynamic, both sides must seek a new arrangement. What has been lost in US-China discord is this: if this rivalry could generate healthy competition fought on an even playing field, the two countries would have more to gain by competing fairly and cooperating where possible than by opposing each other on all fronts. The question now is how we redraw the relationship in a way that recognizes the centrality of commercial competition and the need for that competition to occur fairly and without geopolitical escalation. Let me propose five principles that I believe can guide us to *a new technological relationship.*

Some Purposeful Decoupling Is Necessary

In limited areas—namely, areas with clear security and military applications—some purposeful decoupling is necessary and, in fact, may stabilize the relationship by delineating clear no-go zones. The breakdown of cooperation over medical supply chains is one example. A half-century-long march toward optimizing for efficiency, with "just in time" logistics stretching across global supply chains, left countries around the world facing shortages of critical medical supplies when the pandemic hit. Each nation will have to take careful stock of what it relies on, where that is produced, and how future shocks can be mitigated by combinations of iron-clad supply guarantees, stockpiling, and domestic production capacity. Finding a new set point between efficiency and resiliency in the context of Chinese supply chains, without closing ourselves off to the world or spurning the prosperity that an interconnected economy can deliver, is an important issue for the United States to address. While doing so will not be easy or without costs, the problem is solvable. Similarly, preserving essential state functions, such as telecommunications, necessitates decoupling hardware and services that introduce unacceptable security threats into the network core, as is the case with Huawei.

Harder areas to establish a clear plan for decoupling include technologies such as AI, which are inherently dual use, but we must begin that discussion. It should begin with a basic question: If China halted trade with the United States in a crisis or in response to rising tension, what products or materials key to national security would the United States not be able to build or procure domestically or find elsewhere in the world market? We should not overact, but we must undertake a careful and systematic analysis. Today we might depend on China for personal protective equipment and ventilators. We must make sure, though, that it is never an electronic chip or any other critical technology that leaves us in a position of being coerced or having to concede a vital interest because of our dependence.

Decoupling, seen through this lens, is not just about disconnecting from China. It is about revitalizing America's own productivity in critical areas and building up allies' and partners' capacities. Done right, purposeful decoupling could spur a commercial renaissance in particular classes of technologies across Western nations and their allies, helping to strengthen the liberal world order.

Continuing Cooperative Research, Which Produces Significant Joint Benefit

Advocates for much stronger prohibitions on commercial interchange have pushed US leadership to take steps toward more fully decoupling the international research system, especially on AI and biology but also in other areas of technology too. They cite China's well-documented espionage, intellectual property theft, and talent recruitment programs, which are unquestionably disadvantaging our companies, our universities, and our military.[10] It is certainly true that particular types of joint ventures between Chinese and US firms do need to be placed off limits due to national security concerns. Greater policing of intellectual property theft in industry and academia is necessary, on a scale appropriate to the size of the problem. Also needed in policy is a more careful demarcation of the dynamics of cooperation, competition, and mutual benefit across different kinds of research— fundamental, applied, product development. But it would be a catastrophic mistake to make unfortunate and serious edge cases the basis for undoing a system that has on the whole yielded impressive joint gains and driven the accrual of enormous economic value.

Take AI as an example. Analysis by Schmidt Futures of top AI research submitted to conferences shows that research collaborations between American and Chinese institutions are, by a wide margin, the most productive AI research pairings in the world. Two-thirds of the research papers published by US-based institutions at top AI conferences have a coauthor of Chinese descent. Additionally, the United States has benefited enormously from its ability to attract top Chinese technical talent. A recent analysis indicated that of a group of 128 high-level researchers with undergraduate degrees from Chinese universities whose papers were presented at AI conferences, more than half currently work in the United States. Among international students majoring in computer science and math at US universities, nearly 20% were Chinese nationals.[11] At the same time, the Chinese tech ecosystem has prospered as well, since a sizable number of China's technology and research leaders educated in the United States return home to take leadership roles. The community of Chinese American technologists and their immediate American colleagues know best the fruits of global technological collaboration. Their voices are necessary to help us confront the challenges we face and find additional ways that cooperation can be sustained and encouraged. We must not lose sight of how competition in research, in peaceful application, and in commercial markets is healthy, normal, and most often accelerates technological progress for everyone.

CLEAR COMMITMENT TO COMMERCIAL INTERCHANGE BETWEEN TECH SECTORS

Anyone with an Amazon account, or really any American consumer, grasps the kind of economic value being generated in China in response to US consumer demand. The vital role that the US export market plays for China, along with Chinese ownership of US Treasury securities and the value of the US dollar, is widely understood to have powered both economies to unprecedented heights. What is less known is the value that accrues to US firms selling goods and services to China, especially in the technology market.

Today China accounts for about 45% of global semiconductor demand but relies on imports for more than 90% of its chip needs. Semiconductors are China's single largest import ($241 billion), followed by oil ($228 billion)—leading to the oft-repeated and stunning fact that China spends more on silicon than it does on hydrocarbons.[12] These foreign semiconductors are critical components for China's national champion companies, including ZTE in telecom. Although moves to decouple the chip ecosystem have already begun, with US government restrictions on particular classes of hardware leading the Chinese to accelerate their own domestic design and production capacity, companies based in the United States and its allies, including Taiwan, will continue to supply the majority of this crucial hardware, at least in the short term. Apple's hardware and services are another easily identifiable illustration of beneficial interchange; in the hands of one in five Chinese smartphone users are iPhones designed in California and loaded with tools and services from Apple's App Store.

Human capital is perhaps an even more significant aspect of how entrepreneurial technology companies have been founded and grown. It is hard to find an arrangement that has had more mutual benefit to the development of technology and wealth on both sides of the Pacific than the influx of high-skilled Chinese talent to the United States. Just as leading American technology firms have executive teams that are internationally diverse, especially on the engineering and product development side, Baidu, Alibaba, and Tencent all have US-educated executives within their ranks. It is not just the old guard either. Colin Huang, China's new second-richest man and the founder of the rapidly growing e-commerce company Pinduoduo, was educated in the United States and has written publicly about his formative experience starting his career at Google.[13] These high-profile "sea turtles" act not only as crucial carriers of value in US-China interchange. Having a stake in each society, they are also a beachhead from which further dialogue and stronger cooperation can be built.

The United States is an overwhelming winner as well. In fact, multiculturalism is arguably our deepest competitive moat in the development of technology, protecting the lead that many US firms have built over global competitors. Just as teams of international talent within US firms have been the biggest driver of commercial breakthroughs in the last generation, the primary determining factor for whether the future of technology will be defined in the United States or China in the coming generation is human capital. The ability to attract and retain top-tier talent from around the world drives a flywheel spinning continuously faster in which the best talent comes to the United States to work at the best institutions on the most cutting-edge intellectual property. High-skilled immigration and diversity power our nation's competitive advantage in technology. Continuing to draw the best talent here is a core competency for our country, and we should be doing everything we can to reinforce it.

Ultimately, both the United States and China would be harmed if their economic and technological systems decouple fully. Imagine a world with two wholly different internets—How much would that set us back in the creation of new products, services, and technologies? How much would two separate internets set back cooperation in health care, science, and research? How much would it increase the risk of a miscalculation militarily between the two greatest powers in the world system? When viewed in this light, it is easier to see how deliberately splitting the "tech stacks" upon which our modern lives are built will much more likely make the world smaller, not bigger.

GREATER COLLABORATION IN SHARED CHALLENGE AREAS

The scope of possible cooperation between the United States and China is growing in concert with the promise of technology. AI, machine learning, and expanding digital connectivity provide a rich arena for cooperation to solve the world's hardest challenges. The outbreak of COVID-19 spotlights the importance of making progress in health care and global health security and in channeling modern machine learning techniques toward fighting a pandemic. Others challenge areas, such as climate change, are ripe for cooperation and in urgent need of solutions that scale. There are still other areas such as AI safety—that is, ensuring AI systems do only what they are designed to do—where cooperation would benefit both countries and many others as well. The world would be a better place if China and the United States found a way to meet these challenges together, even as they continued to compete in global markets.

A great question before policy makers is how to call attention to these shared challenge areas more explicitly to reaffirm the mutual benefits of cooperation and to make progress together. One could imagine both top-down and bottom-up approaches. A commission of prominent Chinese and American political and business leaders could, for instance, craft a joint strategy to maximize cooperation in specific areas. We could similarly pull a page from the Cold War handbook for US-Soviet cooperation and boost bottom-up approaches driven by young people, whether through new incarnations of student exchanges that build on existing successes (e.g., the Schwarzman scholars program) or more modern takes such as a youth competition on major US and Chinese social media platforms. Whatever approaches we pursue, we must act now, as one can sense a turning tide. News that broke in mid-June 2020 about Baidu, the Chinese internet search giant, withdrawing from the Partnership on AI, a US-industry-based effort to address the ethical challenge of AI, is illustrative of the kind of cooperation that could be lost if the break between the two nations accelerates.[14]

Gearing Up to Win the Platform Competition

While greater cooperation is essential to realizing the benefits of the US-China relationship, we must also remain clear-eyed that we are in a fierce competition with China. Forcing action through engagement will only produce mutual benefits if we stay ahead or at parity in this competition. With the intensification of the competition after breakout progress made by the Chinese on multiple fronts, we must take action now to keep from falling behind.

Indeed, the trends are stark. Absent change, we will soon be competing with a country that has a bigger economy, more investment in R&D, better quality research, wider application of new technologies, and stronger computing infrastructure. As the 2020s begin, we should be gearing our policy and legislation to compete effectively in a 2030s world that may look very different. We must devise a comprehensive national strategy to win. That strategy must see the range of technologies emerging today as interconnected opportunities. Advances in quantum computing will spur developments in AI, progress in AI will help accelerate discoveries in biotechnology, 5G networks will open up new opportunities to leverage AI applications, and so on. Such a strategy could embrace the following elements.

Funding. Overall federal R&D spending has not kept pace with technological change. Simply put, we need to place big bets. US government funding for R&D has seen a decades-long decline and is now at pre-Sputnik levels as a percentage of gross domestic product.[15]

Nationwide Infrastructure. Given the interconnected nature of emerging technologies, we must invest in foundational infrastructure. This includes supporting a competitive and secure global alternative to Huawei in 5G, ensuring that the US microelectronics supply chain is resilient and assured, and investing in next-generation and high-performance computing.

Flexible Grants. The United States graduates the largest number of science and engineering doctorates of any country. We need new mechanisms to accelerate expert research in the postdoc and junior faculty phases. Congress should consider more models for multiyear investments in promising researchers, not just funding specific projects.

Government-Industry-Academia Collaborations. Because the commercial sector outspends the government on R&D in many important areas, the government must partner more closely with private companies to shape technology development. Partnerships can help researchers overcome technical and financial barriers. Congress should also explore tax incentives for companies that share data and provide computing capabilities to research institutions, and it should accelerate efforts to make government data sets more widely available.

Talent Development. The United States needs major new STEM (science, technology, engineering, and mathematics) education initiatives at the K–12, college, and graduate levels. This includes expanding the existing STEM scholarship programs and designing new ones. We also need to attract more global expertise to America. That helps our competitiveness.

A New Rivalry and Relationship

With COVID, unexpected hardship took hold in Wuhan and soon spread the world over. Hardships are now affecting our families, our communities, and our nation. No corner of the world will escape. An even bigger and more far-reaching setback is the prospect that the intensification of the US-China rivalry in a moment of global crisis will produce a permanent condition. A sharp break between the two dominant actors in the global system, at a time when all of humanity should be reaching for cooperation against a mutual threat, would be a costly setback.

The future—if managed by prudent leaders—must transcend the present confrontation. If market and platform dominance really is synonymous with geopolitical dominance, then we must prepare for a great power relationship with China that could risk outright confrontation. It will be a future much closer to the Cold War paradigm of "peaceful coexistence," only one with potentially devastating consequences to our own economic trajectory. But if we pursue fierce technological competition on a transparent, open, and reciprocal playing field, then I welcome the challenge of "competitive cooperation."

Today, the Chinese are competing to become the world's leading innovators. The United States is not playing to win. That must change. Our way to technology leadership is a dual path: better protect our innovations and out-innovate our competitors. Decoupling completely is not a viable option. We must embrace the core notion that competition produces benefits for both nations—that it spurs us both to be better.

What must we do to win in such a world? We must reassert our own American system, preserving the democratic values at its core. This means addressing deep fissures and inequalities and remembering that immigrants give us our strength; alliances, our scale; ideas and creativity, our power. If we lead in this way—the American way—our allies, and ultimately the rest of the world, will join us.

NOTES

1. Josh Zumbrun, "China a Bright Spot for U.S. in Gloomy Global Trade Picture," *Wall Street Journal*, June 14, 2020, https://www.wsj.com/articles/china-a-bright-spot-for-u-s-i n-gloomy-global-trade-picture-11592127001.

2. This essay expands upon an earlier work: Eric Schmidt, "China as Worthy Competitor—Working toward Shared Success in 2021 and Beyond" (paper presentation, Belfer Center US-China dialogue Managing the US-China Rivalry after the Pandemic, June 19, 2020).

3. Dusan Stojanovic, "China's 'Mask Diplomacy' Wins Support in Eastern Europe," Associated Press, April 14, 2020, https://apnews.com/76dff4b113e82d85716262895909f151.

4. David Welna, "General Tapped to Lead 'Operation Warp Speed' Vaccine Drive Faces Skeptical Senators," National Public Radio, June 18, 2020, https://www.npr.org /2020/06/18/880592090/general-tapped-to-lead-operation-warp-speed-vaccine-drive-fac es-skeptical-senato.

5. Niall Ferguson, "The New Cold War? It's with China, and It Has Already Begun," *New York Times*, December 2, 2019, https://www.nytimes.com/2019/12/02/opinion/china -cold-war.html.

6. Stu Woo, "In the Race to Dominate 5G, China Sprints Ahead," *Wall Street Journal*, September 7, 2019, https://www.wsj.com/articles/in-the-race-to-dominate-5g-china-has-an -edge-11567828888.

7. Field Cady and Oren Etzioni, "China May Overtake US in AI Research," Allen Institute AI2 (blog), March 13, 2019, https://medium.com/ai2-blog/china-to-overtake-us -in-ai-research-8b6b1fe30595.

8. "2018 Global R&D Funding Forecast," special issue, *R&D*, Winter 2018.

9. See James Manyika and William McRaven, *Independent Task Force Report No. 77: Innovation and National Security: Keeping Our Edge* (New York: Council on Foreign Relations, 2019), https://www.cfr.org/report/keeping-our- edge/pdf/TFR_Innovation_Strategy .pdf.

10. US Senate Permanent Subcommittee on Investigations, *Threats to the U.S. Research Enterprise: China's Talent Recruitment Plans*, November 18, 2018, https://www.hsgac.sen ate.gov/imo/media/doc/2019-11-18%20PSI%20Staff%20Report%20-%20China's%20Tal ent%20Recruitment%20Plans.pdf.

11. Tracy Qu and Coco Feng, "Beijing's Hopes for AI Dominance May Rest on How Many US-Educated Chinese Want to Return Home," *South China Morning Post*, December 6, 2019, https://www.scmp.com/tech/big-tech/article/3040797/beijings-hopes-ai-domi nance-may-rest-how-many-us-educated-chinese.

12. Cheng Ting-Fang "China's Upstart Chip Companies Aim to Topple Samsung, Intel and TSMC," *Nikkei Asian Review*, April 25, 2018, https://asia.nikkei.com/Spotlight/The -Big-Story/China-s-upstart-chip-companies-aim-to-topple-Samsung-Intel-and-TSMC.

13. See Colin Huang, "My First Job—Google," December 5, 2016, https://colinhuang .com/my-first-job-google-4268e09578a2.

14. Will Knight, "Baidu Breaks Off an AI Alliance amid Strained US-China Ties," *Wired*, June 18, 2020, https://www.wired.com/story/baidu-breaks-ai-alliance-strained -us-china-ties.

15. In 1953, the United States spent 0.72% of its GDP on R&D. In 1957, when the then-Soviet Union launched Sputnik, it had grown to 1.3%. R&D spending peaked at 1.86% in 1964. In 2017, it declined below 1953 levels to 0.61%. "Federal R&D Budget Dashboard," American Association for the Advancement of Science, https://www.aaas.org/programs /r-d-budget-and-policy/federal-rd-budget-dashboard.

Chapter Twenty-Three

From COVID War to Cold War

The New Three-Body Problem

Niall Ferguson

I n Liu Cixin's extraordinary science fiction novel *The Three-Body Problem*, China recklessly creates, then ingeniously solves, an existential threat to humanity. During the chaos of Mao Zedong's Cultural Revolution, Ye Wenjie, an astrophysicist, discovers the possibility of amplifying radio waves by bouncing them off the sun and in this way beams a message to the universe. When, years later, she receives a response from the highly unstable and authoritarian planet Trisolaris, it takes the form of a stark warning not to send further messages. Deeply disillusioned with humanity, she does so anyway, betraying the location of Earth to the Trisolarans, who are seeking a new planet because their own is subject to the chaotic gravitational forces exerted by three suns (hence the book's title). So misanthropic that she welcomes an alien invasion, Ye cofounds the Earth-Trisolaris Organization as a kind of fifth column, in partnership with a radical American environmentalist named Mike Evans. Yet their conspiracy to help the Trisolarans conquer Earth and eradicate humankind is ingeniously foiled by the dynamic duo of Wang Miao, a nanotechnology professor, and Shi Qiang, a coarse but canny Beijing cop.[1]

The nonfictional threat to humanity we confront today is not, of course, an alien invasion. The coronavirus SARS-CoV-2 does not come from outer space,

Niall Ferguson is the Milbank Family Senior Fellow at the Hoover Institution, Stanford University, and a senior faculty fellow of the Belfer Center for Science and International Affairs at Harvard University.

though it shares with the Trisolarans an impulse to colonize us. The fact, however, is that the first case of COVID-19—the disease the virus causes—was in China, just as the first messages to Trisolaris were sent from China. Similar to *The Three-Body Problem*, the Chinese Communist Party (CCP) caused this disaster—first by covering up how dangerous SARS-CoV-2 was, then by delaying measures that might have prevented its worldwide spread. Yet now—again, as in Liu Cixin's novel—China wants to claim credit for saving the world from it. Liberally exporting testing kits, face masks, and ventilators, the Chinese government has sought to snatch victory from the jaws of a defeat it inflicted. Not only that, but the deputy director of the Chinese Foreign Ministry's Information Department has gone so far as to endorse a conspiracy theory that the coronavirus originated in the United States. On March 12, Zhao Lijian tweeted: "It might be [the] US army who brought the epidemic to Wuhan."[2] Zhao also retweeted an article claiming that an American team had brought the virus with them when they participated in the World Military Games in Wuhan last October.

It was already obvious early in 2019 that a new cold war—Cold War II, between the United States and China—had begun. What started out in early 2018 as a trade war—a tit for tat over tariffs while the two sides argued about the American trade deficit and Chinese intellectual property theft—had by the end of the year metamorphosed into a technology war over the global dominance of the Chinese company Huawei in 5G (fifth generation) network telecommunications; an ideological confrontation, in response to Beijing's treatment of the Uyghur minority in China's Xinjiang region and the pro-democracy protesters in Hong Kong; and an escalation of old frictions over Taiwan and the South China Sea. Henry Kissinger himself acknowledged last November that we are "in the foothills of a Cold War."[3]

The COVID-19 pandemic has merely intensified Cold War II, at the same time revealing its existence to those who last year doubted it was happening. Chinese scholars such as Yao Yang, a professor at the China Center for Economic Research and dean of the National School of Development at Peking University, now openly discuss it.[4] Proponents of the era of US-China "engagement" since 1972 are now writing engagement's obituary, ruefully conceding (in Orville Schell's words) that it foundered "because of the CCP's deep ambivalence about the way engaging in a truly meaningful way might lead to demands for more reform and change and its ultimate demise."[5] Critics of engagement are eager to dance on its grave, urging instead that the People's Republic be economically "quarantined," with its role in global supply chains drastically reduced. To quote Daniel Blumenthal and Nick Eberstadt, "The maglev from 'Cultural Revolution' to 'Chinese Dream' does not make stops at Locke Junction or Tocqueville Town, and it has no connections to Planet Davos."[6] Moves in the direction of economic quarantine are already happening. The European Chamber of Commerce in China says that more than half its member companies are considering moving supply chains out of China. Japan has earmarked 240 billion yen ($2.2 billion) to help manufacturers leave China. "People are worried about our supply chains," Prime Minister Shinzo Abe said in April.[7] "We should try to relocate high added value items to Japan. And for everything else, we should diversify to countries like those in ASEAN." In the words of Republican senator Josh Hawley of Missouri: "The international order as we have known it for thirty years is breaking. Now imperialist China seeks to remake the world in its own image, and to bend the global economy to its own will . . . [W]e must recognize that the economic system designed by Western policy makers at the end of the Cold War does not serve our purposes in this new era."[8] In early May, Missouri's attorney general, Eric Schmitt, filed a lawsuit in federal court seeking to hold Beijing responsible for the outbreak.

To be sure, many voices have been raised to argue against Cold War II. Yao Yang has urged China to take a more conciliatory line toward Washington, by acknowledging what went wrong in Wuhan in December and January and eschewing nationalistic "wolf warrior" diplomacy. A similar argument for reconciliation to avoid the "Thucydides Trap" has been made by Yu Yongding and Kevin Gallagher. Eminent architects of the strategy of engagement, notably Hank Paulson and Robert Zoellick, have argued for its resurrection.[9] Wall Street remains as addicted as ever to the financial symbiosis that Moritz Schularick and I christened "Chimerica" in 2007, and Beijing's efforts to attract big US financial firms such as American Express, Mastercard, J. P. Morgan, Goldman Sachs, and BlackRock into the Chinese market are proving successful.[10] Nevertheless, the political trend is quite clearly in the other direction. In the United States, public sentiment toward China has become markedly more hawkish since 2017, especially among older voters. There are few subjects these days about which there is a genuine bipartisan consensus in the United States. China is one of them.

It is therefore stating the obvious to say that Cold War II will be the biggest challenge to world order, whoever is sworn in as president of the United States next January, for most of that person's term in office. Armed with John Bolton's new memoir—which reveals President Donald J. Trump to be privately a good deal more conciliatory toward his Chinese counterpart, Xi Jinping, than he has been in public—Joe Biden's campaign can now claim that their man would be tougher on China than Trump.[11] According to the Beijing-controlled *Global Times*, Chinese netizens have taken to mocking the American president as Chuan Jianguo, or "Build-up-the-country Trump"—a kind of parodic Manchurian Candidate.[12] By contrast, the language of some potential cabinet-level appointees in a Biden administration is so tough in places as to be indistinguishable from that of Secretary of State Mike Pompeo. Michèle Flournoy's recent *Foreign Affairs* article featured fighting words that might equally well have been spoken by the late senator John McCain.[13] Indeed, they echo arguments made by McCain's former aide, Christian Brose, in his new book, *The Kill Chain*.[14]

Commentators (and there are many) who doubt the capacity of the United States to reinvigorate and reassert itself imply, or state explicitly, that this is a cold war the Communist power can win. "Superpowers expect others to follow them," Kishore Mahbubani told *Der Spiegel* in April.[15] "The United States has that expectation, and China will too, as it continues to get stronger." In an interview with the *Economist*, he went further: "History has turned a corner. The era of Western domination is ending."[16] This view has long had its supporters among left-leaning or sinophile Western intellectuals, such as Martin Jacques[17] and Daniel Bell.[18] The COVID-19 crisis has made it more mainstream. Yes, the argument runs, the fatal virus may have originated in Wuhan, whether in one of the local "wet markets" where live wild animals are sold for their meat or in one of two biological research laboratories located in the city. Nevertheless, after an initially disastrous sequence of events, the Chinese government has been able to get the contagion under control with remarkable speed, illustrating the strengths of the "China model," and then to bend the global narrative in its favor, recasting itself as the savior rather than scourge of mankind.[19]

By contrast, the United States has badly bungled its pandemic response. "America is first in the world in deaths, first in the world in infections and we stand out as an emblem of global incompetence," retired diplomat William Burns told the *Financial Times* in May.[20] "The damage to America's influence and reputation will be very hard to undo."[21] The editor in chief at Bloomberg, John Micklethwait, and his coauthor Adrian Wooldridge wrote in a similar vein in April. "If the 21st century turns out to be an Asian century as the 20th was an American one," wrote Lawrence Summers in May, "the pandemic may well be remembered as the turning point."[22] Nathalie Tocci, who advises the high representative (foreign minister) of the European Union (EU), Josep Borrell, has likened this moment to the 1956 Suez Crisis. The American journalist and historian Anne Applebaum has written: "there is no American leadership in the world . . . [T]he outline of a very different, post-

American, post-coronavirus world is already taking shape . . . A vacuum has opened up, and the Chinese regime is leading the race to fill it."[23] Those who take the other side of this argument—notably Gideon Rachman and Joseph Nye—are in a distinct minority. Even Richard Haass, who argues that "the world following the pandemic is unlikely to be radically different from the one that preceded it," sees a dispiriting future of "waning American leadership, faltering global cooperation, great-power discord."[24]

Meanwhile, those who believe in historical cycles, such as hedge-fund-manager-turned-financial-historian Ray Dalio, are already writing the obituary for a dollar-dominated world economy. The historian Peter Turchin has made a similar argument on the basis of "structural demographic theory," predicting in 2012 that the year 2020 would be "the next instability peak [of violence] in the United States."[25] Who, given the circumstances of 2020, can blame the playwright David Mamet for being haunted by Cassandra's prophecies?

As Henry Kissinger has argued, the pandemic "will forever alter the world order . . . the world will never be the same after the coronavirus."[26] But how exactly will the international system change? One possible answer is that COVID-19 has reminded many countries of the benefits of self-reliance. In Kissinger's words: "Nations cohere and flourish on the belief that their institutions can foresee calamity, arrest its impact and restore stability. When the Covid-19 pandemic is over, many countries' institutions will be perceived as having failed. Whether this judgment is objectively fair is irrelevant."[27] Not everyone shares Daniel Bell's ecstatic assessment of the performance of the Chinese Communist Party. True, this may not be Xi Jinping's Chernobyl. Unlike its Soviet counterpart in 1986, the Chinese Communist Party has the ability to weather the storm of a disaster and to restart the industrial core of its economy. Yet there is no plausible way that Xi can now meet his cherished goal of having China's 2020 gross domestic product be double that of 2010: COVID-19 has necessitated the abandonment of the growth target that was necessary to achieve that. In an effort to keep down unemployment, the government has ended the prohibition against street vendors in major cities. Nor should Xi be regarded as politically unassailable. On reflection, it may prove to be somewhat naïve to have assumed that China was likely to be the net beneficiary of the pandemic.

However, that is not to say that the United States will somehow emerge from the pandemic panic with its global primacy intact. It is not just that Trump himself bungled his response to the crisis, though he certainly did. Much more troubling is the realization that the parts of the federal government that are responsible for handling a crisis such as this also bungled it. The Department of Health and Human Services (HHS) is a mansion with many houses, but the ones that were charged with pandemic preparedness appear to have failed abjectly: not only the Centers for Disease Control and Prevention but also the Food and Drug Administration, the Public Health Service, as well as the National Disaster Medical System. This was not for want of legislation. In 2006 Congress passed a Pandemic and All-Hazards Preparedness Act, in 2013 a reauthorization act of the same name, and in June 2019 a Pandemic and All-Hazards Preparedness and Advanced Innovations Act. In October 2015, the bipartisan Blue Ribbon Study Panel on Biodefense, cochaired by Joe Lieberman and Tom Ridge, published its first report, calling for better integration of the agencies responsible for biodefense. In 2019 it was renamed the Bipartisan Commission on Biodefense "to more accurately reflect its work and the urgency of its mission."[28]

Since August 2017, Robert Kadlec, a career US Air Force doctor, has been assistant secretary for preparedness and response at HHS. On October 10, 2018, Kadlec gave a lecture at the University of Texas's Strauss Center on the evolution of biodefense policy in which he quoted from Nassim Taleb's *Black Swan* as part of his argument for an insurance policy against a pandemic. "If we don't build this," concluded Kadlec, "we're gonna be 'SOL' [shit out of luck] should we ever be confronted with it . . . We're whistling in the dark, a little bit."[29] The previous month, the Trump administration had published a thirty-six-page report, *National Biodefense Strategy* (2018). Its implementation plan included as one of its five goals: "Assess the risks posed by research, such as with potential pandemic pathogens, where biosafety lapses could have very high consequences."[30]

As a consequence of the failure of the public health bureaucracy during the pandemic, the United States has fallen back on the 1918–19 playbook of pandemic pluralism (states do their own thing; in some states a lot of people die) but has combined it with the 2009–10 playbook of financial crisis management. A significant part of the national economy was shut down by state governors in March and April; meanwhile the national debt exploded, along with the Federal Reserve system's balance sheet. By May, lockdowns had become intolerable for most Republicans, but state governments were nowhere near having the integrated systems of testing and contact tracing necessary for economic reopening to be anything other than "dumb," in the formulation of John Cochrane.[31] As this debacle has played out, it has been like watching all my earlier visions of the endgame of American empire—in the trilogy *Colossus* (2004), *Civilization* (2011), and *The Great Degeneration* (2012)—but speeded up.

The truth is that this crisis has exposed the weaknesses of all the big players on the world stage: not only the United States but also China and, for that matter, the European Union. This should not surprise us. History shows that plagues are generally bad for big empires, especially those with porous frontiers (witness the reigns of the Roman emperors Marcus Aurelius and Justinian);[32] city-states are generally better at limiting the spread of pathogens. In 2019 the new Global Health Security Index ranked the United States first and the United Kingdom second in the world in terms of their "global health security capabilities."[33] It proved otherwise. A league table of coronavirus health safety published in early April by the Deep Knowledge Group puts Israel, Singapore, New Zealand, Hong Kong, and Taiwan at the top. (Iceland deserves an honorable mention, too. And some second-tier great powers—notably Germany and Japan—have also done well, minimizing infections and deaths without inflicting protracted lockdowns on their economies.) The key point is that there are diseconomies of scale when a new pathogen is on the loose. Four of those countries, in their different ways, had reasons to be paranoid in general as well as focused on the specific danger of a new coronavirus. Israel, Singapore, Hong Kong, and Taiwan had learned the lessons of SARS and MERS. By contrast, the big global players—China, the United States, and the EU—have all done quite badly, each in its own distinctive way. (Among members of the Organisation for Economic Co-operation and Development, the United States rates below Austria, Denmark, and Germany in one recent assessment, but above Belgium, Italy, and Spain.)[34] The winners in the short run are none of the above empires. The winners are today's equivalents of city-states.

The question is, Who gains from this stunning demonstration in Israel, Singapore, and Taiwan that, in a real crisis, small is beautiful? On balance, I would say that the centrifugal forces unleashed by the pandemic are a much bigger threat to a monolithic one-party state than to a federal system that was already in need of some decentralization. To which of the three empires do the successful city-states feel most loyalty? That is the question.

As Kissinger observes, "No country . . . can in a purely national effort overcome the virus . . . The pandemic has prompted an anachronism, a revival of the walled city in an age when prosperity depends on global trade and movement of people." Ultimately, Taiwan cannot prosper in isolation; no more can South Korea. "Addressing the necessities of the moment," Kissinger writes, "must ultimately be coupled with a global collaborative vision and program. Drawing lessons from the development of the Marshall Plan and the Manhattan Project, the U.S. is obliged to undertake a major effort . . . [to] safeguard the principles of the liberal world order."

The reputation of the Trump administration is currently at rock bottom in the eyes of most scholars of international relations. The president is seen as a wrecking ball, taking wild swings at the very institutions on which the liberal world order supposedly depends, notably the World Trade Organization and, most recently, the World Health Organization, to say nothing of the Joint Plan of Action on Iran's nuclear program and the Paris Agreement on the climate. Yet reasonable questions may be asked about the efficacy of all of these institutions and agreements with respect to the Trump administration's core strategy of engaging in "strategic competition" with China.[35] If an administration is judged by its actions in relation to its objectives, rather than by presidential tweets in relation to some largely mythical liberal international order, a rather different picture emerges. In four distinct areas, the administration has achieved, or stands a chance of achieving, meaningful success in its competition with China.

The first is financial. For many years, China toyed with the idea of making its currency convertible. This proved to be impossible because of the pent-up demand of China's wealth owners for assets outside China. More recently, Beijing has sought to increase its financial influence through large-scale lending to developing countries, some of it (not all) through its Belt and Road Initiative. The crisis unleashed by the COVID-19 pandemic has presented the United States with an opportunity to reassert its financial leadership in the world. In response to the severe global liquidity crisis unleashed in March, the Federal Reserve created two new channels—swap lines and a repo facility for foreign international monetary authorities—by which other central banks can access dollars. The first already applied to Europe, the United Kingdom, Canada, Japan, and Switzerland and was extended to nine more countries, including Brazil, Mexico, and South Korea. At its peak, the amount of swaps outstanding was $449 billion. In addition, the new repo facility made dollars available on a short-term basis to 170 foreign central banks. At the same time, the International Monetary Fund—an institution the Trump administration has shown little inclination to undermine—has stepped in to manage a spate of requests for assistance from around a hundred countries, canceling six months of debt payments due from twenty-five low-income countries such as Afghanistan, Haiti, Rwanda, and Yemen, while the G20 countries have agreed to freeze the bilateral debts of seventy-six poorer developing countries. As international creditors brace themselves for a succession of defaults by countries such as Argentina, Ecuador, Lebanon, Rwanda, and Zambia, the United States is in a much stronger position than China. Since 2013, total announced lending by Chinese financial institutions to Belt and Road Initiative projects amounted to $461 billion, making China the single biggest creditor to emerging markets. The lack of transparency that characterized these loans long ago aroused the suspicions of Western scholars, notably Carmen Reinhart, now chief economist at the World Bank.[36]

It is one thing to lament the dominance of the dollar in the international payments system; it is another to devise a way to reduce it.[37] Unlike in the 1940s, when the US dollar stood ready to supplant the British pound as the international reserve currency, the Chinese renminbi remains far from being a convertible currency, as Hank Paulson and others have pointed out. Chinese and European experiments with central bank digital currencies pose no greater threat to dollar dominance.[38] As for Facebook's grand design for a digital currency, Libra, it "has about as much chance of displacing the dollar," one wit observed, "as Esperanto has of replacing English."[39] The most that can be said is that the United States now lags worryingly behind Asia, Europe, and even Latin America when it comes to innovations in financial technology. But it is hard to see how even the most ambitious scheme—the projected East Asian digital currency consisting of the Chinese yuan, Japanese yen, South Korean won, and Hong Kong dollar—will come to fruition, in view of the profound suspicions many in Tokyo feel toward the financial ambitions of Beijing.

The second area where US dominance seems likely (though not certain) to be reasserted is in the race to find a vaccine against SARS-CoV-2. According to the Milken Institute, there are over 170 vaccine research projects under way at the time of writing this, ten of which are now in human trials.[40] The most advanced candidate is AZD1222, first developed by researchers at Oxford and Vaccitech. It and six others—including those of Moderna and Pfizer—are being given US government funding as part of the Trump administration's Operation Warp Speed, the White House program for accelerating vaccine development. True, there are also five vaccines in clinical trials in China, but four of them are inactivated whole-virus vaccines, an earlier generation of medical science than Moderna's mRNA-1273. An early April survey in *Nature* noted that "most COVID-19 vaccine development activity is in North America, with 36 (46%) developers of the confirmed active vaccine candidates compared with 14 (18%) in China, 14 (18%) in Asia (excluding China) and Australia, and 14 (18%) in Europe."[41] It is possible that one of the Chinese contenders will beat the odds and produce a vaccine. It is nevertheless worth remembering the recurrent problems the People's Republic has had in recent years with vaccine safety and regulation, most recently in January 2019, when children in the province of Jiangsu received out-of-date polio shots, and before that in July 2018, when 250,000 doses of vaccine for diphtheria, tetanus, and whooping cough were found to be defective. It was only thirteen years ago that Zheng Xiaoyu, the former head of the Chinese State Food and Drug Administration, was sentenced to death for taking bribes from eight domestic drug companies.

Third, the United States is pulling ahead of China in the "tech war." The Trump administration's pressure on allied countries not to use 5G hardware produced by Huawei is yielding results. In Germany, Norbert Röttgen, a prominent member of Chancellor Angela Merkel's Christian Democratic Union, helped draft a bill that would bar any "untrustworthy" company from "both the core and peripheral networks."[42] In Britain, Neil O'Brien, Conservative member of Parliament and founder of the China Research Group, and a group of thirty-eight rebel Tory backbenchers appear to have succeeded in changing Prime Minister Boris Johnson's mind about Huawei, much to the fury of the editors of *China Daily*. Perhaps more significant are the US Commerce Department rules announced on May 15 that would cut Huawei off from using advanced semiconductors produced anywhere in the world using US technology or intellectual property. This includes the chips produced in Taiwan by the Taiwan Semiconductor Manufacturing Company, or TSMC, the world's most advanced manufacturer. The new rules pose a potentially mortal threat to Huawei's semiconductor affiliate HiSilicon.

Finally, the United States' lead in artificial intelligence research, as well as in quantum computing, would appear still to be commanding, although the recent decision by President Trump to restrict visas for computer programmers and other skilled workers who enter the country with H-1B visas could ultimately reduce that lead. One recent study showed that, while "China is the largest source of top-tier AI researchers, . . . a majority of these Chinese researchers leave China to study, work, and live in the United States."[43] Frey and Osborne concluded a recent survey of the tech war as follows: "If we look at the 100 most cited patents since 2003, not a single one comes from China . . . A surveillance state with a censored Internet, together with a social credit system that promotes conformity and obedience, seems unlikely to foster creativity."[44] If Yan Xuetong, dean of the Institute of International Relations at Tsinghua University, is correct in contending that Cold War II will be a purely technological competition, without the nuclear brinkmanship and proxy wars that made the first one so risky and so costly, then the United States is the favorite to win it.

It can hardly be claimed that the Trump administration is "safeguard[ing] the principles of the liberal world order." It would nevertheless be fair to say that, in practice, the administration has been quite effective in at least some of the steps it has taken to execute its stated goal of competing strategically with China.

The great achievement of the various strategies of containment pursued by the United States during the Cold War was to limit and ultimately reverse the expansion of Soviet power without precipitating a World War III. Might strategic competition prove less successful in that regard? It is possible. First, there is a clear and present danger that information warfare and cyberwarfare operations, honed by the Russian government and now being adopted and enacted by China, could cause severe disruption to the US political and economic system.[45]

Second, as Christian Brose has argued, the United States could find itself at a disadvantage in the event of a conventional war in the South China Sea or the Taiwan Strait, because US aircraft carrier groups, with their F-35 fighters, are now highly vulnerable to new Chinese weapons such as the DF-21D, the world's first operational anti-ship ballistic missile ("the carrier killer").[46]

Third, the United States already finds it difficult to back up words with actions. China has signaled that it will impose new national-security laws on Hong Kong, dealing a blow to the territory's autonomy and surely violating the terms of the 1984 Sino-British Joint Declaration, which guarantees a "one country, two systems" model until 2047. Adding various Chinese agencies and institutions to the US Commerce Department's entity list will not deter Beijing from going ahead. Nor will similar economic sanctions threatened by indignant senators. Secretary of State Pompeo has gone out of his way to show friendliness toward the Taiwanese government this year, publicly congratulating President Tsai Ing-Wen on her reelection in January. Yet how effectively could the United States react if Beijing decided to launch a surprise amphibious invasion of the island? Such a step is openly proposed by nationalist writers on Chinese social media as a solution to the threat that Huawei will be cut off from TSMC. One lengthy post on this subject was headlined "Reunification of the two sides, take TSMC!"

The reunification of Taiwan and the mainland is Xi Jinping's most cherished ambition and is one of the justifications for his removal of term limits. Xi may well be asking himself if there will ever again be a more propitious time to force the issue than this year, with the United States in a lockdown-induced recession and just months away from a contentious and decisive election. While the Pentagon is skeptical of China's ability to execute a successful invasion, the People's Liberation

Army is rapidly increasing its amphibious capabilities. With good reason, Graham Allison has warned that the administration's ambition to "kill Huawei" could play a role similar to the sanctions imposed on Japan between 1939 and 1941, culminating in the August 1941 oil embargo.[47] It was economic pressure that ultimately drove the imperial government to gamble on a war that began with a surprise attack on Pearl Harbor.[48] If it were the United States that suddenly found itself cut off from TSMC, the boot would be on the other foot, as the Taiwanese company's new foundry in Arizona will take years to complete and will be no substitute for the much larger facilities it has in Taiwan.[49]

Cold wars can deescalate in a process we remember as détente. But they can also escalate: a recurrent feature of the period from the late 1950s until the early 1980s was fear that brinkmanship might lead to Armageddon. At times, as John Bolton has shown, President Trump inclines to a very crude form of détente. There are important members of his administration who lean in that direction, too. We hear occasional melodious mood music about the phase one trade deal announced late last year,[50] despite abundant evidence that it is being honored by Beijing mainly in the breach.[51] Yet the language of the secretary of state remains consistently combative. To be sure, his meeting with Yang Jiechi, the director of the CCP Office of Foreign Affairs, in Hawaii on June 17 was notable for the uncompromising harshness of the language used in the official Chinese communiqué released afterward.[52] But that might have been exactly what Secretary Pompeo wanted on the eve of his hard-hitting speech to the Copenhagen Democracy Summit, which was clearly intended to galvanize his European audience.

How likely is this appeal to be successful? In some quarters, not at all. The Italian foreign minister, Luigi Di Maio, was one of a number of Italian politicians all too ready to swallow Beijing's aid and propaganda back in March, when the COVID-19 crisis in northern Italy was especially bad. "Those who scoffed at our participation in the Belt and Road Initiative now have to admit that investing in that friendship allowed us to save lives in Italy," Di Maio declared in an interview.[53] The Hungarian prime minister, Viktor Orbán, was equally enthusiastic. "In the West, there is a shortage of basically everything," he said in an interview with Chinese state television. "The help we are able to get is from the East," he continued.[54] "China is the only friend who can help us," gushed the Serbian president, Aleksandar Vučić, who kissed a Chinese flag when a team of doctors flew from Beijing to Belgrade.[55] However, mainstream European reaction, especially in Germany and France, has displayed a rather different sentiment. "Over these months China has lost Europe," Reinhard Bütikofer, a German Green Party member of the Bundestag, declared in an interview in April.[56] "The atmosphere in Europe is rather toxic when it comes to China," said Jörg Wuttke, president of the EU Chamber of Commerce in China.[57] On April 17, the editor in chief of Germany's biggest tabloid, *Bild*, published an open letter to General Secretary Xi Jinping titled "You are endangering the world."[58] In France, too, "wolf warrior diplomacy" has been a failure.

One reason for its failure is that, after an initial breakdown in early March, when *sauve qui peut* was the order of the day, European institutions have risen to the challenge posed by COVID-19.[59] In a remarkable interview published on April 16, the French president declared that the EU faced a "moment of truth" in deciding whether it was more than just a single economic market. "You cannot have a single market where some are sacrificed," he told the *Financial Times*.[60] "It is no longer possible . . . to have financing that is not mutualized for the spending we are undertaking in the battle against Covid-19 and that we will have for the economic recovery."[61] He continued: "If we can't do this today, I tell you the populists will win—today, tomorrow, the day after, in Italy, in Spain, perhaps in France and elsewhere."[62] His German counterpart agreed. Europe, declared Angela Merkel, was a "community of fate" (*Schicksalsgemeinschaft*). To the surprise of skeptical commentators, the result was very different from the cheese-paring that characterized the German response to the global financial crisis.[63] The Next Generation EU plan, presented by the European Commission on May 27, proposed 750 billion euros of additional EU spending, to be financed through bonds issued by the EU and to be allocated to the regions hardest hit by the pandemic.[64] Perhaps even more significantly, the German federal government adopted a supplementary budget of 156 billion euros (4.9% of gross domestic product) followed by a second fiscal stimulus package worth 130 billion euros (or 3.8% of gross domestic product), which—along with large-scale guarantees from a new economic stabilization fund—was intended to ignite recovery with a "ka-boom," in the words of Finance Minister Olaf Scholz.[65] Such large-scale fiscal measures, combined with large-scale asset purchases by the European Central Bank, have done much to dampen support for the populist right in most EU member states.

Yet this successful reassertion of European solidarity—made easier by the departure of the United Kingdom from the EU negotiating table—has had an unexpected consequence from the vantage point of Washington. Europeans, especially young Europeans and especially Germans, have never since 1945 been more disenchanted with the transatlantic relationship. In one pan-European survey conducted in mid-March, 53% of young Europeans said they had more confidence in authoritarian states than democracies when it came to addressing the climate crisis.[66] In a German poll published by the Körber Foundation in May, 73% of Germans said that their opinion of the United States had deteriorated—more than double the number of respondents who felt that way toward China.[67] Just 10% of Germans considered the United States to be their country's closest partner in foreign policy, compared with 19% in September 2019. And the proportion of Germans who prioritized close relations with Washington over close relations with Beijing has decreased significantly, from 50% in September 2019 to 37%, roughly the same share as those who preferred China to the United States (36%).

In the Cold War with the Soviets, it is sometimes forgotten that there was a Non-Aligned Movement (NAM), which had its origins in the 1955 Bandung Conference hosted by Indonesian president Sukarno and attended by the Indian prime minister Jawaharlal Nehru, the Egyptian president Gamal Abdel Nasser, his Yugoslav counterpart Josip Broz Tito, and the Ghanaian president Kwame Nkrumah, as well as the North Vietnamese president Ho Chi Minh, the Chinese premier Zhou Enlai, and the Cambodian prime minister Norodom Sihanouk. Formally constituted in 1956 by Tito, Nehru, and Nasser, the NAM's goal was (in the words of one of Nehru's advisers) to enable the newly independent countries of the Third World to preserve their independence in the "face of [a] complex international situation demanding allegiance to either of the two warring superpowers." For most Western Europeans and many East and Southeast Asians, however, nonalignment was not an attractive option. That was partly because the choice between Washington and Moscow was a fairly easy one—unless the Red Army's tanks were rolling into a country's capital city. It was also because the NAM's geopolitical nonalignment was not matched by a comparable ideological nonalignment, a feature that became more prominent with the ascendancy of the Cuban dictator Fidel Castro in the 1970s, finally leading to a near breakup of the movement over the Soviet invasion of Afghanistan.

Today, by contrast, the choice between Washington and Beijing looks to many Europeans like a choice between the frying pan and the fire or, at best, the kettle and the pot. As the Körber poll mentioned above strongly suggests, "The [German] public is leaning toward a position of equidistance between Washington and Beijing." Even the government of Singapore has made it clear that it "fervently hope[s] not to be forced to choose between the United States and China." Moreover, "Asian countries see the United States as a resident power that has vital interests in the region," the Singaporean prime minister wrote in a recent issue of *Foreign Affairs*.

"At the same time, China is a reality on the doorstep. Asian countries do not want to be forced to choose between the two. And if either attempts to force such a choice—if Washington tries to contain China's rise or Beijing seeks to build an exclusive sphere of influence in Asia—they will begin a course of confrontation that will last decades and put the long-heralded Asian century in jeopardy . . . Any confrontation between these two great powers is unlikely to end as the Cold War did, in one country's peaceful collapse."[68]

Lee Hsien Loong is right in one respect at least. The fact that both world wars of the 20th century had the same outcome—the defeat of Germany and its allies by Britain and its allies—does not mean that Cold War II will have the same outcome as it predecessor: the victory of the United States and its allies. Cold wars are usually regarded as bipolar; in truth, though, they are always three-body problems, with two superpower alliances and a third nonaligned network in between. This may indeed be a general truth about war itself: that it is seldom simply a Clausewitzian contest between two opposing forces, each bent on the other's subjugation, but more often a three-body problem in which winning the sympathies of the neutral third parties can be as important as inflicting defeat on the enemy.[69]

The biggest problem facing the president of the United States today, and for years to come, is that many erstwhile American allies are seriously contemplating nonalignment in Cold War II. And without a sufficiency of allies, to say nothing of sympathetic neutrals, Washington may well find Cold War II to be unwinnable.

NOTES

1. Cixin Liu, *The Three-Body Problem*, trans. Ken Liu (New York: Tor Books, 2014).

2. Lijian Zhao (@zlj517), "2/2 CDC was caught on the spot. When did patient zero begin in US? How many people are infected?," Twitter, March 12, 2020, https://twitter.com/zlj517/status/1238111898828066823.

3. Andrew Browne, "Foothills of a Cold War," *Bloomberg*, November 21, 2020, https://www.bloomberg.com/news/newsletters/2019-11-21/-foothills-of-a-cold-war?sref=ojq9DljU.

4. Yao Yang, "Is a New Cold War Coming?," interview with the *Beijing Cultural Review*, April 28, 2020, https://www.readingthechinadream.com/yao-yang-the-new-cold-war.html.

5. Orville Schell, "The Death of Engagement," *The Wire China*, June 7, 2020, https://www.thewirechina.com/2020/06/07/the-birth-life-and-death-of-engagement/.

6. Dan Blumenthal and Nicholas Eberstadt, "China Unquarantined," *National Review*, June 4, 2020, https://www.nationalreview.com/magazine/2020/06/22/our-disastrous-engagement-of-china/#slide-1.

7. Katsuji Nakazawa, "Xi Fears Japan-Led Manufacturing Exodus from China," *Nikkei Asian Review*, April 16, 2020, https://asia.nikkei.com/Editor-s-Picks/China-up-close/Xi-fears-Japan-led-manufacturing-exodus-from-China.

8. Dave Lawler, "Josh Hawley Crafts the Case against China," *Axios*, May 20, 2020, https://www.axios.com/josh-hawley-china-policy-f9e1fc01-2883-4db7-a721-fbb3f7aeacb8.html.

9. Robert B. Zoellick, "The U.S. Doesn't Need a New Cold War," *Wall Street Journal*, May 18, 2020, https://www.wsj.com/articles/the-u-s-doesnt-need-a-new-cold-war-11589842987.

10. "China Opens $45 Trillion Financial Market as U.S. Closes," *People's Daily*, June 15, 2020, http://en.people.cn/n3/2020/0615/c90000-9700486.html.

11. John Bolton, *The Room Where It Happened*, excerpt quoted in "John Bolton: The Scandal of Trump's China Policy," *Wall Street Journal*, June 17, 2020, https://www.wsj.com/articles/john-bolton-the-scandal-of-trumps-china-policy-11592419564?.

12. David Rennie as "Chaguan," "Elites in Beijing See America in Decline, Hastened by Trump," *Economist*, June 11, 2020, https://www.economist.com/china/2020/06/11/elites-in-beijing-see-america-in-decline-hastened-by-trump.

13. Michèle A. Flournoy, "How to Prevent a War in Asia," *Foreign Affairs*, June 18, 2020, https://www.foreignaffairs.com/articles/united-states/2020-06-18/how-prevent-war-asia.

14. Christian Brose, *The Kill Chain: Defending America in the Future of High-Tech Warfare* (New York: Hachette, 2020).

15. Bernhard Zand, "There Are Better Ways to Deal with Asia and China," interview with Kishore Mahbubani, *Der Spiegel*, August 4, 2020, https://www.spiegel.de/international/world/political-scientist-kishore-mahbubani-on-the-asian-century-a-79680d54-17be-4dd2-bc8c-796101581f31.

16. Kishore Mahbubani, "Kishore Mahbubani on the Dawn of the Asian Century," *Economist*, April 20, 2020, https://www.economist.com/by-invitation/2020/04/20/kishore-mahbubani-on-the-dawn-of-the-asian-century.

17. Martin Jacques, *When China Rules the World: The End of the Western World and the Birth of a New Global Order*, 2nd ed. (London: Penguin, 2012).

18. Daniel Bell, *The China Model: Political Meritocracy and the Limits of Democracy* (Princeton, NJ: Princeton University Press, 2016).

19. See, e.g., "Pro-people Policies, Dutiful Citizens Effective in China's COVID-19 Fight," interview with Daniel Bell, *Global Times*, May 2, 2020, https://www.globaltimes.cn/content/1187304.shtml.

20. Edward Luce, "Inside Trump's Coronavirus Meltdown," *Financial Times*, May 14, 2020, https://www.ft.com/content/97dc7de6-940b-11ea-abcd-371e24b679ed?shareType=nongift.

21. Luce, "Inside Trump's Coronavirus Meltdown."

22. Lawrence Summers, "Covid-19 Looks Like a Hinge in History," *Financial Times*, May 14, 2020, https://www.ft.com/content/de643ae8-9527-11ea-899a-f62a20d54625.

23. Anne Applebaum, "The Rest of the World Is Laughing at Trump," *Atlantic*, May 3, 2020, https://www.theatlantic.com/ideas/archive/2020/05/time-americans-are-doing-nothing/611056/.

24. Richard Haass, "The Pandemic Will Accelerate History Rather Than Reshape It," *Foreign Affairs*, April 7, 2020, https://www.foreignaffairs.com/articles/united-states/2020-04-07/pandemic-will-accelerate-history-rather-reshape-it.

25. Peter Turchin, "Dynamics of Political Instability in the United States, 1780–2010," *Journal of Peace Research* 49, no. 4 (2012), https://doi.org/10.1177/0022343312442078. See also Peter Turchin, *Ages of Discord: A Structural-Demographic Analysis of American History* (Chaplin, CT: Beresta Books, 2016), esp. 241f.

26. Henry Kissinger, "The Coronavirus Pandemic Will Forever Alter the World Order," *Wall Street Journal*, April 3, 2020, https://www.wsj.com/articles/the-coronavirus-pandemic-will-forever-alter-the-world-order-11585953005.

27. Kissinger, "Coronavirus Pandemic Will Forever Alter the World Order."

28. "Blue Ribbon Study Panel on Biodefense Is Now the Bipartisan Commission on Biodefense," Bipartisan Commission on Biodefense, September 17, 2019, https://biodefense commission.org/blue-ribbon-study-panel-on-biodefense-is-now-the-bipartisan-commission -on-biodefense/.

29. Robert Kaldec, "Evolution of Biodefense Policy" (lecture, Robert Strauss Center for International Security and Law, Austin, Texas, October 10, 2018), https://www.youtube .com/watch?list=UUPLAYER_RobertStraussCenter&v=6U4e4029SpE.

30. *National Biodefense Strategy*, White House, 2018, https://www.whitehouse.gov/wp -content/uploads/2018/09/National-Biodefense-Strategy.pdf.

31. John Cochrane, "Dumb Reopening Might Just Work," *The Grumpy Economist* (blog), May 4, 2020, https://johnhcochrane.blogspot.com/2020/05/dumb-reopening-might-just -work.html.

32. Kyle Harper, *The Fate of Rome: Climate, Disease, and the End of an Empire* (Princeton, NJ: Princeton University Press, 2017).

33. "GHS Index: About" Global Health Security Index, accessed July 10, 2020, https:// www.ghsindex.org/about/.

34. *Economist* Intelligence Unit, "How Well Have OECD Countries Responded to the Coronavirus Crisis?," June 17, 2020, https://www.eiu.com/n/campaigns/oecd-countries -responded-to-the-coronavirus-crisis/.

35. *National Security Strategy*, White House, December 2017, https://www.whitehouse .gov/wp-content/uploads/2017/12/NSS-Final-12-18-2017-0905.pdf.

36. Sebastian Horn, Carmen M. Reinhart, and Christoph Trebesch, "China's Overseas Lending" (NBER working paper no. 26050, May 2020), http://papers.nber.org/tmp/15188 -w26050.pdf.

37. Gita Gopinath et al., "Dominant Currency Paradigm" (NBER working paper no. 22943, December 2016), https://www.nber.org/papers/w22943.pdf.

38. Huw van Steenis, "The New Digital-Payments Race," *Project Syndicate*, April 21, 2020, https://www.project-syndicate.org/onpoint/central-banks-digital-payments-by-huw-van -steenis-2020-04?barrier=accesspaylog.

39. John Paul Koning (@jp_koning), "Facebook isn't a real threat. It has introduced a number of payments products over the years. None of them have attracted wide usage," February 6, 2020, https://twitter.com/jp_koning/status/1225418083323568129.

40. "Covid-19 Treatment and Vaccine Tracker," Milken Institute, July 9, 2020, https:// covid-19tracker.milkeninstitute.org/.

41. Tung Thanh Le, Zacharias Andreadakis, Arun Kumar, Raul Gomez Roman, Stig Tollefsen, Melanie Saville, and Stephen Mayhew, "The COVID-19 Vaccine Development

Landscape," *Nature*, April 9, 2020, https://www.nature.com/articles/d41573-020-00073
-5?utm_source=Nature+Briefing&utm_campaign=98c3a376d1-briefing-dy-20200409
&utm_medium=email&utm_term=0_c9dfd39373-98c3a376d1-43976957.

42. Natalie Liu, "German Decision on Huawei 5G 'Imminent,' Says Ambassador," *Voice of America*, February 11, 2020, https://www.voanews.com/europe/german-decision-hua wei-5g-imminent-says-ambassador.

43. Ishan Banerjee and Matt Sheehan, "America's Got AI Talent: US' Big Lead in AI Research Is Built on Importing Researchers," Macro Polo, June 9, 2020, https://macropolo .org/americas-got-ai-talent-us-big-lead-in-ai-research-is-built-on-importing-researchers/.

44. Carl Benedikt Frey and Michael Osborne, "China Won't Win the Race for AI Dominance," *Foreign Affairs*, June 19, 2020, https://www.foreignaffairs.com/articles/united -states/2020-06-19/china-wont-win-race-ai-dominance.

45. Ariel E. Levite and Lyu Jinghua, "Travails of an Interconnected World: From Pandemics to the Digital Economy," *Lawfare Blog*, April 30, 2020, https://www.lawfareblog .com/travails-interconnected-world-pandemics-digital-economy.

46. Brose, *Kill Chain*.

47. Salvatore Babones, "Boris Johnson's Huawei 5G Decision Is a Massive Mistake," *National Interest*, January 28, 2020, https://nationalinterest.org/blog/buzz/boris-johns ons-huawei-5g-decision-massive-mistake-118016.

48. Graham Allison, "Could Donald Trump's War against Huawei Trigger a Real War with China?," *National Interest*, June 11, 2020, https://nationalinterest.org/feature/could -donald-trump%E2%80%99s-war-against-huawei-trigger-real-war-china-162565.

49. Steve Blank, "The Chip Wars of the Twenty-First Century," *War on the Rocks*, June 11, 2020, https://warontherocks.com/2020/06/the-chip-wars-of-the-21st-century/.

50. Jenny Leonard, "Lighthizer Says He Feels 'Very Good' about Phase One China Deal," *Bloomberg*, June 4, 2020, https://www.bloomberg.com/news/articles/2020-06-04 /lighthizer-says-he-feels-very-good-about-phase-one-china-deal-kb16qm1v.

51. "China Halts Some U.S. Farm Imports Threatening Trade Deal," *Bloomberg*, June 2, 2020, https://www.bloomberg.com/news/articles/2020-06-01/china-halts-some-u-s-farm -imports-threatening-trade-deal?sref=ojq9DljU.

52. "Foreign Spokesperson Zhao Lijian's Remarks on Yang Jiechi's Meeting with US Secretary of State Michael R. Pompeo," Ministry of Foreign Affairs of the People's Republic of China, June 18, 2020, https://www.fmprc.gov.cn/mfa_eng/xwfw_665399/s2510 _665401/t1789798.shtml.

53. "Luigi Di Maioospite a TG2 Post Rai 2 24 03 2020," YouTube, March 24, 2020, https://www.youtube.com/watch?v=oW7JRf6qaog.

54. John Micklethwait and Adrian Wooldridge, "The Virus Should Wake Up the West," *Bloomberg Opinion*, April 12, 2020, https://www.bloomberg.com/opinion/articles/2020-04-13 /coronavirus-pandemic-is-wake-up-call-to-reinvent-the-state?sref=ojq9DljU.

55. Mattia Ferraresi, "China Isn't Helping Italy: It's Waging Information Warfare," *Foreign Policy*, March 31, 2020, https://foreignpolicy.com/2020/03/31/china-isnt-helping-italy -its-waging-information-warfare/.

56. Alan Crawford and Peter Martin, "China's Coronavirus Diplomacy Has Finally Pushed Europe Too Far," *Taipei Times*, April 26, 2020, https://www.taipeitimes.com/News /editorials/archives/2020/04/26/2003735306.

57. Crawford and Martin, "China's Coronavirus Diplomacy."

58. Joseph de Weck, "China's COVID-19 Diplomacy Is Backfiring in Europe," *Foreign Policy Research Institute*, April 21, 2020, https://www.fpri.org/article/2020/04/chinas-covid-19-diplomacy-is-backfiring-in-europe/.

59. Joseph de Weck and Dimitris Valatsas, "The European Union Will Survive COVID-19," *Foreign Policy Research Institute*, April 30, 2020, https://www.fpri.org/article/2020/04/the-european-union-will-survive-covid-19/.

60. Victor Mallet and Roula Khalaf, "Macron Warns of EU Unravelling Unless It Embraces Financial Solidarity," *Financial Times*, April, 16, 2020, https://www.ft.com/content/d19dc7a6-c33b-4931-9a7e-4a74674da29a.

61. Mallet and Khalaf, "Macron Warns of EU Unravelling."

62. Mallet and Khalaf, "Macron Warns of EU Unravelling."

63. Wolfgang Munchau, "How to Think about the EU's Rescue Fund," *Financial Times*, April 26, 2020, https://www.ft.com/content/854b21dc-8637-11ea-b872-8db45d5f6714.

64. "Europe's Moment: Repair and Prepare for the Next Generation," European Commission, May 27, 2020, https://ec.europa.eu/commission/presscorner/detail/en/ip_20_940.

65. Guy Chazan, "German Stimulus Aims to Kick-Start Recovery with a Ka-boom," *Financial Times*, June 4, 2020, https://www.ft.com/content/335b5558-41b5-4a1e-a3b9-1440f7602bd8.

66. Timothy Garton Ash and Antonia Zimmermann, "In Crisis, Europeans Support Radical Positions," *Eupinions Brief*, May 6, 2020, https://eupinions.eu/de/text/in-crisis-europeans-support-radical-positions.

67. Ronja Scheler and Joshua Webb, "Keeping an Equidistance," *Berlin Policy Journal*, May 18, 2020, https://berlinpolicyjournal.com/keeping-an-equidistance/.

68. Lee Hsien Loong, "The Endangered Asian Century: America, China, and the Perils of Confrontation," *Foreign Affairs*, July/August 2020, https://www.foreignaffairs.com/articles/asia/2020-06-04/lee-hsien-loong-endangered-asian-century.

69. Emile Simpson, *War from the Ground Up: Twenty-First Century Combat as Politics* (Oxford: Oxford University Press, 2012).

Index

unemployment rates in, 56, 316; unilateralism vs. multilateralism in foreign policy of, 76, 144, 170–71, 363n11. *See also* inequality; international cooperation; state and local governments; unpreparedness; US-China relations; *specific presidents*
United States–Mexico–Canada Agreement, 268
unpreparedness, 223–37, 317; congressional legislation on preparedness and, 424; EU, 230–32, 425; how to fix the system, 232–35, 354; inertia and, 232; international institutions, 224–25; medical unpreparedness, 53; misleading ratings of "global health security capabilities," 425; transnational supply chain vulnerabilities, 241; UN and WHO, 227–30; US failure to provide leadership, 227–28, 323, 423–24, 425
US-China Cyber Agreement (2015), 381
US-China relations, 2, 8, 9; Americans viewing China as threat to American well-being, 311, 421; China as largest US trading partner, 407; climate change action and, 136, 141, 289, 290, 383, 399–400, 414; "coopetition" and "coevolution" of, 371, 380–81; COVID-19's effect on, 42, 136, 144, 193, 201, 260, 298, 300, 304, 349, 370, 388–89, 390–91, 395–96, 408, 414; decoupling US economy to decrease vulnerability to China, 200, 326, 328, 378, 407, 411–12, 414; deepening conflict, 259, 260–62, 377–80, 408–10; effect on US economy, 194–95, 325; exceptionalism of China and, 344; financial firms entering Chinese market, 421; One-Worldism and, 193–96; other countries finding way around US-China conflict, 270, 322, 336, 380, 430, 432–33; pharmaceutical manufacture and medical equipment, US reliance on China, 169, 177–82, 408; Phase One (US-China) trade deal (2019), 198–99, 214, 220n16, 301, 430; at pivot point to rethink relations, 199–200, 321–23, 349, 407–10, 422; R&D collaboration, 410–15; rebordering of the world and, 262–63; "rivalry partnership," 10, 13, 327, 371, 377, 380–81, 389, 397–402; technological relationship and rivalry in aftermath of COVID-19, 10, 169–70, 180–81, 260–62, 391, 406–18; Trump-Xi relations, 319–20; visa ban imposed on

Chinese graduate students and researchers, 181, 241, 337, 428; world order framed by, 259, 270, 279, 288–92, 334, 336–37, 351, 361, 370–71, 382–83, 407; zero-sum approach to all issues, 13, 301, 410. *See also* great-power competition; new cold war, emergence of; origins of COVID-19 pandemic
US Special Trade Representative (USTR), 218, 333

vaccines: availability and distribution of, 77, 88, 127, 202, 242, 247, 307; AZD1222 development, 427; compulsory vaccination law, 97; considered as end of pandemic, 29–30; development, 2, 16, 20n28, 28–29, 44, 81, 82–84, 88, 127; funding for development of, 333; international cooperation in development of, 59, 75, 82, 181, 220n14, 233, 305, 400, 406; local public health providing immunizations, 103; Operation Warp Speed, 359, 408, 427; refusal to get immunized, 86, 126; urgency of development, 127; US-China relations and vaccine development, 181, 202, 241, 397, 408, 427. *See also specific pandemics*
Venezuela, 148, 319
ventilators, shortage of, 81, 84–85, 115–16
Vienna Convention against Illicit Traffic in Narcotic Drugs and Psychotropic Substances, 283
Vietnam, 262, 353, 357, 374, 375, 378
Vietnam War, 51, 325
Volcker, Paul A., 208

Wang Yi, 379
war and conflicts: end dates of, 25–26; ethnic conflicts after demise of Soviet Union, 353; hunger in war-torn countries, 148, 151; likelihood of future international conflict, 67; social impacts of, 26. *See also specific wars*
Warsaw Pact, 198
water shortages, 136, 155, 355
West Africa, 28, 76, 104, 224
West Nile virus, 152
Westphalian system, 64, 66, 278
Wilson, Woodrow, 3, 401
World Bank: alignment with G20 Leaders, 216; changes in role and responsibilities of, 11, 198, 220n19; creation of, 3, 52, 162, 192;